ESSENTIALS OF CLINICAL PHARMACOLOGY AND DOSAGE CALCULATION

ESSENTIALS OF CLINICAL PHARMACOLOGY AND DOSAGE CALCULATION

MARGARET C. LANNON, R.N., M.S.
Instructor, Boston University School of Nursing
Boston, Massachusetts

VIRGINIA POOLE ARCANGELO, R.N., M.S.N.
Instructor, Helene Fuld School of Nursing
Camden, New Jersey

CONSULTANT
FREDDY A. GRIMM, B.A., M.S., Pharm. D.
Assistant Director, Pharmacy Service, Hospital of the University of Pennsylvania
Philadelphia, Pennsylvania

SECOND EDITION

J. B. LIPPINCOTT COMPANY
Philadelphia
London • Mexico City • New York • St. Louis • São Paulo • Sydney

Manuscript Editor: Margaret E. Maxwell
Indexer: Maria Coughlin
Design Director: Tracy Baldwin
Design Coordinator: Anne O'Donnell
Designer: Pat Pennington
Production Supervisor: J. Corey Gray
Production Coordinator: Kathleen R. Diamond
Compositor: Maryland Composition Co., Inc.
Printer/Binder: The Murray Printing Company
Cover Printer: Philips Offset Company, Inc.

Second Edition

6 5 4 3 2 1

Library of Congress Cataloging-in-Publication Data

Lannon, Margaret C.
   Essentials of clinical pharmacology and dosage
calculation.

   Rev. ed. of: Essentials of pharmacology
   Bibliography: p.
   Includes index.
   1. Pharmacology. 2. Chemotherapy. 3. Nursing.
I. Arcangelo, Virginia Poole. II. Grimm, Freddy A.
III. Cibulskis, Margaret M.   Essentials of pharmacology.
IV. Title. [DNLM: 1. Drug Therapy—nurses' instruction.
2. Pharmacology—nurses' instruction.   QV 4 L292e]
RM300.L27 1986   615'.1   85-23066
ISBN 0-397-54531-2

The authors and publisher have exerted every effort to ensure that drug selection and dosage set forth in this text are in accord with current recommendations and practice at the time of publication. However, in view of ongoing research, changes in government regulations, and the constant flow of information relating to drug therapy and drug reactions, the reader is urged to check the package insert for each drug for any change in indications and dosage and for added warnings and precautions. This is particularly important when the recommended agent is a new or infrequently employed drug.

For Erica

Preface

In recent years the practice of nursing has undergone tremendous change. The structure of nursing care has changed, in both the hospital and outpatient settings. With the implementation of primary nursing, more nurses are administering medications to their patients. Although increasing numbers of graduate nurses are expected to give medications, few feel they have been adequately prepared to assume this responsibility. They lack confidence in their ability to apply the principles of pharmacology and drug administration safely in the clinical setting.

As one who taught first-level pharmacology for a number of years, I have been frustrated by the lack of an appropriate textbook for this population of nursing students. It has been my experience that existing first-level texts, in an effort to simplify pharmacologic principles and dosage calculations, often omit information that is pertinent to a thorough understanding of drug action. Those texts that do contain complete drug information are often unnecessarily detailed or difficult for the average first-level student or new graduate to understand. Texts that contain adequate and appropriately detailed information often lack a comprehensive review of mathematics and dosage calculation.

Essentials of Clinical Pharmacology and Dosage Calculation, Second Edition, was written in response to the need for a first-level pharmacology text that includes information about drug action in a readable, understandable format; explains possible adverse effects; gives particulars of dosage, route, and use; and gives specific nursing implications for each drug discussed in detail.

Special attention has been given to nursing implications. A thorough understanding of this aspect of medication administration enables the nurse to become a safer practitioner. Often, it is not enough to know simply what adverse effects may occur with the administration of a particular drug. The nurse must be aware of what she must do to check for adverse effects. With this text as a guide, the student can begin to consider the nursing implications associated with each drug. With this preparation and constant reinforcement during her student experience, the graduate nurse who encounters a new or unfamiliar drug should feel more comfortable with its administration. She will be prepared to review the adverse effects listed by the manufacturer and then, on the basis of her experience with this text, realize that certain nursing implications need to be considered.

Part One of the text gives general drug information, principles of pharmacology, and arithmetic review—necessary background for the study of medications and medication administration. In this second edition, Part One has been expanded to include a thorough review of elementary arithmetic functions and dosage calculation. In addition, practice problems that use realistic, pertinent clinical situations have been added throughout the text to reinforce both chapter content and dosage calculation skills. Parts Two through Seven are intended to encourage the student or graduate nurse to view each patient as a system interacting with his environment as well as his own internal mechanisms. Each part focuses on one of humankind's survival needs and the medications given to help meet this need. It is hoped that this format will encourage the student to view each patient as a unique individual with many interacting needs. Part Eight contains brief chapters on drugs used in special circumstances, such as obstetrics, pediatrics, diagnostic testing, and treatment of heavy metal poisoning.

As in the previous edition, each chapter begins with an overview of the material to be covered. Chapter content is then presented in the following manner. First, the category of drugs to be discussed—their general use—is introduced. Second, the pharmacologic action (basic anatomy and physiology are reviewed where indicated) is described. Third, subgroups of the category are detailed and their action and use—important adverse effects, drug and food interactions, changes brought about by drug use, and potential problems—are discussed. Finally, nursing implications are given.

Most chapters contain tables that give particulars of nomenclature, usual dosage range and routes, use, a summary of adverse effects, and nursing implications. The student should use these tables as a quick reference in the administration of medications to her patients.

In this second edition, Chapter 16, Vitamins, Minerals, Fluids, and Electrolytes, has been considerably expanded to include information on intravenous therapy. Principles of fluid and electrolyte balance have been stressed, as well as the principles underlying safe administration of intravenous fluids. Content has been added in Chapter 38, Drugs Used in Pediatrics, to familiarize the student with different methods of dosage calculation

for the pediatric patient. Many practice problems are included.

All of the chapters in this second edition have been updated with current information. Groups of drugs introduced into widespread use since the publication of the first edition, such as the calcium channel blockers, transdermal systems for administering nitroglycerin, and human insulins (Chapter 34), are now included. Over 75 new drug entries have been added to the comprehensive chapter tables, and those medications no longer in use have been deleted.

In listing drug names, generic names are always mentioned first, followed by the trade name in parentheses. When more than one trade name is used, those included have been picked arbitrarily. No bias or preference is intended.

Drugs with more than one use are listed in the chapter in which their most common use is discussed. No attempt has been made to include possibly effective or experimental uses.

The routes of administration and dosage ranges listed are those suggested by the drug manufacturer for administration to adults. Pediatric dosage is not listed unless the drug is given exclusively or primarily to children.

In a text of this nature, it is not possible to include all the information that is known about every drug. Every effort has been made, however, to include all the information the student or graduate needs to know to safely administer the drug in question.

The use of "she" and "her" in reference to the nurse, and of "he" and "him" in reference to the patient is not intended as any assignation of sex, but is meant solely for convenience and clarity.

Margaret C. Lannon, R.N., M.S.

Preface
to the first edition

Today's nurses are undergoing tremendous role changes. The structure of nursing care is also changing, in both the hospital and outpatient settings. With the implementation of primary nursing, more and more nurses are administering medications to their patients. Although increasing numbers of graduate nurses are expected to give medications, few feel they have been adequately prepared to assume this responsibility. They lack confidence in their ability to apply the principles of pharmacology and drug administration safely in the clinical setting.

As one who has taught first-level pharmacology for a number of years, I have been frustrated by the lack of an appropriate textbook for this population of nursing students. It has been my experience that existing first-level texts, in an effort to simplify, often omit information pertinent to a thorough understanding of drug action. Those texts that do contain complete drug information are often unnecessarily detailed or difficult for the average first-level student or new graduate to understand.

Essentials of Pharmacology was written in response to the need for a first-level pharmacology text that includes information about drug action in a readable, understandable format; explains possible adverse effects; gives particulars of dosage, route, and use; and, most important, gives specific nursing implications for each drug discussed in detail.

Special attention should be given to nursing implications. It is through a thorough understanding of this aspect of medication administration that the nurse becomes a safer practitioner. Often, it is not enough to simply know what adverse effects are possible with administration of a particular drug. The nurse must be aware of what she must do to check for adverse effects. With this text as a guide, the student begins to consider nursing implications associated with each drug. With this preparation and constant reinforcement during her student experience, the graduate nurse who encounters a new or unfamiliar drug should feel more comfortable with administration. She will review the adverse effects listed by the manufacturer and then, on the basis of her experience with this text, realize that certain nursing implications need to be considered.

Part One of the text gives general drug information, principles of pharmacology, and arithmetic review—necessary background for the study of medications and medication administration. Parts Two through Seven are arranged to reflect my view of each person as a system interacting with his environment as well as his own internal mechanisms. Each part focuses on one of humankind's survival needs and the medications given to help meet this need. It is hoped that this format will encourage the student to view each patient as a unique individual with many interacting needs. Part Eight contains brief chapters on drugs used in special circumstances, such as obstetrics, pediatrics, diagnostic testing, and treatment of heavy metal poisoning.

Each chapter begins with an overview of the material to be covered. Chapter content is then presented in the following manner: 1, introduction to the category of drugs to be discussed—their general use; 2, pharmacologic action (basic anatomy and physiology are reviewed where indicated); 3, subgroups of the category with general discussion of their action and use—important adverse effects, drug and food interactions, changes brought about by drug use, and potential problems; and 4, nursing implications.

Most chapters contain tables that give particulars of nomenclature, usual dosage range and routes, use, a summary of adverse effects, and nursing implications. The student should utilize these tables as a quick reference as she administers medications to her patients.

In listing drug names, generic names are always mentioned first, followed by the trade name in parentheses. When more than one trade name is used, those included have been picked arbitrarily. No bias or preference is intended.

Drugs with more than one use are listed in the chapter in which their most common use is discussed. No attempt is made to include possibly effective or experimental uses.

The routes and dosage ranges listed are those suggested by the drug manufacturer for administration to adults. Pediatric dosage is not listed unless the drug is given exclusively or primarily to children.

In a text of this nature, it is not possible to include all information on every drug. Every effort has been made, however, to include all the information the student or graduate needs to know to safely administer the drug in question.

The use of "she" and "her" in reference to the nurse, and of "he" and "him" in reference to the client is not intended as any assignation of sex, but is meant solely for convenience and clarity.

Margaret M. Cibulskis, R.N., M.S.

Acknowledgments

Special thanks to David W. DePiero, M.S., R.Ph. for his independent review and suggestions, and to Lorraine Bonanno for her invaluable help with the manuscript.

Contents

PART

1 Introduction to Pharmacology   1

1 General Principles of Pharmacology   *3*
2 Drug Action   *5*
3 Systems of Measurement   *11*
4 Arithmetic Review   *15*
5 Drug Administration and Calculation of Dosage   *29*

2 Drugs Used to Help Meet Patients' Needs for Comfort, Safety, and Hygiene   41

6 Psychotropic Drugs   *43*
7 Anti-infectives   *55*
8 Dermatologic Drugs   *77*
9 Serums and Vaccines   *83*
10 Alcohol   *87*
11 Analgesics and Anesthetics   *91*

3 Drugs Used to Help Meet Patients' Needs for Activity, Exercise, Rest, and Sleep   103

12 Stimulant Drugs   *105*
13 Anti-inflammatory, Antirheumatic, and Uricosuric Drugs   *109*
14 Skeletal Muscle Relaxants and Antiparkinsonian Drugs   *117*
15 Sedatives and Hypnotics   *125*

4 Drugs Used to Help Meet Patients' Needs for Intake and Utilization of Nutrients and the Elimination of Waste   131

16 Vitamins, Minerals, Fluids, and Electrolytes   *133*
17 Antacids, Digestants, Demulcents, and Carminatives   *143*
18 Antispasmodics   *147*

19 Emetics and Antiemetics   *153*
20 Diuretics   *157*
21 Cathartics and Stool Softeners, Enemas, and Antidiarrheals   *165*

5 Drugs Used to Help Meet Patients' Needs for the Intake, Transportation, and Utilization of Oxygen   171

22 Oxygen   *173*
23 Respiratory Stimulants   *175*
24 Bronchodilators   *177*
25 Mucolytics, Expectorants, and Antitussives   *183*
26 Antihistamines   *187*
27 Blood Products   *191*
28 Antianemics   *193*
29 Drugs That Affect Blood Clotting   *197*
30 Antilipemics   *201*
31 Cardiac Stimulants and Cardiac Depressants   *203*
32 Vasodilators and Vasoconstrictors   *211*
33 Antihypertensives   *219*

6 Drugs Used to Help Meet Patients' Needs for the Maintenance of Regulatory Mechanisms and Functions   227

34 Hormones   *229*
35 Antineoplastic Drugs   *245*

7 Drugs Used to Help Meet Patients' Needs for the Maintenance of Sensory and Motor Mechanisms and Functions   255

36 Anticonvulsants   *257*
37 Eye and Ear Medications   *263*

8 Drugs Used in Special Circumstances   269

38 Drugs Used in Pediatrics   *271*
39 Drugs Used in Obstetrics   *275*
40 Diagnostic Agents   *279*
41 Heavy Metal Antagonists   *281*

Answers to Practice Problems   283

Bibliography   285

Index   287

PART 1
Introduction to pharmacology

CHAPTER 1
General principles of pharmacology

Pharmacology is the study of the actions of drugs on a living system. A drug is any chemical substance taken into the body for the purpose of affecting body function.

Pharmacology was being studied as far back as 2000 B.C. Early cultures experimented with the chemical substances found in naturally occurring plants. Through years of experience and much trial-and-error testing, a grouping of helpful natural substances evolved. This information was handed down from generation to generation and eventually written down in books called *pharmacopeias*.

In the early 19th century chemists began to add knowledge to pharmacology by discovering and isolating active ingredients from various plants and animals. This activity led to the development of synthetic (man-made) drugs.

The drugs we use today come from many sources. From plants we obtain such medications as digitalis and quinine. Insulin and corticosteroids are obtained from animals. Minerals such as iron and calcium are often given as medications to supplement dietary intake. Chemical substances such as the synthetic drugs are now available as pharmacologic agents.

LAWS GOVERNING DRUG USE

With the introduction of so many substances that can affect body function, it became necessary to pro-tect the consumer's health. The *Pure Food and Drug Act*, passed in 1906, was the first attempt by government to control the unrestricted sale of drugs or substances alleged to affect the body. The act established two references, the *United States Pharmacopeia* (USP) and the *National Formulary* (NF), as the official criteria by which all drugs were to be standardized. This law also required that the labels of medications containing narcotics list what and how much of the specific narcotic each dose contained.

In 1938 the *Federal Food, Drug and Cosmetic Act* added more regulations to the manufacture and distribution of drugs. It required that all new drugs be tested in animals and judged "safe" before being made available to the general public. This act also added many provisions to ensure accurate, honest labeling of all drug products. Amendments to this act in 1951 and 1965 further controlled the use of habit-forming and other dangerous drugs.

The *Harrison Act* of 1914 was the first law passed that dealt with the problem of drug abuse by regulating the use of narcotic drugs. As a result of the rapid increase in drug abuse, the comprehensive *Controlled Substances Act* was passed in 1970. This law, which became effective May 1, 1971, defines the "drug-dependent" person and the drug "addict." It provides for both education of the public about the problem of drug abuse and rehabilitation programs for the abuser. Enforcement power is given to the Drug Enforcement Agency (DEA) of the United States Department of Justice.

The Controlled Substances Act classifies all drugs that have the potential for causing dependence into "schedules." These are designated as Schedule I, II, III, IV, and V. Drugs are categorized according to their medical usefulness, their potential for abuse, and the severity of the dependence produced. A drug such as heroin, which has no approved medical use in the United States yet can cause severe dependence, is classified in Schedule I. The Controlled Substances Act also establishes penalties for all drug-related illegal acts. It requires that careful records be kept for all Schedule medications and that every dose administered be accounted for. The law also includes regulations about the writing and filling of prescriptions.

Laws similar to those discussed above govern drug use in Canada. International agencies are responsible for controlling drug use, especially of narcotics, in international transactions.

DRUG NAMES

In the study of drugs, the first confusing issue is the names of drugs. Each drug you will study has several names. The two names we shall be concerned with are those you will encounter when you give medications. The generic name is a name used worldwide for the particular drug. The trade (or brand) name is a name given the drug by its manufacturer. The generic name is usually listed first, with an initial lowercase letter; trade names are usually capitalized and found in parentheses following the generic name, for example, erythromycin (Ilotycin). Although there is only one generic name for a drug, there may be many trade names, depending on the number of drug manufacturers. Carbenicillin, for example, may be packaged as Geocillin, Geopen, or Pyopen. All are the same drug, differing only in trade name.

In recent years the trend has been to order and refer to all drugs by their generic rather than trade name. Until this becomes a uniform practice, however, it will be necessary for nurses to be familiar with both the generic name and trade names for each drug they administer.

Knowledge about drugs is constantly changing as research on old drugs continues and new drugs are introduced. Anyone involved in administering medication must refer to current drug handbooks for the information needed to do so safely. The most complete and reliable sources of drug information in the United States are the two official publications, the USP and the NF. These books are revised regularly so that their information will always be current. In Britain the *British Pharmacopeia* (BP), which is similar to the USP, is used. Canada uses both the USP and the BP. Another source of drug information is the *Physicians' Desk Reference*, or PDR. It contains manufacturers' descriptions of drugs and is published yearly. *Drug Facts and Comparisons** contains detailed information on over 10,000 prescription and nonprescription drugs. It is available in loose-leaf and microfiche formats, which are updated monthly, and it is available as a bound volume, which is published annually. Other sources of drug information are the package inserts that accompany many medications, the pharmacist, and the many pharmacology textbooks available.

* *Drug Facts and Comparisons* is published by the J. B. Lippincott Company.

CHAPTER 2
Drug action

The action of a particular drug in the human body is affected by many variables. The variables we discuss in this chapter are physical differences among patients, psychological factors, dosage forms, route of drug administration, and side-effects and adverse reactions.

PHYSICAL DIFFERENCES

The *age* of the patient may have a distinct influence on drug action. Both children and the elderly may need smaller doses of some medications. *Body size* is a related factor that influences drug action. A very large person may need a larger-than-average dose to produce the desired result, whereas a thin, small person would benefit from smaller-than-average doses. Drug dosage for children is usually calculated according to body weight, body surface area, or age (see Chapter 38).

The *amount of food in the stomach* directly affects drug action. Drugs taken on an empty stomach usually reach the bloodstream more quickly than those taken when the stomach is full. Irritating drugs are often ordered to be taken with meals, and other drugs are ordered to be given on an empty stomach.

The *presence of disease* may alter drug action. A change in gastrointestinal function, for example, may delay or accelerate absorption of medications given orally. Altered kidney function may necessitate reduced dosage of medications excreted through the kidneys. If full doses were given, serious cumulative effects could result. In this case, the drug is said to be *contraindicated* in the presence of kidney disease. Contraindications for use are listed along with the other properties of each drug in the various drug information sources.

PSYCHOLOGICAL FACTORS

Much drug action is an outcome of patient beliefs. If a patient believes a drug will work, chances are it will. This effect is documented by research on the "placebo effect."* Conversely, mistrust of the physician, a generally depressed attitude, and feelings of hopelessness may lead to a decrease in drug effectiveness. Those who administer medications should recognize that their attitudes about drugs may influence the patient and, indirectly, the drug action.

DOSAGE FORMS

Many different forms of drugs are available (Fig. 2-1). The dosage form can influence how quickly a drug begins to act (called the *onset of action*), the intensity of its action, and the duration of action.

Solutions are liquids that contain completely dissolved substances. They may be water-based

---

* A placebo is an inactive substance, such as sugar or plain starch, which, when given to some patients, produces results identical to those obtained with medication.

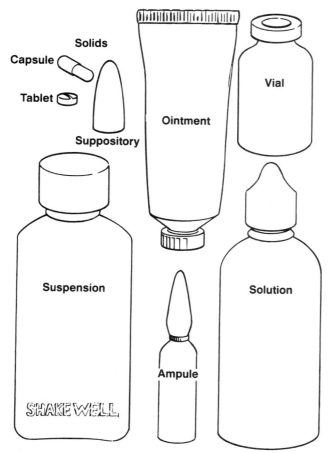

Figure 2-1. Package and dosage forms.

covered with a substance that resists breakdown by stomach enzymes. These medications will be absorbed in the intestine. Most medications administered by mouth are in tablet form, even though people usually refer to all medication as "pills."

For topical administration of medication there are many *lotions, ointments,* and *creams.* These are usually spread over the skin and may or may not be rubbed in.

Suppositories are drugs mixed with a lubricating substance and molded into shapes that can be inserted into body cavities such as the rectum and vagina.

Medications to be injected are usually found in containers called *ampules* or *vials.* An ampule is a small glass container that usually contains just one dose of a drug in solution form. A vial is a small glass container with a rubber stopper that may contain one dose or a number of doses of the drug. Vials containing numerous doses of a drug are referred to as "multiple-dose" vials. Most drugs in vials are in solution form. Occasionally, however, a vial may contain a powdered drug. A certain type and amount of liquid (usually specified on the drug label) must be added to the vial to reconstitute the medication before it is withdrawn into a syringe and administered.

ROUTE OF DRUG ADMINISTRATION

Until relatively recent years most drugs were given orally, and the distinction between foods and drugs was not always clear. In modern medicine oral administration is only one of several ways we can give a drug.

The route of drug administration depends on the form of the drug and the action desired. Drugs with local action affect the area where they are placed. These *topical* applications may be rubbed into or sprayed on the skin or mucous membranes. *Suppositories, inhalations,* and *irrigations* may also lead to local effect.

Drugs with *systemic* action are administered so that the medication enters the bloodstream and is circulated throughout the body. The safest, easiest, and most inexpensive way to achieve systemic drug action is by giving a drug orally (PO). The sublingual (SL, or under the tongue) and rectal (PR) routes also lead to systemic effects.

Parenteral routes of systemic drug administration are any methods other than those involving the gastrointestinal tract. We usually think of par-

(aqueous) or alcoholic solutions such as elixirs, fluid extracts, spirits, or tinctures. Drugs in solution form are easily and quickly absorbed. The more concentrated a solution is, the more rapidly it is absorbed.

Suspensions are liquids in which the particles are mixed, not dissolved. If bottles of suspensions are left on the shelf, they will separate into a sediment, which forms on the bottom, and a liquid, which remains on top. These medications must be shaken to redistribute the particles before the medication is poured.

Medication in *solid* form may be capsules, tablets, or pills. Capsules are usually made of gelatin and hold powdered medication. The gelatin dissolves quickly in the stomach, and the medication is absorbed soon afterward. Tablets and pills come in a variety of colors, shapes, and sizes. Some are coated with sugar or chocolate to disguise an unpleasant taste. Others are enteric-coated, that is,

enteral routes as being those involving *injections*. Drugs given by injection must be sterile, easily absorbed liquids.

The *intradermal* (ID) or *intracutaneous* (IC) injection deposits medication just under the epidermis. *Subcutaneous* (SC) injections are made into the subcutaneous layer of fat. In *intramuscular* (IM) injections the needle passes through the skin and subcutaneous layers into underlying muscle. *Intravenous* (IV) injections, or infusions, deposit medication directly into the bloodstream (Fig. 2-2).

When drugs are administered orally, the onset of action is slower than with parenteral routes, but drug effects may last longer. Drugs administered parenterally are usually more potent. Their onset of action is rapid, but their duration of action may be shorter than after oral administration. The speed of drug action following parenteral injection depends on the blood supply to the injection site. Muscles have the largest number of blood vessels; therefore, IM injections lead to quicker drug action than SC injections. When slower, more prolonged action is desired, as with insulin, the SC route is used. The SC route is contraindicated if there is a decrease in blood supply, such as in cases of shock. Intravenous administration of drugs leads to immediate effect.

PATIENT RESPONSE TO DRUGS

Side-effects and adverse reactions

Some authors distinguish two types of unfavorable patient responses to medications. The generally milder and usually more predictable responses, such as pupillary constriction after narcotic use or nausea with neoplastic agents, are called *side-effects*. The generally more severe and sometimes unexpected responses, such as the appearance of hypertension or cardiac arrhythmias, are called *adverse effects*. This text stresses the importance of recognizing and reporting any unfavorable patient response to medication. Therefore, no distinction is made between them, and they are consistently referred to as adverse effects.

Drug allergy occurs when the administered drug acts as an antigen and the body produces antibodies against it (see Chapter 9). Serious effects may not be seen after the first dose, but subsequent doses may lead to allergic reactions. The reaction may be mild, resulting in hives (urticaria), itching

(pruritus), and congestion, or a serious reaction, called *anaphylaxis*, may occur. Anaphylaxis can occur within seconds of an IV dose of a drug or days later. The reaction may involve shock, loss of consciousness, dyspnea, convulsions, and cardiac arrest. A discussion of anaphylaxis can be found in Chapter 7.

All patients should be carefully questioned about their previous drug-taking experiences. Any unusual effects or allergic reactions they can recall should be reported immediately and noted on the patient's medical record. If the patient is allergic to many nondrug substances (dust, pollen, animals), he may also be allergic to drugs. Whenever a drug reaction or allergy occurs, no matter how mild it is, it must be reported. The next time the same drug is given the effects may be much more serious.

A *drug idiosyncrasy* is an unexpected response to a medication. For example, most people become sleepy after taking antihistamines. An idiosyncratic reaction would occur if the patient became hyperactive instead of sleepy. Drug idiosyncrasy can be either an overresponse or an underresponse.

When the body does not eliminate a drug in the normal fashion (such as when kidney or liver disease is present), the effects will last longer than usual. If the next dose is given as scheduled, cumulative effects may cause serious problems. For example, an antihypertensive drug, if not eliminated before another dose is given, could cause a cumulative *hypo*tensive effect and a severe hypotensive crisis in the patient.

Drug dependence is the single term now used instead of "habituation" or "addiction." A drug-dependent person is unable to control his intake of a drug. Dependence may be physical, psychological, or both. Physical dependence leads to intense physical discomfort if the drug is abruptly withdrawn. Psychological dependence is an emotional problem. It may lead to mild or severe dependence. Drug dependence is an adverse reaction that occurs primarily with use of Schedule medications such as narcotics, barbiturates, and amphetamines.

Drug abuse is the chronic misuse of a drug. It results from too much of the drug, either continually or periodically. Because of the large number of drugs currently available, drug abuse has become a major social issue and health problem in the United States and around the world.

Tolerance is a property of some drugs. It occurs when continued administration of a drug leads to

(*Text continues on p. 10.*)

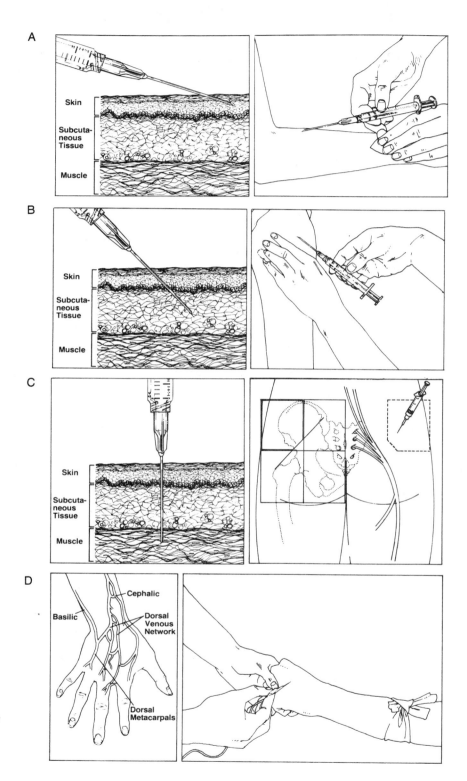

Figure 2-2. Parenteral routes of drug administration. (A) Intradermal. (B) Subcutaneous. (C) Intramuscular. (D) Intravenous.

TABLE 2-1 SOME IMPORTANT THERAPEUTIC DRUG INTERACTIONS

PRIMARY DRUG	KNOWN INTERACTANTS	RESULT
Alcohol	Furazolidone, metronidazole, nitroglycerin, sulfonylureas, disulfiram	Hypotension, nausea, vomiting, diarrhea
Alcohol	CNS depressants, narcotics, tranquilizers	Alcohol potentiates effect of the other drugs
Alcohol	Griseofulvin	Apathy, forgetfulness, impaired cerebral function
Alcohol	Vancomycin	Convulsions
Anticoagulant	Aspirin	Patients controlled on anticoagulant therapy may bleed because of added anticoagulant effect of aspirin.
Chlorpromazine	Orphenadrine	Hypoglycemia
Chlorpromazine	Trifluoperazine	Hypoglycemia
Coumarin anticoagulants	Indomethacin, oxyphenbutazone, phenylbutazone	Patients well controlled on anticoagulant therapy may bleed because of displacement of plasma-bound coumarin.
Coumarin anticoagulants	Anabolic steroids, barbiturates, chloral hydrate, clofibrate, glutethimide, griseofulvin, phenobarbital, primidone, D-thyroxine	Patients well controlled on anticoagulant therapy *plus* one of these drugs may bleed if second drug is discontinued without reduction of anticoagulant dosage. These drugs probably stimulate hepatic microsomal enzymes responsible for coumarin metabolism.
Digitalis	Diuretics	Digitalis intoxication due to diuretic-induced potassium loss
Digitalis	Calcium gluconate	Digitalized patients rapidly develop toxic reactions if given calcium gluconate intravenously; Ca^{++} synergizes the action of glycosides.
Diphenhydramine	Thioridazine	Epistaxis, dry mouth, dizziness, disorientation
Guanethidine	Methylphenidate	Cardiac arrhythmia
Imipramine	Amitriptyline	Alternating drowsiness and agitation leading to convulsions and coma
Insulin	Indomethacin	Hypoglycemia; indomethacin may block catecholamine-induced glycogenolysis
Isoniazid	Para-aminosalicylic acid, ethionamide	Severe side-effects may result from isoniazid in slow inactivators
Methotrexate	Aspirin, sulfonamides	Displacement of methotrexate from its plasma albumin binding
α-Methyldopa	Amitriptyline	Agitation, tremor
Monoamine oxidase inhibitors	Meperidine	Exaggeration of effects of meperidine
Monoamine oxidase inhibitors	*Drugs:* Alcohol, amphetamines, anesthetics (some), antihistamines (some), hypotensives (some), imipramine, metaraminol, α-methyldopa, morphine, muscle relaxants (some), pressor agents (some), reserpine, sympathomimetics (some) *Foods:** Beer, broad beans, cheese, chicken liver, chocolate, game, pickled herrings, wines, yeast extract	Hypertensive crises and visual hallucinations may occur following any one combination
Nondepolarizing muscle relaxants	Bacitracin, colistin, kanamycin, neomycin, polymyxin B, streptomycin	Prolonged neuromuscular block
Phenylbutazone	Acetohexamide	Potentiation of acetohexamide; phenylbutazone blocks renal excretion of chief metabolite of acetohexamide, hydroxyhexamide
Phenylbutazone	Phenobarbital, promethazine	Reduced half-life of phenylbutazone
Phenytoin	Coumarin anticoagulants	Prolonged action of phenytoin

(continued on page 10)

TABLE 2-1   (continued)

PRIMARY DRUG	KNOWN INTERACTANTS	RESULT
Phenytoin	Phenylbutazone, phenyramidol, sulfaphenazole	Prolonged action of phenytoin; possible inhibition of phenytoin metabolism
Probenecid	Salicylates	Hyperuricemia; transient gout
Quinidine	Nondepolarizing and depolarizing muscle relaxants	Prolonged muscle relaxation
Reserpine	General anesthetics	Profound fall in blood pressure due to failure of compensatory mechanisms
Sulfonamides	Para-aminobenzoic acid-containing local anesthetics	Inactivation of sulfonamide
Sulfonylureas	Monoamine oxidase inhibitors, oxyphenbutazone, probenecid, salicylates, sulfonamides	Potentiation of hypoglycemic effect of sulfonylureas
Sympathomimetics (direct acting)	Bretylium, guanethidine	Hypertension
Tetracyclines	Antacids, metals, milk	Decreased tetracycline absorption
Thiazide diuretics	Glucocorticosteroids	Hyperglycemia
Tolbutamide	Sulfonamides	Hypoglycemia due to displacement of tolbutamide from albumin fraction

* Foods containing tyramine. (After Bevans JA: Essentials of Pharmacology, 2nd ed. Hagerstown, Harper & Row, 1976)

decreased drug effect. This necessitates increasing the dose to gain the desired effect. Barbiturates and narcotics are likely to cause tolerance.

Drug overdose is an adverse reaction that occurs when too large a dose is given, or when cumulative effects occur because of a failure in drug metabolism or excretion. The result is an exaggerated response, or drug poisoning. Death can result from untreated drug overdose.

Drug interactions occur when two or more drugs (in medications, foods, or chemicals) are given and the action of one or all is affected. The result is an unfavorable drug response or one that differs from the expected response. Drug interactions may occur with drugs taken previously, concurrently, or afterward. Three broad categories of drug interactions are recognized:

1. *Additive effect.* This occurs when the combined effect of all drugs taken is greater than the effect of each drug given separately.

2. *Inhibition.* This occurs when decreased drug effect is caused by the interaction of two or more medications. Milk, for example, will inhibit (decrease) the effect of tetracyclines in the body. A specific type of inhibition called *antagonism* occurs when each of two drugs cancels the other's actions so that the result is *no action.*

3. *Potentiation.* This occurs when there is increased drug effect. When aspirin is given to patients on anticoagulants, for example, the anticoagulant's action is increased.

Teratogenic effects occur when drugs taken by a pregnant woman cross into the placenta and affect the embryo or fetus. The embryo is especially sensitive to drugs taken during the first 3 months, since this is the period when fetal organs are developing.

Table 2-1 lists some therapeutic drug interactions.

CHAPTER 3
Systems of measurement

Different countries use different systems of measurement. Some countries define the same terms of measurement in different ways. The quart, for example, contains 32 ounces in the United States and 40 ounces in Britain.

In the late 19th century the metric system was established in an attempt to standardize weights and measurements worldwide. Most countries in the world now use the metric system exclusively. The United States is one of the few that do not. The metric system is, however, the official system of the United States, British, and international pharmacopeias, as well as the *National Formulary*.

The United States monetary system is based on the metric system, but measurements of length, volume, and weight are not. In medicine the United States does utilize the metric system. Two other systems of measurement, the apothecaries' and the household, are also used. Until legislation is passed to make the metric system the only one to be followed, nurses will need to be familiar with all three systems so equivalents can be determined.

THE METRIC SYSTEM

The metric system is a decimal system for measuring length, volume, and weight. In a decimal system all measurements are based on ten or a multiple or division of ten.

1.0	= one
10.0	= ten
100.0	= one hundred
1,000.0	= one thousand
10,000.0	= ten thousand
100,000.0	= one hundred thousand
1,000,000.0	= one million
0.1	= one tenth
0.01	= one hundredth
0.001	= one thousandth
0.0001	= one ten-thousandth
0.00001	= one hundred-thousandth
0.000001	= one millionth

The fundamental units of measurement in the metric system are:

length—meter
volume—liter
weight—gram

Latin prefixes are used to indicate divisions of the basic units:

"deci"—divide the basic unit by 10
"centi"—divide the basic unit by 100
"milli"—divide the basic unit by 1000

Greek prefixes are used to indicate multiples of the basic units:

"deca"—multiply the basic unit by 10
"hecto"—multiply the basic unit by 100
"kilo"—multiply the basic unit by 1000

Using these rules, we see that when a basic unit, for example, the meter, is divided by 100, the resulting unit is a centimeter (a meter divided by 100). Likewise, a kilometer is a multiplication (by 1000) of the basic unit. Measurements in the metric system are always given in arabic numbers, followed by the appropriate abbreviation.

In medicine, all measurements of length are expressed metrically. A wound, for instance, may be described as being 5 cm × 3.5 cm in size. Blood pressure is measured in mm of mercury (the rise of the column of mercury in a glass tube), usually expressed as mm Hg.

In metric volume measurements the basic unit is the liter. If a liter is divided by 1000 the result is a milliliter (ml). In the metric system all fluids are measured in milliliters, which are equal to cubic centimeters (cc). Patient intake and output are measured in these units. For example, a patient may have 240 cc of juice for breakfast; his urine output may be 350 cc.

Metric weight, whether people or drugs are being weighed, is based on the gram. When drugs are measured, the unit most frequently used is the milligram (one gram divided by 1000). When a person is weighed, a larger unit is necessary—the kilogram (one gram multiplied by 1000).

In the metric system temperature is measured in degrees centigrade. "Centi" refers to a division (by 100) along the Celsius scale. Degrees centigrade are written °C. The two fixed reference points are the boiling point of water (100°C) and the freezing point of water (0°C). These numbers are equivalent to 212° and 32° on the Fahrenheit (°F) scale. To convert °F to °C (and vice versa) special formulas have been devised:

$$(°F - 32) \times \frac{5}{9} = °C \qquad \left(°C \times \frac{9}{5}\right) + 32 = °F$$

Example 1

Convert a temperature of 37°C to °F.

$$\left(37 \times \frac{9}{5}\right) + 32 =$$

$$\left(\frac{37 \times 9}{5}\right) + 32 =$$

$$\left(\frac{333}{5}\right) + 32 = 66.6 + 32 = 98.6°F$$

Example 2

Convert a temperature of 100°F to °C.

$$(100 - 32) \times \frac{5}{9} =$$

$$68 \times \frac{5}{9} =$$

$$\frac{68 \times 5}{9} = \frac{340}{9} = 37.8°C$$

Example 3

Convert 10°C to °F.

$$\left(10 \times \frac{9}{5}\right) + 32 =$$

$$\left(\frac{10 \times 9}{5}\right) + 32 =$$

$$\frac{90}{5} + 32 = 18 + 32 = 50°F$$

METRIC MEASUREMENTS

Metric length based on the meter
    1 meter = 10 decimeters (dm)
              100 centimeters (cm)
              1000 millimeters (mm)
    1000 meters = 1 kilometer (km)
Metric weight based on the gram
    1 gram (g) = 10 decigrams (dg)
              100 centigrams (cg)
              1000 milligrams (mg)
              1,000,000 micrograms (mcg)
    1000 grams = 1 kilogram (kg)
Metric volume based on the liter
    1 liter = 1000 milliliters (ml)

THE APOTHECARIES' SYSTEM

The apothecaries' system is an ancient system of measurement seldom used in modern medicine. The basic units of measurement in the apothecaries' system are:

Volume—minim (℈)
           fluid dram (f℥)
           fluid ounce (f℥)
Weight—grain (gr)
          dram (℥)
          ounce (℥)

In the apothecaries' system Roman numerals rather than Arabic numbers are used, and the symbol precedes the number. An example of this is "grains X."

Most hospital pharmacies use the metric system, but a few drugs, such as aspirin, morphine, and thyroid preparations, are still ordered (probably out of habit) by apothecaries' units of measurement. A common order for aspirin reads: "Give ASA gr X PO q 4h prn headache," which means: "Give 10 grains of aspirin orally every 4 hours as necessary for headache."

ROMAN NUMERALS

I — 1		X — 10	
II — 2		L — 50	
III* — 3		C — 100	
IV — 4		D — 500	
V — 5		M — 1000	

THE HOUSEHOLD SYSTEM

If medications are administered in the home, neither the apothecaries' nor the metric system is used. Instead, we usually use measures such as the teaspoon, tablespoon, glass, and cup. While these measures are not accurate, they are often sufficient for approximating the metric measurements (see Approximate Household Equivalents).

* Roman numerals may also be written as lowercase letters. For example, 1, 2, and 3 are written i, ii, and iii.

APPROXIMATE HOUSEHOLD EQUIVALENTS

Household	Metric
1 teaspoon (tsp)	5 ml
1 dessert spoon	8 ml
1 tablespoon (Tbl)	15 ml
2 tablespoons	30 ml
1 teacup (6 oz)	180 ml
1 glass (8 oz)	240 ml

CONVERSION

To convert means to change into another form. Thus, by conversion we can describe the same quantity of a substance in different terms. Sometimes it is necessary to convert measurements from one system of measurement to another. We may also need to convert units within the same system, such as changing grams to milligrams and vice versa. Practice problems for converting measurements from one system to another can be found in Chapter 5.

In order to convert, we need to know the equivalents between units of measurement. An equivalent is the same quantity stated in other terms. An example of an equivalent is 4 quarters = \$1.00. Other examples of equivalents include the following:

1 cc	= 1 ml
1000 ml	= 1 liter
1000 mg	= 1 g
1000 g	= 1 kg
2.2 lb	= 1 kg
2.5 cm	= 1 in
30 cc	= 1 oz

Charts are available that list metric and apothecaries' equivalents. The most important equivalents in these two systems include the following:

gr $\frac{1}{60}$	= 1 mg
60 mg	= gr i†
30 mg	= gr $\frac{1}{2}$
15 mg	= gr $\frac{1}{4}$
1 g	= gr xv

† In the apothecaries' system lowercase Roman numerals are used.

CHAPTER 4
Arithmetic review

One of the responsibilities of the nurse who administers medications to patients is the proper calculation of dosage. Because it is essential that the patient receive the amount of medication prescribed, the nurse must have a knowledge of the basics of mathematics to properly determine correct dosages. This chapter provides the basic mathematical principles needed for proper calculation of drug dosage.

ROMAN NUMERALS

In the apothecaries' system, Roman numerals are used. When a smaller Roman numeral follows a larger one, the numbers are added.

Example 1

LII = L for 50 and II for 2

50 + 2 = 52

Example 2

CXV = C for 100, X for 10, and V for 5

100 + 10 + 5 = 115

When a smaller Roman numeral precedes a larger one, the smaller number is subtracted from the larger number.

Example 1

IX = I for 1 and X for 10

10 − 1 = 9

Example 2

XLIV = X for 10, L for 50, I for 1, and V for 5

(50 − 10) + (5 − 1)
40 + 4 = 44

FRACTIONS

A fraction is a portion of a whole number. It consists of a numerator and a denominator. The denominator is the number of equal parts into which the whole is divided. The numerator is the number of those parts to be considered.

$\dfrac{3}{4}$ numerator
denominator

The line separating the numerator and denominator is an indication to divide. For example, in the fraction $\dfrac{3}{4}$, 3 is divided by 4.

Only like things can be expressed in a fraction:

$$\frac{mg}{mg} \ \text{or}\ \frac{cc}{cc}, \ \text{not}\ \frac{mg}{cc} \ \text{or}\ \frac{g}{mg}$$

Lowest terms

A fraction is simplified by being reduced to lowest terms; that is, the numerator and the denominator are divided by the same number. For example, in the fraction $\frac{5}{10}$ we can divide both the numerator and the denominator by the number 5. The result is $\frac{1}{2}$. This fraction is equivalent to (means the same as) the original fraction, but it is reduced to lowest terms, which makes the numbers easier to work with.

Example 1

Reduce $\frac{12}{15}$ to lowest terms.

Numerator and denominator can be divided by 3.

$$\frac{\cancel{12}\ 4}{\cancel{15}\ 5} = \frac{4}{5}$$

$\frac{4}{5}$ cannot be reduced further

Example 2

Reduce $\frac{16}{48}$ to lowest terms.

Numerator and denominator can be divided by 8.

$$\frac{\cancel{16}\ 2}{\cancel{48}\ 6}$$

$\frac{2}{6}$ can be reduced further by dividing both numerator and denominator by 2

$$\frac{\cancel{2}\ 1}{\cancel{6}\ 3} = \frac{1}{3}$$

$\frac{1}{3}$ cannot be reduced further

Always reduce fractions to lowest terms before carrying out any addition, subtraction, multiplication, or division. Answers to problems should also be reduced to lowest terms.

Types of fractions

Proper fractions. A proper fraction consists of a numerator that is less than the denominator and represents a portion of a whole. Examples of proper fractions are $\frac{1}{4}$ and $\frac{2}{5}$.

Improper fractions. An improper fraction consists of a numerator that is greater than or equal to the denominator. An improper fraction represents one or more units. Examples of improper fractions are $\frac{13}{10}$, $\frac{100}{81}$, and $\frac{3}{3}$.

Mixed numbers

An improper fraction can also be expressed as a mixed number—a whole number plus a proper fraction. Examples of mixed numbers are $2\frac{1}{2}$, $5\frac{1}{2}$, and $6\frac{1}{4}$. To change an improper fraction to a mixed number:

1. Divide the numerator by the denominator.
2. Place the remainder over the denominator of the improper fraction.
3. The mixed number is the whole number plus the proper fraction.

Example 1

Change $\frac{10}{4}$ to a mixed number.

1. Divide 10 by 4: $4\overline{)10}$
    $$\begin{array}{r} 2 \\ 4\overline{)10} \\ \underline{8} \\ 2 \end{array}$$

2. The remainder (2) is placed over the denominator (4): $\frac{2}{4}$

3. The mixed number is $2\frac{2}{4}$ which, when reduced to lowest terms, becomes $2\frac{1}{2}$.

Example 2

Change $\dfrac{21}{5}$ to a mixed number.

$$5\overline{)21} \quad \dfrac{4}{} = 4\dfrac{1}{5}$$
$$\dfrac{20}{1}$$

Example 3

Change $\dfrac{175}{126}$ to a mixed number.

First, reduce to lowest terms. Numerator and denominator can be divided by 7.

$$\dfrac{\cancel{175}\,25}{\cancel{126}\,18} = \dfrac{25}{18}$$
$$18\overline{)25} \quad \dfrac{1}{} = 18\dfrac{7}{18}$$
$$\dfrac{18}{7}$$

Improper fractions should always be changed to mixed numbers.

We can also change a mixed number to an improper fraction:

1. Multiply the denominator by the whole number.
2. Add the numerator.
3. Place this number above the denominator of the improper fraction.

Example 1

Change $2\dfrac{1}{2}$ to an improper fraction.

1. $2 \times 2 = 4$
2. $4 + 1 = 5$
3. $\dfrac{5}{2}$ = the improper fraction

Example 2

Change $12\dfrac{3}{4}$ to an improper fraction.

1. $4 \times 12 = 48$
2. $48 + 3 = 51$
3. $\dfrac{51}{4}$ = the improper fraction

Example 3

Change $2\dfrac{6}{18}$ to an improper fraction.

1. Reduce to lowest terms:

$$2\dfrac{\cancel{6}\ 1}{\cancel{18}\ 3} = 2\dfrac{1}{3}$$

2. $2 \times 3 = 6$
3. $6 + 1 = 7$
4. $\dfrac{7}{3}$ = the improper fraction

Addition of fractions

When the denominators of fractions to be added are the same, simply add the numerators together. The resulting number is placed above the denominator.

Example 1

$$\begin{array}{r} \dfrac{3}{5} \\[4pt] +\,\dfrac{1}{5} \\[2pt] \hline \dfrac{4}{5} \end{array}$$

Example 2

$$\begin{array}{r} \dfrac{4}{7} \\[4pt] +\,\dfrac{5}{7} \\[2pt] \hline \dfrac{9}{7} = 1\dfrac{2}{7} \end{array}$$

To add fractions whose denominators are not the same, a common denominator must be found. We look for the lowest common denominator, or the lowest number that can be divided by all denominators in the problem.

Example 1

Add $\frac{2}{5}$ and $\frac{3}{4}$.

In this example the denominators are different. The lowest number that can be divided by both 4 and 5 is 20. This, then, becomes the common denominator. To find equivalent numerators:

1. For each fraction, divide the common denominator by the original denominator.
2. Multiply this number by the numerator of each fraction.
3. The resulting number becomes the numerator for the common denominator.

Example 1 can now be done:

$$\frac{2}{5} = \frac{8}{20}$$
$$+ \frac{3}{4} = \frac{15}{20}$$
$$\frac{23}{20} = 1\frac{3}{20}$$

Example 2

Add $\frac{3}{12}$ and $\frac{3}{4}$.

$$\frac{3}{12} = \frac{3}{12}$$
$$+ \frac{3}{4} = \frac{9}{12}$$
$$\frac{12}{12} = 1$$

In example 2, the number 12 is the lowest common denominator. The answer $\frac{12}{12}$ is equal to 1.

Subtraction of fractions

When the denominators of fractions to be subtracted are the same, simply subtract the numerators. The resulting number is placed above the denominator.

Example 1

Subtract $\frac{1}{5}$ from $\frac{3}{5}$.

$$\frac{3}{5} - \frac{1}{5} = \frac{2}{5}$$

To subtract fractions whose denominators are not the same, a common denominator must be found. Look for the lowest common denominator.

Example 2

Subtract $\frac{3}{8}$ from $\frac{7}{16}$.

$$\frac{3}{8} = \frac{6}{16}$$
$$\frac{7}{16} - \frac{6}{16} = \frac{1}{16}$$

Adding and subtracting with mixed numbers

When both fractions and mixed numbers are to be added or subtracted, the rules for adding and subtracting fractions must be followed first. The whole numbers may then be added or subtracted.

Example 1

Add $2\frac{2}{5}$ and $1\frac{3}{4}$.

$$2\frac{2}{5} = 2\frac{8}{20}$$
$$+ 1\frac{3}{4} = 1\frac{15}{20}$$
$$3\frac{23}{20} = 4\frac{3}{20}$$

Note: When $\frac{23}{20}$ is changed to a mixed number it becomes $1\frac{3}{20}$, which, when added to the whole number in the answer (3), gives us a final answer of $4\frac{3}{20}$.

Example 2

Subtract $1\frac{2}{5}$ from $3\frac{7}{10}$.

$$3\frac{7}{10} = 3\frac{7}{10}$$
$$-1\frac{2}{5} = 1\frac{4}{10}$$
$$2\frac{3}{10}$$

When subtracting mixed numbers, it is necessary to borrow from the whole number when the numerator of the fraction being subtracted from is less than the numerator of the fraction being subtracted.

Example 3

Subtract $1\frac{2}{3}$ from $3\frac{5}{8}$.

$$3\frac{5}{8} - 1\frac{2}{3} =$$
$$3\frac{15}{24} - 1\frac{16}{24} =$$
$$2\frac{39}{24} - 1\frac{16}{24} = 1\frac{23}{24}$$

Multiplication of fractions

Fractions and whole numbers. To multiply a fraction and a whole number:

1. Multiply the whole number by the numerator of the fraction.
2. Divide that number by the denominator.
3. Reduce the fraction to lowest terms.

Example 1

$$4 \times \frac{1}{3} = \frac{4}{3}$$
$$= 1\frac{1}{3}$$

Example 2

$$\frac{2}{3} \times 6 = \frac{\cancel{12}\,4}{\cancel{3}\,1}$$
$$= 4$$

Two fractions. To multiply two fractions:

1. Multiply the numerators.
2. Multiply the denominators.
3. Reduce the new fraction to lowest terms.

Example 1

$$\frac{4}{2} \times \frac{3}{4} = \frac{4 \times 3}{2 \times 4}$$
$$= \frac{\cancel{12}\,3}{\cancel{8}\,2}$$
$$= \frac{3}{2} \text{ or } 1\frac{1}{2}$$

Example 2

$$\frac{3}{4} \times \frac{12}{21} = \frac{3 \times 12}{4 \times 21}$$
$$= \frac{\cancel{36}\,3}{\cancel{84}\,7}$$
$$= \frac{3}{7}$$

Fractions and mixed numbers. To multiply a fraction and a mixed number, or two mixed numbers, change the mixed number to an improper fraction and proceed with the steps for multiplication of two fractions.

Example 1

$$2\frac{1}{3} \times 1\frac{1}{4} = \frac{7}{3} \times \frac{5}{4}$$
$$= \frac{35}{12}$$
$$= 2\frac{11}{12}$$

Example 2

$$\frac{3}{4} \times 3\frac{2}{3} = \frac{3}{4} \times \frac{11}{3}$$
$$= \frac{3 \times 11}{4 \times 3}$$
$$= \frac{33}{12}$$
$$= 2\frac{\cancel{9}\,3}{\cancel{12}\,4}$$
$$= 2\frac{3}{4}$$

Division of fractions

When two fractions are divided the second fraction is inverted (turned upside down). Then the two fractions are multiplied.

Example 1

Divide $2\frac{1}{3}$ by $\frac{2}{3}$.

$2\frac{1}{3}$ as an improper fraction is $\frac{7}{3}$

$$\frac{7}{3} \div \frac{2}{3} = \frac{7}{3} \times \frac{3}{2}$$
$$= \frac{7 \times 3}{3 \times 2}$$
$$= \frac{\overset{7}{\cancel{21}}}{\underset{2}{\cancel{6}}}$$
$$= \frac{7}{2} \text{ or } 3\frac{1}{2}$$

Example 2

Divide $\frac{3}{4}$ by $\frac{3}{5}$.

$$\frac{3}{4} \div \frac{3}{5} = \frac{3}{4} \times \frac{5}{3}$$
$$= \frac{3 \times 5}{4 \times 3}$$
$$= \frac{\overset{5}{\cancel{15}}}{\underset{4}{\cancel{12}}}$$
$$= \frac{5}{4} \text{ or } 1\frac{1}{4}$$

In division problems with fractions and whole numbers, first change the whole number to an improper fraction by placing it above a denominator of 1.

Example 3

Divide 3 by $\frac{1}{2}$.

$$\frac{3}{1} \div \frac{1}{2} = \frac{3}{1} \times \frac{2}{1}$$

$$= \frac{3 \times 2}{1 \times 1}$$
$$= \frac{6}{1} \text{ or } 6$$

To divide a whole number or a fraction by a mixed number, change the mixed number to an improper fraction and proceed as with division of two fractions.

Example 1

$$1\frac{3}{4} \div \frac{2}{3} = \frac{7}{4} \div \frac{2}{3}$$
$$= \frac{7}{4} \times \frac{3}{2}$$
$$= \frac{7 \times 3}{4 \times 2}$$
$$= \frac{21}{8} \text{ or } 2\frac{5}{8}$$

Example 2

$$2\frac{1}{8} \div \frac{1}{5} = \frac{17}{8} \div \frac{1}{5}$$
$$= \frac{17}{8} \times \frac{5}{1}$$
$$= \frac{17 \times 5}{8 \times 1}$$
$$= \frac{85}{8} \text{ or } 10\frac{5}{8}$$

Larger and smaller fractions

When fractions with the same denominator are compared, the fraction with the larger numerator is the larger fraction. For example, $\frac{2}{3}$ is greater than $\frac{1}{3}$. If two fractions have different denominators, to find which is the larger fraction you must first find a common denominator. Once the common denominator is determined, you can find the equivalent numerators. The larger fraction can now be determined by finding the fraction with the larger numerator.

Example 1

Which is larger, $\dfrac{2}{3}$ or $\dfrac{3}{4}$?

1. Find the common denominator:

$$\frac{2}{3} = \frac{8}{12}$$

$$\frac{3}{4} = \frac{9}{12}$$

2. Compare the numerators.

3. The larger fraction is $\dfrac{9}{12}$, or $\dfrac{3}{4}$.

Example 2

Which is larger, $\dfrac{3}{7}$ or $\dfrac{10}{21}$?

$$\frac{3}{7} = \frac{9}{21}$$

$$\frac{10}{21} = \frac{10}{21}$$

The larger fraction is $\dfrac{10}{21}$.

DECIMALS

A decimal is a fraction whose denominator is ten or a multiple of ten (100, 1000, 10,000, etc.). The denominator is not written, but it is expressed by the placement of a decimal point. The first place to the right of the decimal point is tenths, the second hundredths, the third thousandths, and so on.

thousands	hundreds	tens	ones	decimal point	tenths	hundredths	thousandths	ten thousandths
4	3	2	1	·	1	2	3	4

0.1 is one tenth*
0.10 is ten hundredths
0.105 is one hundred five thousandths

With a whole number, the fraction is read as follows:

2.05 is two and five hundredths
10.1 is ten and one tenth

Three tenths can be expressed $\dfrac{3}{10}$ or 0.3

It is essential that the decimal point be placed properly. For instance, if one tenth were written as .01 instead of 0.1, the patient would get only $\dfrac{1}{10}$ of the medication ordered. If one and twenty-five hundredths of a milligram were ordered and were transcribed as 12.5 mg instead of 1.25 mg, the patient would receive ten times the amount of medication ordered.

Addition and subtraction of decimals

When adding or subtracting decimals, it is important to line the numbers up so that those of the same value (tenths, hundredths, ones, tens, etc.) are in the same column. Then, addition or subtraction (as done with whole numbers) can be carried out.

Note: Zeros added to the right of a decimal point (past the fraction) do not change the value of the number. Their function is to help maintain column alignment.

Example 1

0.10 + 1.002 + 50.0651

```
     | 0|.|1|0| | |
     | 1|.|0|0|2| |
  + |5|0|.|0|6|5|1|
  -----------------
   |5|1|.|1|6|7|1|
```

* In order to prevent errors, a zero should be added to the left of a decimal point if there is no whole number.

Example 2

39.762 − 5.0312

$$
\begin{array}{r}
3\,9\,.\,7\,6\,2\,0 \\
-\ \ 5\,.\,0\,3\,1\,2 \\
\hline
3\,4\,.\,7\,3\,0\,8
\end{array}
$$

Multiplication of decimals

In all multiplication problems involving decimals, the number of decimal places in the answer is equal to the total number of decimal places in the numbers multiplied. Numbers are arranged as with multiplication of whole numbers. The decimal points do *not* need to be lined up, one under another.

Example 1

Multiply 0.25 × 4.

$$
\begin{array}{r}
0.25 \\
\times\ \ \ 4 \\
\hline
1.00
\end{array}\ \text{total of 2 decimal places}
$$

Note: A zero is usually put to the left of the decimal point if there is no whole number in the "tens" place.
Since the 2 numbers multiplied have a combined total of 2 decimal places, there must be 2 decimal places in the answer as well.

Example 2

Multiply 1.25 by 0.3.

$$
\begin{array}{r}
1.25 \\
\times\ \ 0.3 \\
\hline
0.375
\end{array}\ \text{total of 3 decimal places}
$$

Example 3

Multiply 0.017 by 0.5.

$$
\begin{array}{r}
0.017 \\
\times\ \ \ \ 0.5 \\
\hline
0.0085
\end{array}
$$

Since the 2 numbers multiplied have a combined total of 4 decimal places, there must be 4 decimal places in the answer, as well.

To multiply a decimal by ten or a multiple of ten (100, 1000, etc.), the decimal point is moved to the *right* as many places as there are zeros in the number.

Example 1

$$
72.35 \times 10 = 72.35
$$
$$
= 723.5
$$

Example 2

$$
0.814 \times 100 = 0.814
$$
$$
= 81.4
$$

Division of decimals

Recall the terms: $\text{divisor}\overline{)\text{dividend}}^{\text{quotient}}$.

If the divisor is a whole number, division is carried out as with whole numbers. The decimal point is placed in the quotient directly above its position in the dividend.

Example 1

Divide 2.5 by 5.

$$
\begin{array}{r}
.5 \\
5\overline{)2.5} = 0.5 \\
2\ 5
\end{array}
$$

A decimal can never remain in the divisor. It must be moved to the right to change the decimal to a whole number. The rules to follow for division of decimals when there is a decimal in the divisor are as follows:

1. Move the decimal in the divisor to the right as many places as necessary to make the decimal a whole number.

2. Move the decimal in the dividend an equal number of places, adding zeros if necessary, to make up the necessary places.

3. Divide the numbers as with whole numbers, placing the decimal point in the quotient directly above the decimal point in the dividend.

Example 2

Divide 33.6 by 1.2.

$$1.2\overline{)33.6}$$

$$12\overline{)336.} = 28.\ \text{or}\ 28$$
$$\begin{array}{r} 28. \\ \underline{24} \\ 96 \\ \underline{96} \end{array}$$

Example 3

Divide 210 by 1.5.

$$1.5\overline{)210.0}$$

$$15\overline{)2100.} = 140.\ \text{or}\ 140$$
$$\begin{array}{r} 140. \\ \underline{15} \\ 60 \\ \underline{60} \end{array}$$

Note: In division of decimals, the answer is usually rounded off to the nearest hundredth.

To divide a decimal or a whole number by ten or a multiple of ten, move the decimal point to the *left* as many places as there are zeros in the number.

Example 1

$$376.201 \div 100 = 3\underset{\smile}{76}.201 = 3.76201$$

Example 2

$$4.21 \div 10 = \underset{\smile}{4}.21 = 0.421$$

To divide a smaller number by a larger number, place the decimal point to the right of the number, add as many zeros as needed to divide, and proceed with division.

Example 1

$$3 \div 12 = 12\overline{)3.00}$$

$$= 12\overline{)3.00}$$
$$\begin{array}{r} .25 \\ \underline{2\ 4} \\ 60 \\ \underline{60} \\ 0 \end{array}$$
$$= 0.25$$

Example 2

$$7.1 \div 220 = 220\overline{)7.1000}$$
$$\begin{array}{r} .0322 \\ \underline{6\ 60} \\ 500 \\ \underline{440} \\ 600 \\ \underline{440} \\ 160 \end{array}$$
$$= 0.032$$

(The answer has been rounded off to the nearest thousandth.)

Changing a fraction to a decimal

To convert a fraction to a decimal, divide the numerator by the denominator. The fraction's numerator is the dividend and the fraction's denominator is the divisor. Add a zero (or two, if necessary) after the whole number in the dividend and place the decimal point directly above its position in the dividend. Then divide as with whole numbers.

Example 1

Change $\frac{4}{5}$ to a decimal.

$$5\overline{)4.0} = 0.8$$
$$\underline{4\ 0}$$

Example 2

Change $\frac{2}{5}$ to a decimal.

$$5\overline{)2.0} = 0.4$$
$$\underline{2\ 0}$$

Changing a decimal to a fraction

In order to change a decimal to a fraction, write the decimal number as the numerator. The denominator is designated by the name given to the number of decimal places.

Example 1

Change 0.5 to a fraction.

1. The numerator is 5.

2. The denominator is "tenths," or $\frac{5}{10}$.

3. $0.5 = \frac{\cancel{5}\ 1}{\cancel{10}\ 2}$, or $\frac{1}{2}$

Example 2

Change 0.125 to a fraction.

1. The numerator is 125.

2. The denominator is "thousandths," or $\frac{125}{1000}$.

3. $0.125 = \frac{\cancel{125}\ 1}{\cancel{1000}\ 8}$, or $\frac{1}{8}$

PERCENTS

Percent means "per 100." Nine percent (9%), for example, means 9 parts per 100. When changed to fractions, all percents have a denominator of 100. In other words, $9\% = \frac{9}{100}$, and $25\% = \frac{25}{100}$ or $\frac{1}{4}$. Fractions are always reduced to lowest terms.

To convert a percent to a decimal, divide by 100 by moving the decimal point two places to the left. This means that $9\% = .09$, or 0.09.

To change a decimal to a percent, multiply by 100 by moving the decimal point two places to the right and adding a percentage sign (%). For example, $0.18 = 0.18 \times 100 = 18\%$.

Percentage of a number

To find the percentage of a number, change the percent to a fraction and multiply the number by this fraction.

Example 1

Find 15% of 500.

1. $15\% = \frac{15}{100}$ or $\frac{3}{20}$

2. $\frac{\overset{25}{\cancel{500}}}{1} \times \frac{3}{\underset{1}{\cancel{20}}} = \frac{25 \times 3}{1 \times 1} = \frac{75}{1}$ or 75

3. 15% of 500 is 75.

Example 2

Find 10% of $\frac{3}{5}$.

1. $10\% = \frac{10}{100}$ or $\frac{1}{10}$

2. $\frac{3}{5} \times \frac{1}{10} = \frac{3 \times 1}{5 \times 10} = \frac{3}{50}$

3. 10% of $\frac{3}{5}$ is $\frac{3}{50}$.

Changing a fraction to a percent

To change a fraction to a percent, divide the numerator by the denominator and multiply the answer by 100.

Example 1

Change $\frac{2}{5}$ to a percent.

1. $5\overline{)2.0}^{\ .4}$

2. $\begin{array}{r} 100 \\ \times\ 0.4 \\ \hline 40.0 \end{array}$

3. $\frac{2}{5} = 40\%$

Example 2

Change $\frac{3}{4}$ to a percent.

1. $\begin{array}{r} .75 \\ 4\overline{)3.00} \\ \underline{2\ 8}\ \ \\ 20 \\ \underline{20} \end{array}$

2.
$$
\begin{array}{r}
100 \\
\times\ \underline{.75} \\
5\ 00 \\
\underline{70\ 0} \\
75.00
\end{array}
$$

3. $\dfrac{3}{4} = 75\%$

Multiplying by percent

When multiplying by percent, first change the percent to a decimal, and then proceed with the multiplication.

Example 1

$$72 \times 3.2\% =$$
$$72 \times 0.032 = 2.304$$

RATIO

A ratio expresses the comparison of one number to another. It is a fraction whose numerator and denominator are separated by a colon.

Example 1

$\dfrac{1}{8}$ expressed as a ratio is $1:8$ and is read "one to eight."

Example 2

$\dfrac{7}{100}$ expressed as a ratio is $7:100$ and is read "seven to one hundred."

To change a ratio to a fraction, the number to the left of the colon (:) becomes the numerator and the number to the right of the colon becomes the denominator.

Example 1

$$3:100 = \frac{3}{100}$$

Example 2

$$3:8 = \frac{3}{8}$$

To change a ratio to a decimal or a percent, the number to the left of the colon is divided by the number to the right of the colon.

Example 1

$$
\begin{aligned}
3:100 &= 3 \div 100 \\
&= 100\overline{)3.00}^{\,.03} \\
&= 0.03,\text{or } 3\%
\end{aligned}
$$

Example 2

$$
\begin{aligned}
3:8 &= 3 \div 8 \\
&= 8\overline{)3.000}^{\,.375} \\
&\quad\ \underline{2\ 4} \\
&\quad\ \ 60 \\
&\quad\ \ \underline{56} \\
&\quad\ \ \ 40 \\
&\quad\ \ \ \underline{40} \\
&= 0.375 \text{ or } 37.5\%
\end{aligned}
$$

To change a ratio to a decimal or percent, the number to the left of the colon is divided by the number to the right of the colon.

Example 1

$$3:100 = 3 \div 100 = 0.03 \text{ or } 3\%$$

Example 2

$$3:8 = 3 \div 8 = 0.375 \text{ or } 37.5\%$$

PROPORTION

A proportion is a statement of equal relationship between two ratios. An example of a proportion is:

$$3:4 = 75:100$$

This proportion can also be expressed as 3:4 :: 75:100, with the double colon (::) replacing the equal sign. Expressed either way, the proportion above is read "three to four is the equivalent of seventy-five to one hundred." It can also be read "three is to four as seventy-five is to one hundred."

In the proportion 1:2 :: 4:8, the first and fourth numbers (the two outside, 1 and 8) are called the *extremes*. The second and third numbers (the two inside, 2 and 4) are the *means*. The product of the extremes always equals the product of the means. Using the above example this means:

$$
\begin{array}{ccc}
1 \times 8 & = & 2 \times 4 \\
(\text{extremes}) & & (\text{means}) \\
8 & = & 8
\end{array}
$$

Using this knowledge, it is possible to determine an unknown term in the proportion. The product of the two known terms is determined and then is divided by the third known term. The unknown is represented by "x." Thus, if one mean is unknown, the product of the extremes is divided by the known mean.

Example 1

$$6: x = 12 : 16$$

$$12x = 96$$
$$\frac{\cancel{12}x}{\cancel{12}} = \frac{\cancel{96}\,8}{\cancel{12}\,1}$$
$$x = 8$$

If one extreme is unknown, the product of the means is divided by the known extreme.

Example 1

$$2:6 :: 3:x$$

$$18 = 2x$$
$$9\ \frac{\cancel{18}}{1\ \cancel{8}} = \frac{\cancel{2}x}{\cancel{2}}$$
$$9 = x$$

Proportions can be used to work conversion problems, as long as one set of equivalents is known.

Example 1

Change 3 g to milligrams.
You already know there are 1000 mg in 1 g; therefore:

$$1000 \text{ mg} : 1 \text{ g} :: x \text{ mg} : 3 \text{ g}$$
$$3000 = 1x$$
$$3000 = x$$
$$3 \text{ g} = 3000 \text{ mg}$$

Example 2

Change 44 lb to kilograms.
You already know there are 2.2 lb in 1 kg; therefore:

$$2.2 \text{ lb} : 1 \text{ kg} :: 44 \text{ lb} : x \text{ kg}$$
$$2.2x = 44$$
$$\frac{\cancel{2.2}x}{\cancel{2.2}} = \frac{44}{2.2}$$

$$2.2\overline{)44.0}$$

$$
\begin{array}{r}
20 \\
22\overline{)440.} \\
\underline{44} \\
0
\end{array}
$$

$$x = 20$$
$$44 \text{ lb} = 20 \text{ kg}$$

PRACTICE PROBLEMS—ARITHMETIC REVIEW

Reduce to lowest terms.

1. $\dfrac{12}{30}$

2. $\dfrac{6}{12}$

3. $\dfrac{7}{21}$

4. $\dfrac{8}{6}$

5. $\dfrac{130}{100}$

Change to an improper fraction.

6. $3\dfrac{10}{11}$

7. $15\dfrac{2}{3}$

Do the following problems:

8. $\dfrac{7}{8} + \dfrac{2}{3} =$

9. $1\dfrac{1}{12} - \dfrac{1}{4} =$

10. $\dfrac{13}{18} - \dfrac{1}{6} =$

11. $4\dfrac{1}{2} + 2\dfrac{1}{3} + \dfrac{1}{4} =$

12. $6 \times \dfrac{1}{6} =$

13. $\dfrac{3}{4} \times \dfrac{1}{21} =$

14. $2\dfrac{1}{3} \times 10\dfrac{2}{5} =$

15. $3\dfrac{7}{8} - \dfrac{2}{3} =$

16. $7\dfrac{1}{4} - \dfrac{3}{16} =$

17. $3.205 + 7.6 =$

18. $0.31 + 1.025 =$

19. $10.67 - 0.356 =$

20. $0.75 \times 11 =$

21. $6.13 \times 0.35 =$

22. $3.7 \div 2.1 =$

23. $62.1 \div 0.025 =$

24. Change $\dfrac{7}{16}$ to a decimal.

25. Change 0.375 to a fraction.

26. What is 45% of 70?

27. What is 0.6% of 12?

28. Change $\frac{4}{5}$ to a percent.

Solve for x.

29. 3:4 :: x : 20

30. 7:49 :: 3 : x

31. x : 10 = 4:12

32. 3 : x = 9:20

Answers are given on p. 283.

CHAPTER 5
Drug administration and calculation of dosage

Drug administration is one of the nurse's most important responsibilities. Although the role of the clinical pharmacist is changing to include increasing involvement with administration of medication, this does not diminish the nurse's responsibilities for teaching patients about their medications.

Laws are in effect to protect the patient in the event a mistake is made involving drug administration. The nurse who administers the medication is held directly responsible for her actions. In order to administer drugs safely (and avoid legal problems), the nurse must always use her knowledge of drug action, follow proper technique in preparing and administering the drug, and question any order that does not appear to be correct.

Each hospital has its particular set of regulations for the storage, administration, and charting of medications. Some hospitals have a large supply of "stock" medications on each patient unit that the nurse uses to prepare each patient's medications. Other hospitals follow the "unit dose" system, in which each patient's medications are sent from the pharmacy in premeasured, individually sealed packets especially prepared for that patient.

Although methods of medication administration may vary from hospital to hospital, the basic principles of medication administration do not. The nurse's responsibilities include the following:

1. Preparing the medication
2. Identifying the patient
3. Administering the medication
4. Observing the patient for medication effect
5. Reporting and recording any adverse effect

PREPARING THE MEDICATION

Drugs should never be given without a specific order written by the physician. In emergency situations a registered nurse (RN) may take a verbal order, but this should be verified by the physician, in writing, as soon as possible.

Be sure you understand exactly what the order says. The order must specify the drug, the amount, the route, and the frequency of administration.

You need to be familiar with the abbreviations commonly used in your particular institution. (See the table on the inside of the front cover.)

Question any order that does not appear to be correct. In order to recognize mistakes, you need to know the usual route, dosage range, and use for each drug you administer.

When you prepare medications, you should be in a quiet place where you will be able to concentrate. Any distractions may lead to mistakes in calculations. When dosage calculations or conversion problems must be done, always ask another nurse to double-check an answer you are unsure of. Always read the medication label three times: (1) when you take the medication from the shelf, (2) before you pour the medication, and (3) before you put the medication back on the shelf (Fig. 5-1). Never give a medication from an unlabeled bottle or container or from one with an illegible label.

Capsules, tablets, and pills should not be handled. Pour the correct dose from the bottle into the cap and from there into the medicine cup. Measure liquids correctly, using a calibrated (marked) medicine cup or syringe held at eye level. Never return unused medication to its original container. If a patient refuses a medication, or if the order is changed before you administer a medication you have already poured, simply discard the medication. After you have poured a patient's medication, label the medicine cup or place the medication card near it in such a way that you are sure no patient will receive another patient's medications by mistake. Prepackaged unit dose medications should be opened *at the patient's bedside* and not before.

PREPARING THE PATIENT

It is your responsibility to teach the patient about the drugs he receives. The patient should understand why he is receiving each drug and what, if any, adverse effects he needs to watch for. If there are adverse effects that may alarm him, such as change in urine color, tell him about these effects before they occur.

ADMINISTERING THE MEDICATION

Verify the patient's identity each time you give a medication. If the patient is not wearing an identification band with his name on it, ask him to state his name. Listen to what the patient has to say. Comments such as, "I thought I was off that drug,"

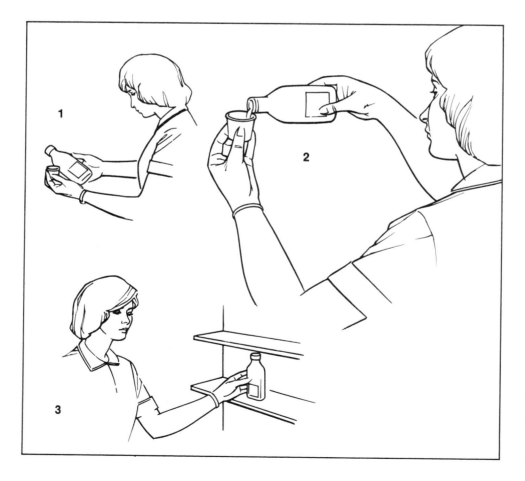

Figure 5-1. Read medication label (1) when removing from shelf, (2) when pouring, and (3) when replacing on shelf.

or "I've never seen this pill before," may alert you to possible errors (Fig. 5-2). Investigate these comments before you give the medication. Never give a medication if you suspect there is an error involved. Many errors may be prevented this way, since the patient is usually much more familiar with his medications than you are. If a drug has an unpleasant taste, agree with the patient as he voices his distaste. Denying the fact may make the patient feel foolish.

Never leave medications at the patient's bedside unless specifically ordered to do so. Always observe to see that the patient actually swallows the medication. This is especially important when giving medications that are frequently abused, such as narcotics or psychotropic drugs. Never leave a tray of medications unattended.

SPECIAL CONSIDERATIONS WHEN ADMINISTERING MEDICATIONS BY INJECTION

Equipment

A needle and a syringe are needed to administer medications by injection. Syringes vary in both size and calibration. A tuberculin syringe holds up to 1 ml and is calibrated in tenths (0.1, 0.2, etc.) with subdivisions in hundredths of a milliliter (0.12, 0.13, 0.14, etc). Syringes for subcutaneous (SC) and intramuscular (IM) injections hold 2 ml to 3 ml and are calibrated in tenths of a milliliter. Insulin syringes, specially designed for insulin, contain up to 1 ml and are calibrated in units. Figure 5-3 shows the three different types of syringes.

Needles are measured in length, expressed in inches, and diameter, or gauge. The larger the gauge, the smaller the needle's diameter. For example, a 19-gauge, 1-inch needle is a short, large-diameter needle suitable for injecting viscous liquids into intravenous tubing. A 25-gauge, 5/8-inch needle is a short, small-diameter needle used for subcutaneous injections. A 22-gauge, 1½-inch needle is suitable for intramuscular injections.

Method

Once the appropriate needle and syringe have been selected, medication can be drawn into the syringe. If the drug to be used is contained in an ampule, carefully break the neck of the ampule. Place the needle at the bottom of the ampule and withdraw all medication into the syringe. Hold the syringe with the needle pointing upward to measure correct dosage. Push any extra medication out of the syringe over a waste receptacle.

If the medication to be used is contained in a vial, first wipe the rubber stopper with an alcohol sponge. Then draw air in the amount equal to that of medication to be withdrawn into the syringe. Introduce the needle into the rubber stopper and inject the air. Then invert the vial so medication can

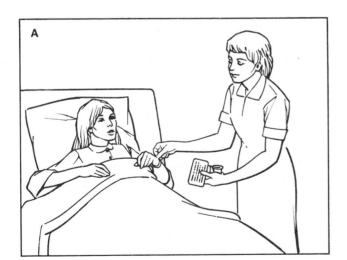
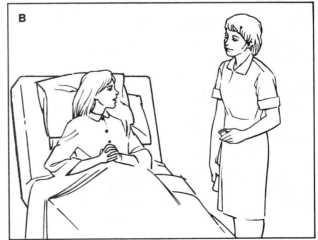

Figure 5-2. (A) Verify medication and patient. (B) Listen to patient.

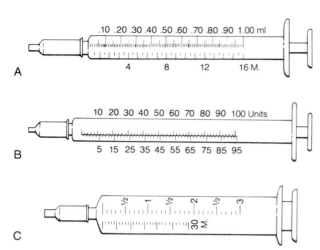

Figure 5-3. Types of syringes. (A) The tuberculin syringe is a narrow 1-ml syringe that is marked off in 1/10 ml, 1/100 ml, and minims. (B) The insulin syringe is a narrow 1-ml syringe that is marked off in single units to a total of 100 units. It is used only for insulin that contains 100 units/ml. (C) The hypodermic syringe most commonly used is a 3-ml syringe that is marked off in 1/10 ml and minims. (Weaver ME, Koehler VJ: Programmed Mathematics of Drugs and Solutions, 5th ed. Philadelphia, JB Lippincott, 1984)

be withdrawn. Be sure the needle is always covered with fluid; otherwise, air, not medication, will fill the syringe.

No matter what type of needle/syringe combination is used, all air must be expelled from the syringe before accurate measurement and administration of the medication can take place.

Mixing medications in the same syringe

It may be appropriate in some cases to mix two medications in one syringe. Preoperative medications are often mixed in the same syringe to lessen the number of injections the patient must receive. Two types of insulin may also be mixed in one syringe. *No more than two medications should be mixed in one syringe.*

When mixing medications, it is necessary to check their compatibility. If the drugs form a precipitate in the syringe, discard the mixture and inject each drug separately.

To mix two drugs in the same syringe:

1. Draw an amount of air into the syringe equal to the amount of solution to be withdrawn from the first vial (vial A).

2. Inject the air into vial A, being careful to keep the needle out of the medication.

3. Remove the empty needle and syringe from vial A.

4. Draw an amount of air equal to the amount of the second medication needed into the syringe.

5. Inject this air into the second vial (vial B).

6. Withdraw the correct amount of medication from vial B and remove the needle and syringe containing the medication.

7. Change the needle.

8. Insert the syringe with the new needle into vial A.

9. Withdraw the solution needed from vial A.

10. Remove the needle and syringe containing both medications from vial A.

If a single-dose vial or ampule is used, withdraw the medication from the multidose vial first.

Example

A preoperative order reads: meperidine (Demerol) 50 mg IM and atropine 0.4 mg IM on call to the operating room.

The vial of meperidine contains 50 mg/ml.

$$\frac{D}{H} \times A = \frac{50 \ \cancel{mg}}{50 \ \cancel{mg}} \times 1 \ ml = 1 \ ml \ of \ meperidine$$

The vial of atropine contains 1 mg/ml.

$$\frac{D}{H} \times A = \frac{0.4 \ \cancel{mg}}{1 \ \cancel{mg}} \times 1 \ ml = 0.4 \times 1 \ ml$$

$$= 0.4 \ ml \ of \ atropine.$$

To draw up the correct amount of each medication:

1. Inject 1 ml of air into the meperidine vial.

2. Withdraw the empty syringe and needle.

3. Inject 0.4 ml of air into the atropine vial.

4. Withdraw 0.4 ml of atropine and remove the syringe and needle from the vial.

5. Change the needle.

6. Place the syringe containing the atropine and the new needle into the meperidine vial.

7. Withdraw 1 ml of meperidine to a total of 1.4 ml of medication in the syringe.

8. Remove the syringe from the vial and inject the medications into the patient.

Injection sites

Intradermal injections. Intradermal injections are given just under the dermis at an angle in the inner surface of the forearm or in the back in the scapular area (see Fig. 5-4).

Subcutaneous injections. Injections of medication can be given into the subcutaneous tissues (see Fig. 2-2). Vaccines, insulin, and heparin are administered subcutaneously. The sites for administration of subcutaneous injections include the outer aspect of the upper arms, the scapular area, the anterior aspect of the thighs, and the abdomen (Fig. 5-5). These sites must be rotated to prevent tissue damage and discomfort. The site should be recorded after each injection to prevent repeated injections in the same site.

Subcutaneous injections are given at either a 45° or a 90° angle. If there is a good amount of subcutaneous tissue, the needle can be inserted at a 90° angle. If the patient is thin, the needle is injected at a 45° angle.

No more than 1 ml of solution should be given subcutaneously.

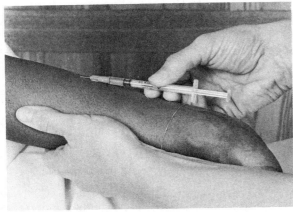

Figure 5-4. The forearm is used here for an intradermal injection. Notice that the needle is held almost parallel to the skin. (Lewis LW: Fundamental Skills in Patient Care, 3rd ed. Philadelphia, JB Lippincott, 1984)

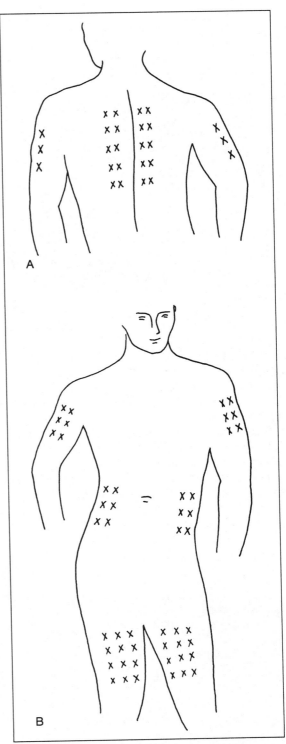

Figure 5-5. Sites for subcutaneous injections. (A) Outer aspect of upper arms and scapular area. (B) Outer aspect of upper arms, abdomen, and anterior thighs. (Lewis LW: Fundamental Skills in Patient Care, 3rd ed. Philadelphia, JB Lippincott, 1984)

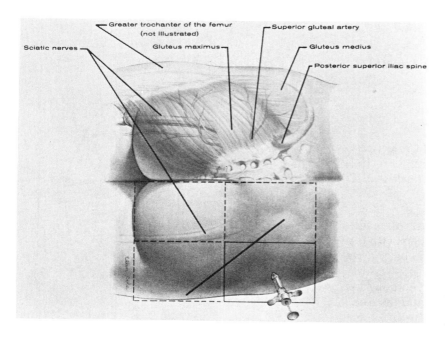

Figure 5-6. Landmarks used to determine location of dorsogluteal intramuscular injection site. (Lewis LW: Fundamental Skills in Patient Care, 3rd ed. Philadelphia, JB Lippincott, 1984)

Intramuscular injections.   Injections are given intramuscularly if the patient is NPO or is nauseated and vomiting or if the medication is unavailable in an oral form. There are five different sites used to give IM injections.

The *dorsogluteal injection* is given in the upper outer aspect of the upper outer quadrant of the gluteal muscle of the buttocks. There are two methods of determining the correct spot to give this injection: The first approach is to divide the buttocks into quarters (see Fig. 5-6). A vertical line is drawn from the iliac crest to the gluteal fold. A horizontal line is drawn from the medial fold to the lateral aspect of the buttocks. The second approach is to palpate the posterior iliac spine and draw a line from this point to the greater trocanter of the femur. The injection is given laterally and superiorly to this line (see Fig. 5-6).

To use the gluteal muscle, the patient should be in a prone position with his toes pointing medially (toward the midline). This site is used for adults and for children over 3 years of age.

The *ventrogluteal injection* is given in the gluteus medius muscle 2 to 3 inches (5 cm to 8 cm)

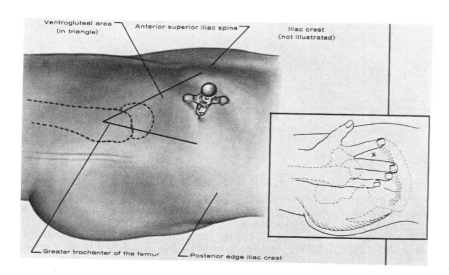

Figure 5-7. Landmarks used to determine location of ventrogluteal intramuscular injection site. (Inset) Example of how hand is used to determine injection site (x). (Lewis LW: Fundamental Skills in Patient Care, 3rd ed. Philadelphia, JB Lippincott, 1984)

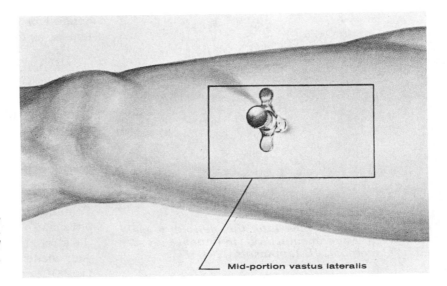

Mid-portion vastus lateralis

Figure 5-8. Injection into the vastus lateralis muscle. (Lewis LW: Fundamental Skills in Patient Care, 3rd ed. Philadelphia, JB Lippincott, 1984)

below the iliac crest. To locate the correct spot, have the patient lie either prone or on his side with his hips and knees flexed. The heel of the hand is placed over the greater trochanter with the fingers toward the patient's head. (The right hand is used for the left hip, and the left hand is used for the right hip.) The index finger is placed on the anterior-superior iliac spine, and the middle finger is

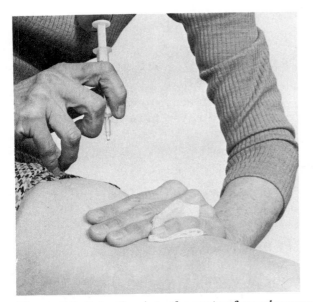

Figure 5-9. Injection into the rectus femoris muscle. (Lewis LW: Fundamental Skills in Patient Care, 3rd ed. Philadelphia, JB Lippincott, 1984)

stretched dorsally and placed just below the iliac crest. The injection is given in the V formed by the index and middle fingers (see Fig. 5-7).

The *vastus lateralis injection* is administered in the middle third of the muscle, which is located on the anterolateral aspect of the thigh. The area between the greater trochanter of the femur and the lateral femoral condyle is divided into thirds, and the injection is given in the middle third (see Fig. 5-8). The patient may be lying or sitting to receive an injection in this location.

The *rectus femoris injection* is given in the muscle located in the anterior aspect of the thigh. This site is a good one for the patient who must administer his own injections. The patient can be lying or sitting to receive an injection in this location (see Fig. 5-9).

The *deltoid injection* is seldom used because the deltoid, which is located in the lateral aspect of the upper arm, is small in most patients. To locate the correct site (the thickest part of the muscle), the lower edge of the acromial process is palpated and the midpoint on the lateral aspect of the arm in line with the axilla is located. A rectangle is drawn in the area about 2 inches below the acromial process. Injections are given in this area (see Fig. 5-10).

When a drug is administered by the SC or IM route, be sure to withdraw the plunger after inserting the needle but before pushing the medication. This aspiration ensures that you have not entered a blood vessel; if you had, the aspiration would show blood.

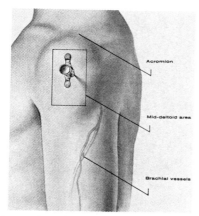

Figure 5-10. Injection into the deltoid muscle. (Lewis LW: Fundamental Skills in Patient Care, 3rd ed. Philadelphia, JB Lippincott, 1984)

Whichever the route, the most important points to remember are the "Five Rights":

Right drug
Right dose
Right route
Right time
Right patient

OBSERVING, REPORTING, AND RECORDING

Observe the patient for any sign of adverse effects, such as drug allergy, cumulative effect, and drug idiosyncrasy. Report any signs of adverse reactions immediately. Also report if the drug is not effective, such as if an analgesic you administered does not lessen your patient's pain within a reasonable time (see Fig. 5-11).

Medications must be recorded as given only after they have been taken. Any refusal should be noted in the chart, as well as on the medication sheet. Never chart a medication as given unless you actually gave it.*

CALCULATION OF DRUG DOSE

Computing drug dosage is necessary whenever the physician's order for a medication differs from the strength of the medication you have on hand. The

* Except: You draw up a medication for the physician to administer. After you see the medication given, you may sign the physician's initials, or write "given by MD" in the medication record.

general formula when computing drug dosage problems is as follows:

$$\frac{\text{Drug Dose Desired}}{\text{Drug Dose You Have}} = \text{Drug Dose You Give}$$

This can be abbreviated as $\dfrac{\text{Desired}}{\text{Have}} = \text{Give}$ or, even more simply, as $\dfrac{D}{H} = G.$

Drugs in solid form

The amount ordered is the amount of drug in the physician's written order. The amount you have is the strength listed on the container of this drug in your medicine closet. The amount you give is expressed in terms of the quantity that you will actually give to the patient, as tablets, capsules, or milliliters.

Example 1

Physician's order reads: "Give phenytoin (Dilantin) 200 mg PO qd."

The label on the bottle of phenytoin capsules you have states: "phenytoin 100 mg."

Drug problem:

$$\frac{\text{Desired}}{\text{Have}} = \text{Give}$$

$$\frac{200 \text{ mg}}{100 \text{ mg}} = x$$

$$\frac{200 \text{ mg}}{100 \text{ mg}} = \frac{2}{1} \text{ or 2 capsules}$$

Answer: In order to carry out the physician's order, you must give the patient 2 capsules.

Example 2

Physician's order reads: aspirin gr X PO stat

You have: aspirin tablets gr V

Drug problem:

$$\frac{\text{Desired}}{\text{Have}} = \text{Give}$$

$$\frac{X}{V} = \frac{10}{5}\frac{2}{1} \text{ or 2 tablets}$$

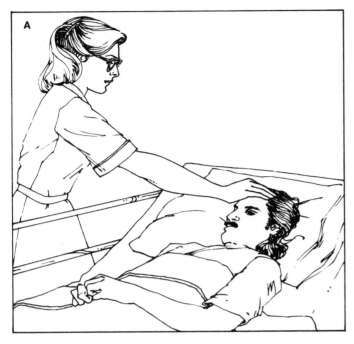

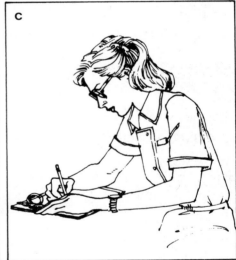

Figure 5-11. (A) Observe, (B) report, and (C) record all adverse reactions.

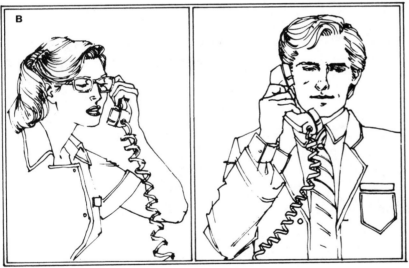

If the written order is expressed in the same units as those of the "on hand" medication, you can set up the problem as in the examples above. Suppose the physician's order reads: "cephalexin (Keflex) 1 g PO" and you have on hand cephalexin 500 mg per capsule. The problem, $\frac{1\text{ g}}{500\text{ mg}} = x$, cannot be solved because the numerator and the denominator are not expressed in the same units. But,

since you know that there are 1000 mg in 1 g, you can substitute the equivalent:

$$\frac{1\text{ g}}{500\text{ mg}} = \frac{1000\text{ mg}}{500\text{ mg}}$$

Now proceed with the problem as in the two preceding examples:

$$\frac{1000 \text{ mg}}{500 \text{ mg}} = x$$

$$\frac{2 \; \cancel{1000} \; \cancel{\text{mg}}}{1 \; \cancel{500} \; \cancel{\text{mg}}} = \frac{2}{1} \text{ or 2 capsules}$$

Drugs in liquid form

For liquid medications given by mouth, a specific amount of drug is contained in a specific amount of liquid. These amounts are listed on the label. The label on suspension of phenytoin reads:

phenytoin suspension (Dilantin)
125 mg/5 ml

The physician usually orders that a specific number of milligrams of the medication be given. For this type of medication order, the following formula can be used:

$$\frac{\text{Drug Dose Desired}}{\text{Drug Dose You Have}} \times \text{Amount of Liquid}$$
$$= \text{Dose You Give}$$

This can be abbreviated as

$$\frac{\text{Desired}}{\text{Have}} \times \text{Amount} = \text{Give}$$

or even more simply as $\dfrac{\text{D}}{\text{H}} \times \text{A} = \text{G}$.

Example 1

Order: phenytoin suspension (Dilantin) 100 mg PO tid

You have: phenytoin suspension 125 mg/5 ml

Drug problem:

$$\frac{\text{Desired}}{\text{Have}} \times \text{Amount} = \text{Give}$$

$$\frac{4 \; \cancel{100} \; \cancel{\text{mg}}}{5 \; \cancel{125} \; \cancel{\text{mg}}} \times 5 \text{ ml} = x$$

$$\frac{4}{5} \times 5 \text{ ml} = x$$

$$\frac{4}{1} \; \frac{\cancel{20}}{\cancel{5}} \text{ or 4 ml}$$

Example 2

Ordered: ascorbic acid (Vitamin C) 500 mg PO qid

You have: ascorbic acid 100 mg/ml

Drug problem:

$$\frac{\text{Desired}}{\text{Have}} \times \text{Amount} = \text{Give}$$

$$\frac{500 \; \cancel{\text{mg}}}{100 \; \cancel{\text{mg}}} \times 1 \text{ ml} = x$$

$$\frac{5}{1} \times 1 \text{ ml} = x$$

$$x = 5 \text{ ml}$$

Since all drugs injected must be in liquid form, the same formula can be used:

Example 3

Ordered: prochlorperazine (Compazine) 10 mg IM

You have: prochlorperazine 5 mg/ml

Drug problem:

$$\frac{\text{Desired}}{\text{Have}} \times \text{Amount} = \text{Give}$$

$$\frac{10 \text{ mg}}{5 \text{ mg}} \times 1 \text{ ml} = x$$

$$\frac{2 \; \cancel{10} \; \cancel{\text{mg}}}{1 \; \cancel{5} \; \cancel{\text{mg}}} \times 1 \text{ ml} = x$$

$$\frac{2}{1} \times 1 \text{ ml} = x$$

$$2 \text{ ml} = x$$

Note: Be sure to read labels for injectable medications very carefully. The strength listed may refer to a part of the ampule or vial, rather than to the whole. For example, 10 mg/ml and 20 mg/2 ml are identical strengths but are expressed differently.

Conversion

Occasionally, medication orders require conversion from one system of measurement to another before the correct dosage can be determined. To convert from one system to another:

1. Refer to the conversion chart for the equivalent (see inside back of cover).
2. Convert to the same system.
3. Proceed with the calculation.

Example 1

The order reads: Codeine gr ¼ PO q4h prn pain.

You have: 30-mg tablets

Drug problem:

1. $1 \text{ gr} = 60 \text{ mg}$

2. $1 \text{ gr}:60\text{mg} :: \frac{1}{4} \text{ gr}:x$

$$x = \frac{1}{4} \times 60 \text{ mg}$$

$$x = \frac{\cancel{60}\; 15}{\cancel{4}\; 1} = 15 \text{ mg}$$

3. $\dfrac{D}{H} = G$

$$\frac{\cancel{15}}{\cancel{30}} = \frac{1}{2} \text{ tablet}$$

Answer: You will give the patient ½ tablet of codeine.

Example 2

The order reads atropine gr $\dfrac{1}{100}$ IM on call to OR. Atropine is dispensed in vials of 1 mg/ml. How much would the patient receive?

Drug problem:

1. $\text{gr i} = 60 \text{ mg}$

2. $\text{gr i} : 60 :: \dfrac{1}{100} : x$

$$1x = 60 \times \frac{1}{100}$$

$$x = \frac{60}{100} = \frac{\cancel{6}\; 3}{\cancel{10}\; 5} = \frac{3}{5}$$

3. $\dfrac{D}{H} \times A = G$

$$\frac{3}{5} \times 1 \text{ ml} = \frac{3}{5} \text{ ml}$$

$$x = 0.6 \text{ ml}$$

Answer: The patient would receive 0.6 ml of atropine.

PART 2
Drugs used to help meet patients' needs for comfort, safety, and hygiene

CHAPTER 6
Psychotropic drugs

Psychotropic drugs are those that affect mental function. In addition to the drugs to be discussed in this chapter, hallucinogens, narcotics, alcohol, sedatives, and hypnotics may also be considered psychotropic because they affect the mind. In this chapter we will be concerned with drugs used in the treatment of patients with psychiatric disturbances. Drugs cannot cure psychiatric illness. However, they modify or lessen symptoms of disease. This often allows the patient to benefit from other treatment, such as psychotherapy or behavior modification.

CLASSIFICATION OF PSYCHOTROPIC DRUGS

The psychotropic drugs are divided into two main categories. *Tranquilizers* decrease anxiety and hyperactivity without causing a marked decrease in the level of consciousness. The tranquilizers are divided into two categories, major and minor. The major tranquilizers, also known as antipsychotics, are used to treat the psychoses; the minor are used to treat the less severe neurotic and psychosomatic (mind–body) disorders. The second group of psychotropic drugs is called the *antidepressants*. They are used to treat depression that has become severe enough to interfere with a person's ability to function normally.

Major tranquilizers

A person suffering from a psychosis is unable to recognize reality. He may have hallucinations and delusions and may display bizarre behavior. If he is able to communicate at all, two-way communication becomes extremely difficult. The major tranquilizers are given to lessen these symptoms. They help to decrease confusion, delusions, and hyperactivity.

Phenothiazines are the drugs most commonly used to treat psychoses. They are used in both acute and chronic treatment of psychotic states, especially those accompanied by increased agitation, panic, fear, hostility, and violent behavior. They also help to decrease anxiety and fear in patients who are scheduled for electroconvulsive therapy (ECT). Drugs in this group are used to treat organic brain disease and alcohol withdrawal symptoms. They are occasionally used to treat psychosomatic disorders, but because of their dangerous adverse effects, this use is limited.

Chlorpromazine (Thorazine), introduced in 1951, is probably the best known of the phenothiazine group. There are other drugs that are more potent than chlorpromazine, such as prochlorperazine (Compazine), trifluoperazine (Stelazine), and fluphenazine (Prolixin), but they also produce more severe adverse effects. There are also phenothiazines of different potencies from chlorpromazine. These drugs, such as acetophenazine maleate (Tindal) and thioridazine (Mellaril), are prescribed to reduce the incidence of certain side-effects that are seen with chlorpromazine and its derivatives.

There are drugs besides the phenothiazines that are used to treat psychoses. Haloperidol (Haldol) is an antipsychotic drug that was first used in the late 1960s. It is especially effective in treating manic states of hyperactivity. Lithium carbonate (Lithane, Eskalith) is a more recent drug. It is used specifically in the treatment of manic-depressive states. Its chief drawback is the small margin of safety between therapeutic and toxic doses.

The major tranquilizers have adverse effects that are worthy of special note, including parkinsonism, dyskinesias, and extreme restlessness. These distressing adverse effects, found with many of these drugs, are caused by stimulation of the extrapyramidal (motor) system. They are often referred to collectively as *extrapyramidal symptoms* and may occur very suddenly. Parkinsonism takes the form of symptoms that would be seen in a patient with true Parkinson's disease: muscles appear weak; there is a tremor and rigidity of muscles, especially those of the extremities; and the facial muscles become frozen in an expressionless (mask-like) appearance. Dyskinesias are sudden involuntary movements or muscle spasms. These may occur in the extremities, or in isolated muscle groups in the face, or they may involve the entire body in what looks like a convulsion. Tardive dyskinesia is an adverse effect of phenothiazines that may occur after long-term therapy. The mouth, tongue, lips, and occasionally the entire body are involved in repetitive, involuntary actions, such as chewing, lip smacking, tongue protrusion, and generalized writhing. In addition to being extremely upsetting and frightening to both patient and family, some extrapyramidal symptoms may be nonreversible. Although the symptoms of parkinsonism will disppear if antiparkinsonian drugs are given, or if the phenothiazine is discontinued, there is no treatment known to prevent or cure tardive dyskinesia other than careful use of the phenothiazines.

Minor tranquilizers

A neurosis is less severe than a psychosis. The neurotic patient is in touch with reality. He can communicate with others but cannot cope adequately with his environment. He is extremely anxious. Drugs used to treat neurotic patients are called minor tranquilizers, antineurotic, or antianxiety drugs.

Drugs belonging to the benzodiazepine group are the most commonly used minor tranquilizers. In addition to reducing anxiety, they also relax muscles and prevent convulsions. For these reasons, they are used to treat muscle spasticity, seizures, and alcoholic withdrawal, as well as anxiety. Benzodiazepines are most effective in short-term therapy; if given over a period of months, they become less effective. Alprazolam (Xanax), chlorazepate (Tranxene), chlordiazepoxide (Librium), diazepam (Valium), lorazepam (Ativan), oxazepam (Serax), and prazepam (Centrax) are examples of benzodiazepine drugs.

Meprobamate (Equanil, Miltown) is another minor tranquilizer effective as an antianxiety agent, anticonvulsant, and muscle relaxant. It decreases anxiety, tension, and abnormal fears in the neurotic patient. Psychosomatic and sleep disorders also respond well to meprobamate.

Two other minor tranquilizers are hydroxyzine hydrochloride (Atarax) and hydroxyzine pamoate (Vistaril). These related compounds also have antiemetic and antihistaminic actions. See Table 6-1 for detailed information on psychotropic drugs.

NURSING IMPLICATIONS

Psychotropic drugs are usually ordered according to the patient's major symptoms. Careful initial assessment of patient behavior is therefore a necessity. The physician will usually order a low dose of the tranquilizer at first, then increase the amount until the patient's behavior shows the desired change. Your assessment of behavioral changes during this process, and communication of what you observe, are important to the success of the drug therapy.

Patients with psychiatric disturbances should be watched as they take their medications. It is not uncommon for such patients to pretend they have taken their pills, only to save them up or throw them away after the nurse leaves the room. You must not only stay with these patients as they take the medication but also check to see that medications have, indeed, been swallowed.

The major tranquilizers can produce both reversible and nonreversible extrapyramidal symptoms. Close observation and reporting of the earliest signs of these disturbances may save the patient and

(*Text continues on p. 50.*)

TABLE 6-1 PSYCHOTROPIC DRUGS

DRUG	ROUTE AND DOSAGE RANGE	USE	ADVERSE EFFECTS	NURSING IMPLICATIONS
MAJOR TRANQUILIZERS				
Phenothiazines Chlorpromazine (Thorazine)	PO—10 mg–50 mg bid to qid PR—50 mg–100 mg tid to qid IM—25 mg–50 mg q3h–4h	To treat psychotic disorders, the manic phase of manic-depressive illness; to control nausea and vomiting, to treat nonpsychotic anxiety, severe tension, or hyperactivity; to relieve intractable hiccoughs, restlessness, and anxiety; to relieve restlessness and apprehension before surgery; to treat acute intermittent porphyria	*CNS:* drowsiness, abnormal posturing, convulsions, Parkinson-like symptoms, restlessness, nightmares, tardive dyskinesias *ANS:* dry mouth, nasal congestion, constipation, urinary retention, pupillary changes *Endocrine:* breast engorgement, gynecomastia, decreased libido, weight changes, menstrual irregularities *Skin:* rashes, darkening of skin color *Eyes:* blurred vision, photosensitivity, lens opacities *Others:* Postural hypotension, blood disorders, jaundice, tachycardia	Make sure patient takes the medication. Assess, record, and report changes in behavior. Warn patient to avoid dangerous activities and driving. Encourage fluids or sucking on hard candy. Keep stool chart. Note any unusual muscle movements—warn the patient of possible extrapyramidal symptoms. Take orthostatic BP. Evaluate patient's appetite. Check skin for rashes. Warn patient to avoid brightly lit areas and direct sun. Check blood at regular intervals. Check weight periodically. Warn patient of possible changes in sexual drive and function, menstrual irregularities, and possible impotence.
fluphenazine HCl (Prolixin)	PO—0.5 mg–20 mg qd in divided doses q6h–8h IM—2.5 mg–10 mg qd in divided doses q6h–8h	To treat psychotic disorders	See chlorpromazine.	See chlorpromazine.
lithium carbonate (Lithane, Eskalith, Lithobid)	PO—300 mg–600 mg tid (adjust to ensure blood levels between 0.5–1.5 mEq/liter	To control manic episodes in manic-depressive illness	*CNS:* dizziness, drowsiness, lethargy, ataxia, tremor, abnormal muscle movements, seizures, slurred speech, headache, incontinence, vertigo, restlessness, confusion *ANS:* blurred vision, dry mouth *GI:* anorexia, nausea, vomiting, diarrhea *GU:* frequent or no urination, sugar or albumin in urine *Skin:* dry, thinning hair, skin anesthesia, itching, rash *Others:* dehydration, weight loss or gain, thyroid disorders	Evaluate mental status. Ambulate with assistance if necessary. Note any abnormal muscle movements. Evaluate speech and vision. Keep accurate I&O. Check weight daily. Assess appetite. Test urine for sugar and albumin. Keep stool chart. Check skin for rashes. Frequent blood tests must be done to determine lithium level. Encourage patient to maintain adequate PO intake and to use salt liberally.

(continued on page 46)

TABLE 6-1 (continued)

DRUG	ROUTE AND DOSAGE RANGE	USE	ADVERSE EFFECTS	NURSING IMPLICATIONS
reserpine (Serpasil)	PO—0.1 mg–1 mg qd IM—For psychiatric emergencies—2.5 mg–5 mg For hypertensive crisis—0.5 mg–1 mg, then at 3-hr intervals 2 mg to 4 mg	To treat agitated psychotic states (usually given for its antihypertensive effect)	*CNS:* dizziness, sedation, headache, anxiety, nightmares, extrapyramidal symptoms *Endocrine:* weight gain, edema, decreased sex drive, impotence *Cardiovascular:* hypotension, bradycardia *GI:* anorexia, nausea, vomiting, diarrhea, increased GI secretions *Skin:* rash, itching *Others:* nasal congestion, deafness, glaucoma	Ambulate with assistance when necessary. Evaluate mood and sleep patterns. Check weight periodically. Check apical pulse and BP at regular intervals. Evaluate appetite. Check skin for rashes. Keep stool chart. Note any unusual muscle movements. Warn patients of possible changes in sexual drive and function. Evaluate vision and hearing.
MINOR TRANQUILIZERS				
alprazolam (Xanax)	PO—0.5 mg–4.0 mg/day in divided doses	See prazepam, plus used for treatment of anxiety associated with depression	*CNS:* confusion, blurred vision, headache, dizziness or lightheadedness, drowsiness *ANS:* dry mouth, increased thirst	Caution patient against engaging in potentially dangerous activities. Evaluate mental status and visual acuity. Note complaints of dry mouth and increased fluid intake.
chlordiazepoxide (Librium, Libritabs)	PO—5 mg–25 mg bid to qid IM, IV—initial dose—50 mg–100 mg; repeat in 2 hr–4 hr if necessary Maintenance—25 mg–50 mg q6h–8h	To manage anxiety disorders; short-term relief of anxiety symptoms, and acute alcohol withdrawal	*CNS:* ataxia, drowsiness, confusion, extrapyramidal symptoms, physical and psychological dependence *GI:* nausea, constipation *Endocrine:* edema, minor menstrual irregularities, changes in sex drive *Others:* skin rashes, blood disorders, EEG changes, liver dysfunction	Caution patients not to engage in potentially dangerous activities. Evaluate mental status. Assist with ambulation if necessary. Keep stool chart. Record I&O. Warn patient of possible changes in sexual drive, function, and menstruation. Note any unusual muscle movements. Check skin for rashes. Blood tests should be done at regular intervals. Watch for dependence.
chlordiazepoxide + clidinium (Librax)	PO—1–2 capsules tid or qid; varies with diagnosis and individual patient	To relieve anxiety and tension and to use with other medications in the treatment of the irritable bowel syndrome and acute enterocolitis	See chlordiazepoxide, *plus:* Dry mouth, blurred vision, urinary hesitation	See chlordiazepoxide, *plus:* Assess visual acuity. Evaluate ease of urination. Administer medication before meals.
clorazepate dipotassium (Tranxene)	PO—15 mg–90 mg qd in divided doses	To treat anxiety disorders; for short-term relief of anxiety	*CNS:* drowsiness, dizziness, nervousness, blurred vision, dry mouth, headache, mental confusion, insomnia, fatigue, ataxia, irritability, diplopia, depression, slurred speech *Others:* GI and GU disturbances, transient skin rashes, hypotension	Evaluate mental status. Assist with activities as necessary. Assess visual acuity. Note changes in sleep patterns. Evaluate speech. Check skin for rashes. Record I&O. Keep stool chart. Monitor blood pressure.

(continued on page 47)

TABLE 6-1 (continued)

DRUG	ROUTE AND DOSAGE RANGE	USE	ADVERSE EFFECTS	NURSING IMPLICATIONS
diazepam (Valium)	PO—2 mg–10 mg bid to qid IM, IV—2 mg–20 mg (IV not to exceed 5 mg/min)	To treat skeletal muscle spasms, anxiety, tension, acute alcohol withdrawal, and status epilepticus; preoperative medication	*CNS:* drowsiness, fatigue, ataxia, headache, confusion, depression, slurred speech, physical or psychological dependence, syncope *Endocrine:* changes in sex drive *Cardiovascular:* hypotension, bradycardia, phlebitis at site of injection *Others:* blurred or double vision, skin rash, hiccoughs	Ambulate with assistance as necessary. Evaluate mental status, speech, and vision. Take BP and apical pulse at regular intervals. Warn patient of possible changes in sex drive. Watch for irritation at injection sites. Check skin for rashes. Watch for dependence. Be sure patient takes medication.
hydroxyzine (Atarax, Vistaril)	PO—10 mg–100 mg qid IM—25 mg–100 mg q4–6h	To treat nausea, vomiting, anxiety, tension, acute and chronic allergic skin reactions; preoperative medication	Drowsiness, dry mouth	Ambulate carefully. Keep siderails up when patient is in bed. Offer fluids if indicated to alleviate dry mouth.
lorazepam (Ativan)	PO—1 mg–10 mg qd in divided doses IM, IV—0.05 mg/kg to a maximum of 4 mg/day	To manage anxiety disorders; use for short-term relief of the symptoms of anxiety or anxiety associated with depressive symptoms	*CNS:* sedation, dizziness, weakness, ataxia, disorientation, depression, nausea, changes in appetite, headache, sleep disturbances, agitation, physical and psychological dependence *Others:* skin rash, changes in vision	Evaluate mental status. Assist with activities as necessary. Note changes in sleep pattern and appetite. Watch for dependence. Check skin for rashes. Assess visual acuity.
meprobamate (Equanil, Miltown)	PO—300 mg–400 mg tid or qid, to a maximum of 2400 mg/day	To treat anxiety and tension; to promote sleep in the anxious, tense person	*CNS:* drowsiness, dizziness, weakness, ataxia, headache, slurred speech, increased EEG activity, euphoria, physical and psychological dependence *Cardiovascular:* arrhythmias, hypotension *GI:* nausea, vomiting, diarrhea *Other:* allergic reactions	Ambulate with assistance if necessary. Avoid any dangerous activities. Keep stool chart. Evaluate speech. Take BP and apical pulse at regular intervals. Evaluate mental status. Watch for dependence. Be sure patient takes medication. Check for any signs of allergic reaction.
oxazepam (Serax)	PO—10 mg–30 mg tid to qid	To manage anxiety disorders; for short-term relief of symptoms of anxiety	Drowsiness, dizziness, ataxia, slurred speech, headache, fainting, nausea, skin rashes, changes in sex drive	Ambulate with assistance if necessary. Avoid hazardous activities. Evaluate speech. Check skin for rashes. Warn patients about possible changes in sex drive.

(continued on page 48)

TABLE 6-1 (continued)

DRUG	ROUTE AND DOSAGE RANGE	USE	ADVERSE EFFECTS	NURSING IMPLICATIONS
prazepam (Centrax)	PO—10 mg–60 mg/ day in divided doses or one single dose at hs	To manage anxiety disorders or for short-term relief of symptoms of anxiety	*CNS:* fatigue, dizziness, drowsiness, light-headedness, ataxia, headache, confusion, tremor, vivid dreams, slurred speech, blurred vision, syncope, physical and psychological dependence *ANS:* dry mouth, increased perspiration *Cardiovascular:* palpitations *Others:* skin rashes, swelling of feet, joint pains	Caution patient against engaging in potentially dangerous activities. Evaluate mental status speech, and visual acuity. Take apical pulse. Check skin for rashes. Check for swelling in feet.
ANTIDEPRESSANTS				
MAO Inhibitors phenelzine (Nardil)	PO—15 mg–90 mg qd in divided doses	To treat atypical, neurotic, or nonendogenous depression (usually given after other antidepressants have failed)	*CNS:* dizziness, weakness, fatigue, restlessness, mania, insomnia *Cardiovascular:* hypotension, flushing, paradoxical hypertensive crisis *GI:* anorexia, nausea, dry mouth, constipation *Musculoskeletal:* muscle tremors and spasms *Others:* tinnitus, skin rashes, urinary retention, impotence, edema	Teach the patient about foods to avoid. Drug interactions may occur with tyramine in foods. Serious reactions can occur even 2 weeks after the last dose of a MAO inhibitor. Ambulate with assistance as necessary. Evaluate appetite. Keep stool chart. Evaluate mental status. Check skin for rashes and flushing. Keep record of I&O. Note any unusual muscle movements. Check BP at regular intervals. Warn patients about possible changes in sexual function.
Tricyclics amitriptyline (Elavil)	PO—40 mg–150 mg qd in divided doses or at hs as a single dose IM—20 mg–30 mg qid	To treat depression of psychosis, neurosis, and depression accompanied by anxiety	*CNS:* drowsiness, dizziness, weakness, ataxia, tremor, paresthesias of extremities, extrapyramidal symptoms, manic reaction, disorientation, hallucinations, delusions, nightmares, seizures *Cardiovascular:* hypotension, hypertension, arrhythmias, myocardial infarction, stroke *Endocrine:* changes in sex drive, breast enlargement *GI:* anorexia, dry mouth and throat, constipation, nausea, vomiting, weight gain or loss, diarrhea	Caution patients not to engage in potentially dangerous activities. Ambulate with assistance as necessary. Offer fluids to alleviate dry mouth and throat. Keep stool chart. Check BP and take apical pulse at regular intervals. Note any abnormal muscle movements. Evaluate appetite. Chart weights periodically. Evaluate mental status. Check skin for rash. Avoid brightly lit areas and direct sun. Evaluate vision. Blood tests should be done at regular intervals.

(continued on page 49)

TABLE 6-1 (continued)

DRUG	ROUTE AND DOSAGE RANGE	USE	ADVERSE EFFECTS	NURSING IMPLICATIONS
amitriptyline (*continued*)			*Others:* skin rash, photosensitivity, edema of the face and tongue, blurred vision, furry tongue, urinary retention, blood disorders	Warn patients of possible changes in sex drive and breast enlargement (in both male and female). Maximum effect may not occur until 1–3 weeks after initial dose. Keep a record of output.
amitriptyline + perphenazine (Triavil, Etrafon)	PO—combination therapy is highly individualized	To treat moderate to severe anxiety or depression and agitation; to treat patients with depression in whom anxiety is severe; to treat patients with depression and anxiety associated with chronic physical disease; to treat schizophrenic patients with depressive symptoms	See amitriptyline and perphenazine.	See amitriptyline and perphenazine.
chlordiazepoxide + amitriptyline (Limbitrol)	PO—2–6 tablets qd in divided doses	To treat moderate to severe depression associated with moderate to severe anxiety	See chlordiazepoxide and amitriptyline.	See chlordiazepoxide and amitriptyline.
desipramine (Norpramin, Pertofrane)	PO—25 mg–300 mg qd in divided doses or one single dose	To treat depression, especially endogenous	See amitriptyline.	See amitriptyline.
doxepin (Sinequan, Adapin)	PO—25 mg–300 mg qd in divided doses (up to 150 mg may be taken in one dose)	To treat depression or anxiety associated with psychoneurosis, alcoholism, and organic disease; to treat psychotic depressive disorders with associated anxiety, including involutional depression and manic-depressive disease	See amitriptyline.	See amitriptyline.
imipramine (Tofranil)	PO—25 mg–300 mg qd in divided doses or one single dose IM—up to 100 mg qd in divided doses	To treat depression, especially endogenous; to treat enuresis	See amitriptyline.	See amitriptyline.
Others maprotiline HCl (Ludiomil)	PO—25 mg–300 mg/ day in divided doses or a single dose at hs	To treat depressive neurosis, manic-depressive illness (depressed type), and anxiety associated with depression	*CNS:* nervousness, anxiety, insomnia, agitation, confusional states, decreased memory, drowsiness, dizziness, tremor,	Evidence of therapeutic effect may take up to 3 weeks. Assess, record, and report behavioral changes. Keep stool chart. Evaluate visual acuity.

(continued on page 50)

TABLE 6-1 (continued)

DRUG	ROUTE AND DOSAGE RANGE	USE	ADVERSE EFFECTS	NURSING IMPLICATIONS
maprotiline HCl (continued)			weakness, fatigue, headache ANS: dry mouth, constipation, blurred vision GI: nausea, vomiting, epigastric distress, abdominal cramps Cardiovascular: hypotension, hypertension, tachycardia, palpitations, arrhythmias, syncope Endocrine: changes in libido, impotence, changes in blood sugar levels Others: skin rash, itching, photosensitization, edema, fever	Monitor temperature, BP, pulse, and blood sugar. Warn patient of possible changes in sexual drive or function. Check for skin rashes.
trazodone (Desyrel)	PO—150 mg–600 mg/day in 3–4 divided doses	To treat moderate to severe depression, with or without prominent anxiety	CNS: anger, hostility, nightmares, confusion, decreased concentration, drowsiness, lightheadedness, excitement, headache, insomnia, paresthesias, tremor Cardiovascular: hyper- or hypotension, shortness of breath, fainting, tachycardia, palpitations GI: bad taste in mouth, dry mouth, nausea, vomiting, diarrhea, constipation, anorexia Others: decreased libido, blurred vision, red eyes, sinus congestion, muscle aches and pains, · dysuria, urinary frequency, sweating, weight gain or loss	Note changes in behavior and/or mood. Evaluate mental status. Caution patient to avoid potentially dangerous activities. Ambulate with assistance as necessary. Evaluate sleep/wake pattern. Note any unusual muscle movements or complaints of muscle discomfort. Check BP and take apical pulse at regular intervals. Offer fluids to alleviate dry mouth. Keep stool chart. Monitor I&O. Evaluate appetite. Chart weights periodically. Warn patient of possible changes in sex drive. Assess visual acuity. Note any complaints of changes in urinary flow.

his family unnecessary trauma. The earliest signs of tardive dyskinesia are abnormal movements of the tongue muscles.

Patients receiving tranquilizers should be cautioned not to drive or perform potentially dangerous activities, since their judgment, coordination, and muscle tone may be affected by the medications. They should also be warned not to change body positions quickly, since postural hypotension and fainting are possible. The body usually adapts to the drug after a few days, and this will no longer be a danger.

Hypersensitivity reactions can occur, so it is important to observe the patient for allergic skin reactions. Many major tranquilizers also cause photosensitivity. Patients need to be warned not to stay outside in bright sunlight, because this may lead to eye damage. Patients who are taking phenothiazines should be warned that prolonged exposure to the sun may cause changes in pigmentation as well.

Patients and their families may become alarmed at changes in body appearance and sexual function caused by the effect of major tranquilizers on the endocrine system. The possibility of weight gain, gynecomastia (breast enlargement) in men, and changes in menstruation and the occurrence of galactorrhea (leakage of milk from the breast of a non-nursing woman) should be explained as expected effects. Decreased libido (sex drive) and male impotence are also common. These problems should be discussed with the patient and the patient's partner.

The patient may have an idiosyncrasy to a particular tranquilizer, and this may aggravate his depression. Thus, you must be alert to the possibility that he may attempt suicide. Precautionary measures, such as the use of window locks and the assistance of special attendants, may be necessary.

High doses of some tranquilizers can cause convulsions. The patient with epilepsy who is taking tranquilizers should be watched carefully for any increase in seizure activity. Be sure the necessary emergency equipment (airway, oxygen, and suction) is at the bedside.

It sometimes happens that the benzodiazepines give rise to nightmares, violent behavior, and extreme agitation and excitement. Because these are opposite to the "tranquil" state expected, they are called *paradoxical states*. If this occurs, you will need to protect the patient and others from injury and report it immediately.

There is little evidence of physical or psychological dependence on the major tranquilizers. Physical and psychological dependence, tolerance, and withdrawal symptoms have, however, occurred after treatment with the minor tranquilizers. Abuse of diazepam, especially, has increased dramatically in recent years. Overdose can lead to coma and, if untreated, death.

Both fluid loss and sodium loss potentiate the effects of lithium. Diuretics are, therefore, absolutely contraindicated in patients on lithium. These patients should be encouraged to use salt liberally and maintain an adequate intake of water.

There are many potentially life-threatening drug interactions that a nurse must be aware of when administering either a major or a minor tranquilizer. One general interaction to watch for is the additive central nervous system (CNS) depression that may occur when tranquilizers are given along with other drugs that also cause CNS depression. Examples are alcohol, anesthetics, antihistamines, aspirin, barbiturates, hypnotics, narcotics, and sedatives. Combinations of these drugs plus tranquilizers can cause excessive sedation, coma, and death. Seizures, excitement, and rage reactions are also possible.

Antidepressants

It is normal to be depressed after certain life experiences, such as serious illness, divorce, death, and the loss of job or home. The depressed person often becomes apathetic and easily fatigued. He may take less and less care of his appearance and may eat and sleep poorly. There may be feelings of worthlessness, hopelessness, and guilt. Often these persons withdraw from social contacts. If depression does not clear within a reasonable time, this type of exogenous (due to outside causes) depression, which is normal, goes on to abnormal depression called a *reactive depression*. In some cases a person is severely depressed with no apparent cause. This is called endogenous (due to internal causes) or psychotic depression. The antidepressant drugs, also called *psychostimulants* or *psychic energizers*, seem most effective when the problem is endogenous depression, although drug therapy is used with both types of depression.

As with other psychotropic medications, the antidepressants do not treat the underlying cause of disease. What they do is increase alertness and physical activity that usually leads to better sleep patterns and appetite. They lift the patient's spirits so he is less preoccupied with depressing thoughts. In this state, the patient is more likely to benefit from other therapy for his depression.

There are two major groups of antidepressant drugs. The monoamine-oxidase (MAO) inhibitors are a group of drugs that stimulate the central nervous system, thereby increasing activity and appetite. They are used to treat both reactive and endogenous depression. These drugs have many adverse effects, some severe enough to cause death. Of special note is the paradoxical hypertension that may occur if certain foods are ingested while the patient is on the drug. It is the tyramine found in certain cheeses (brie, camembert, cheddar), bananas, avocados, canned figs, beer, Chianti wine, sherry, coffee, tea, cola, pickled herring, chicken livers, and sour cream that can bring about this hypertensive crisis. If the blood pressure continues to rise, the small blood vessels in the brain may rupture and death may follow. The first features of this potentially fatal reaction are headache, a stiff neck, nausea, vomiting, increased perspiration, dilated pupils with photophobia, changes in pulse rate, and chest pain.

Tranylcypromine (Parnate) and phenelzine sulfate (Nardil) are two of the commonly prescribed antidepressants of the MAO inhibitor group. Phenelzine is used in both endogenous and reactive depression. Tranylcypromine is prescribed only for severe depression that has not been helped by any other therapy.

The second group of antidepressant drugs are the *tricyclic* antidepressants. These are the most commonly prescribed antidepressants. They have both an antidepressant and a mild tranquilizing effect; moreover, they only slightly depress the central nervous system. They are considered safer to use than the MAO inhibitors because there is less likelihood that hypertensive crisis will develop. Imipramine (Tofranil) is used to treat both endogenous and reactive depression. Amitriptyline (Elavil), desipramine (Norpramin), and nortriptyline (Aventyl) are other commonly used tricyclic antidepressants.

Maprotiline (Ludiomil) is a new antidepressant that belongs to neither group.

NURSING IMPLICATIONS

As with any psychotropic drug, you need to observe that the patient actually takes the ordered medication. Depressed patients may be contemplating suicide; some have been known to save their pills to take all at once and thus overdose. Remember, too, that antidepressants do not treat the underlying problem, so changes in mood (mood swings) should be communicated to the therapist in charge.

The patient receiving an MAO inhibitor should be taught the dangers of eating foods that contain tyramine. His family and visitors need to be aware of this, as well. These foods must not be eaten while the medication is being taken or for 2 to 3 weeks after it has been discontinued. Caution them to avoid medications such as analgesic compounds that may contain caffeine as well. Do not overlook complaints of headache, since this could be the first sign of an impending paradoxical hypertensive crisis. Like patients taking tranquilizers, those receiving antidepressants should be warned about driving, operating dangerous machinery, and possible bodily changes related to hormonal imbalances, as described earlier.

As a rule, tranquilizers and antidepressants are not given together. Even two tranquilizers, or two antidepressants, or one of either plus another drug with a different action but similar chemical make-up, given together can be fatal. An exception is combination therapy, which makes use of interactions for the patient's benefit. An example is the giving of phenothiazines plus an MAO inhibitor to decrease the adverse effects of both. Obviously, patients on combination therapy need extremely close supervision.

PRACTICE PROBLEMS—PSYCHOTROPIC DRUGS

1. The order reads: prochlorperazine (Compazine) 10 mg IM q4h prn nausea. The label reads: prochlorperazine 5 mg/ml. How much prochlorperazine would you give to the patient when he complains of nausea?

$$\frac{D}{H} \times A = G$$

$$\frac{10 \text{ mg}}{5 \text{ mg}} \times 1 \text{ ml} = G$$

$$\frac{2\ \cancel{10}}{1\ \cancel{5}} \times 1 \text{ ml} = 2 \text{ ml}$$

You will give 2 ml of prochlorperazine (Compazine).

2. Your patient is agitated. There is an order that reads haloperidol (Haldol) 1 mg PO q6h for agitation. The pharmacy has sent tablets of 2 mg each. How much haloperidol will you give?

$$\frac{D}{H} = G$$

$$\frac{1}{2} = \frac{1}{2}$$

You will give $\frac{1}{2}$ tablet of haloperidol (Haldol).

3. A preoperative order reads hydroxyzine (Vistaril) 50 mg IM on call to the OR. Hydroxyzine comes in an ampule labeled 100 mg/2 ml. How much will you give?

$$\frac{D}{H} \times A = G$$

$$\frac{1}{2} \frac{\cancel{50} \text{ mg}}{\cancel{100} \text{ mg}} \times 2 = G$$

$$\frac{1}{2} \times 2 \text{ ml} = 1 \text{ ml of hydroxyzine (Vistaril)}$$

to be given.

Work the following problems:
1. The order reads: chlorpromazine (Thorazine) elixir 25 mg PO q4h.
   The label reads: chlorpromazine 10 mg/5 ml.
   How much will you administer every 4 hours?

2. Perphenazine (Trilafon) 7.5 mg IM is ordered. It comes in a vial labeled 5 mg/ml. How much will you give?

3. The order reads promazine (Sparine) 50 mg PO q6h. It comes in a syrup containing 10 mg/5 ml. What volume will you administer?

4. The order is for thioridazine (Mellaril) 75 mg PO tid. The tablets available are 25 mg each. How many will you give?

Answers are given on p. 283.

CHAPTER 7
Anti-infectives

The anti-infectives are a large group of drugs used to treat pathogenic (disease-producing) bacterial, fungal, viral, and parasitic infections. The term *anti-infective* is, therefore, a broad one since it includes drugs that attack *all* pathogenic organisms. An invasion of infective organisms can overwhelm the body's natural defense systems. Anti-infective drugs are given to reduce the number of pathogens to the point that the body's defenses can deal with the remainder and eliminate them. Most anti-infectives are selective in their action. They act on a particular type of organism (or organisms) and are not effective if used against other organisms. They are called *narrow-spectrum* anti-infectives. If an anti-infective is effective against many different pathogens, it is called a *broad-spectrum* anti-infective.

The first step in treating any infection is identifying the causative organism. The way to do this is to obtain a culture specimen from the infected area. The specimen is then taken to the laboratory, where the organisms grow under special conditions. Once the pathogen has been identified, it is tested for sensitivity to many different anti-infectives. If the organism is sensitive to a drug, this means the drug is effective, whereas resistant organisms are not affected by the drug. The drug that is found to be most effective is the one usually ordered by the physician. If there are many different organisms present, or if the organisms cannot be identified quickly, a broad-spectrum anti-infective may be ordered.

It is also necessary to evaluate the patient's overall condition—his ability to fight the organisms. The patient may already be debilitated by another disease; he may be elderly; or he may be receiving drugs that weaken his natural defenses.

Anti-infectives can be applied directly to the infected site (locally) or reach it through the circulation (systemically). When the agent is given systemically, it is common for the physician to order an initial *loading dose*—a dose much greater than the *maintenance dose*. Giving a loading dose ensures that a high blood concentration of drug is quickly achieved. For the drug to be effective, it must always be present in the bloodstream at a concentration specific for that drug. Some anti-infectives need to be given at regular intervals around the clock, while other (newer) products require only once-a-day dosing. Treatment is usually continued until the patient feels well and has had a normal temperature for at least two days, and a culture taken from the infected area shows that few pathogens remain.

ANTIBACTERIAL DRUGS

The first anti-infectives discussed are those for bacterial infections. This group of drugs includes sulfonamides, urinary tract antiseptics, penicillins and cephalosporins, antitubercular drugs, and broad-spectrum anti-infectives. Table 7-1 details

(*Text continues on p. 67.*)

TABLE 7-1 ANTI-INFECTIVES (ANTIBACTERIAL DRUGS)

DRUG	ROUTE AND DOSAGE RANGE	USE	ADVERSE EFFECTS	NURSING IMPLICATIONS
SULFONAMIDES				
sulfisoxazole (Gantrisin)	PO—initial dose—2 g–4 g Maintenance—2 g–8 g qd in 3–6 divided doses SC, IV, IM—50 mg–100 mg/kg/24 hr in 2–4 divided doses	To treat acute, recurrent, or chronic urinary tract infections; to treat cystitis, pyelonephritis, and pyelitis; to treat acute otitis media, trachoma, chancroid, and meningococcal meningitis	*CNS:* ataxia, headache, mental depression *GI:* nausea, vomiting, anorexia, diarrhea, abdominal pain, stomatitis *Others:* blood disorders, muscle weakness, allergic reactions characterized by rash, itch, fever, chills, periorbital edema, tinnitus, or photosensitivity. (Specific allergic reactions include the Stevens-Johnson syndrome and anaphylaxis.)	Blood tests should be done at regular intervals. Keep record of stools. Assess appetite and mouth condition. Evaluate mental status. Assist with ambulation if necessary. Check for rash. Take temperature at regular intervals. Avoid brightly lit areas and direct sunlight. Encourage patients to drink at least 3000 ml of fluid every day. Keep accurate I&O records.
sulfisoxazole + phenazopyridine (Azo Gantrisin)	PO—initial dose—4–6 tablets Maintenance—2 tablets qid	To treat the acute, painful stage of urinary tract infections	See sulfisoxazole, *plus:* red-orange urine color	See sulfisoxazole, *plus:* Warn the patient of a red-orange urine color.
sulfamethoxazole (Gantanol)	PO—2 g–3 g qd in 2–3 divided doses	See sulfisoxazole.	See sulfisoxazole.	See sulfisoxazole.
sulfamethoxazole + trimethoprim (Bactrim, Septra, Bactrim DS, Septra DS)	PO—2 tablets q12h DS (double strength) 1 tablet q12h	To treat urinary tract infections, acute otitis media, shigellosis, and pneumonitis	See sulfisoxazole.	See sulfisoxazole, *plus:* A combination drug is less apt to lead to bacterial resistance than either ingredient alone.
mafenide acetate (Sulfamylon)	Topical—1/16 in (thickness) applied qd to bid	To reduce the bacterial count in tissues of second- and third-degree burns; to prevent wound sepsis	Pain or burning sensation on application, allergic reactions characterized by rash, itching, swelling of the face, hives, or blisters	Check skin carefully for signs of allergic reaction. Apply with a sterile-gloved hand. Keep wound covered with medication at all times.
silver sulfadiazine (Silvadene)	See mafenide acetate.	See mafenide acetate.	See mafenide acetate.	See mafenide acetate.
dapsone (DDS)	PO—50 mg–100 mg qd	To treat Hansen's disease (leprosy)	*CNS:* headache, dizziness, lethargy, muscle weakness, tinnitus, blurred vision *GI:* nausea, vomiting, anorexia, abdominal pain *Others:* fever, blood disorders, edema of the hands and feet, skin and mucous membrane lesions	Assess appetite. Assist with activities as necessary. Evaluate hearing and vision. Check skin and mucuous membranes for lesions. Look for signs of edema in hands or feet. Blood tests should be done at regular intervals. Give with meals to decrease stomach upset. Full drug effect may take up to 6 months. Check temperature at regular intervals.

(continued on page 57)

TABLE 7-1 (continued)

DRUG	ROUTE AND DOSAGE RANGE	USE	ADVERSE EFFECTS	NURSING IMPLICATIONS
sulfanilamide + aminacrine (AVC)	Intravaginal Cream—1 applicatorful qd or bid; suppository—1 qd or bid	To relieve vaginitis when the causative organism is unknown; to treat trichomoniasis, and vulvovaginal candidiasis	See sulfisoxazole, *plus:* systemic effects rarely occur	Treatment should continue through one complete menstrual cycle. A vaginal pad may be worn to prevent stained clothing.
sulfasalazine (Azulfidine)	PO—2 g–8 g qd in evenly divided doses	To treat mild to moderately severe ulcerative colitis and regional enteritis; to treat severe ulcerative colitis (in combination with other medications)	See sulfisoxazole, *plus:* *GU:* crystals, blood, or protein in the urine; kidney damage *Others:* hair loss, male infertility, may turn skin and urine a yellow-orange color	See sulfisoxazole, *plus:* Check urine regularly for presence of blood, crystals, and protein. Warn male patients about possible infertility. Watch for hair loss, and warn patient this may occur. Warn patient about the possible changes in color of skin and urine.
sulfathiazole + sulfacetamide + sulfabenzamide (Sultrin)	Intravaginal Cream—1 applicatorful bid for 4–6 days; then ½–¼ the dose Tablets—1 inserted at hs and 1 in AM for 10 days; repeat course if necessary	To treat vaginitis	See sulfanilamide + aminacrine.	A vaginal pad may be worn to avoid stained clothing.

URINARY TRACT ANTISEPTICS

DRUG	ROUTE AND DOSAGE RANGE	USE	ADVERSE EFFECTS	NURSING IMPLICATIONS
nitrofurantoin (Furadantin)	PO—50 mg–100 mg qid	To treat cystitis, pyelitis, and pyelonephritis caused by susceptible organisms	*CNS:* headache, dizziness, drowsiness, nystagmus *Cardiovascular:* blood disorders *Respiratory:* cough, dyspnea *GI:* anorexia, nausea, vomiting, diarrhea, abdominal pain *GU:* superimposed infections of the urinary tract, brownish color urine *Others:* hair loss, fever, rash, anaphylaxis	Give medication with food or milk to decrease GI upset. Keep stool chart. Assist with activities as necessary. Assess eye movement. Blood tests should be done at regular intervals. Reassure patients who lose hair that this is a temporary effect. Watch for superimposed infections. Evaluate respiratory status. Check skin for any rash. Encourage fluid intake to help flush the urinary tract. Keep accurate I&O records. Warn patient to expect urine to turn brown.
nitrofurantoin macrocrystals (Macrodantin)	PO—50 mg–100 mg qid	See nitrofurantoin.	See nitrofurantoin.	See nitrofurantoin.
methenamine hippurate (Hiprex)	PO—1 g bid (morning and night)	To prevent or treat frequently recurring urinary tract infections when long-term therapy is necessary	Nausea, GI upsets, dysuria, rashes	Evaluate voiding pattern. Observe skin for rash. Encourage patient to avoid meals and medications with high alkali content, as Hiprex works best in an acid urine. Test *p*H of urine at regular intervals. An acidifying agent, such as ascorbic acid, is often given along with Hiprex.

(continued on page 58)

TABLE 7-1   (continued)

DRUG	ROUTE AND DOSAGE RANGE	USE	ADVERSE EFFECTS	NURSING IMPLICATIONS
methenamine mandelate (Mandelamine)	PO—1 g qid	To sterilize the urine and stop bacteriuria associated with cystitis, pyelonephritis, and other chronic urinary tract infections; to sterilize the urine in the neurogenic bladder	Rashes, GI disturbances	Observe skin for rash. Encourage patient to avoid meals and medications with high alkali content; Mandelamine works best in an acid urine. Mandelamine is usually given along with an acidifying agent, such as ascorbic acid.
nalidixic acid (NegGram)	PO—1 g qid	To treat urinary tract infections caused by susceptible organisms	*CNS:* headache, dizziness, drowsiness, vertigo, visual difficulties, convulsions *GI:* nausea, vomiting, diarrhea, abdominal pain *Skin:* rash, itch, photosensitivity *Other:* joint swelling	Give with meals to avoid GI upset. Keep stool chart. Assist with activities as necessary. Assess balance and vision. Take seizure precautions. Check skin for rash or itching. Observe joints. Encourage patient to stay out of brightly lit areas and direct sunlight. Use method other than Clinitest to check for sugar in the urine.
trimethroprim (Proloprim, Trimpex)	PO—50 mg–100 mg q12h or 200 mg qd in one dose	To treat initial episodes of simple urinary tract infections caused by susceptible organisms	*GI:* nausea, vomiting, glossitis *Skin:* rash, itching, dermatitis *Others:* fever, blood disorders, abnormal liver function	Note complaints of GI upset and nausea. Inspect mouth. Check skin for rash, itch, or inflamed areas. Monitor temperature. Blood tests should be done at regular intervals. Liver function tests should be done at regular intervals.
PENICILLINS				
penicillin G potassium (Pentids)	PO—600,000 U–2 million U qd IM, IV—5 U–80 million U qd	To treat moderate to severe infections caused by susceptible organisms including: anthrax; actinomycosis; diphtheria; gingivitis; meningitis; endocarditis; venereal disease; and streptococcal, pneumococcal, staphylococcal, and lower respiratory tract infections; used as prophylaxis for bacterial endocarditis	*GI:* nausea, vomiting, diarrhea, epigastric distress, black tongue *Skin:* rash, itch *Others:* fever, chills, fatal anaphylactoid reaction, superimposed infections, blood disorders	Careful drug history must be obtained to determine any past sensitivity to penicillin or other anti-infective. Give medication on time and on an empty stomach whenever possible (1 hr before or 2 hr after meals). Watch patient closely, especially after the first dose. Check skin for rash. Sensitivity reactions are much more likely to appear after parenteral administration. Take temperature at regular intervals. Keep stool chart. Watch for superimposed infections. Blood tests should be done at regular intervals. Reconstituted solutions must be refrigerated and used within 1 week. **(continued on page 59)**

TABLE 7-1 (continued)

DRUG	ROUTE AND DOSAGE RANGE	USE	ADVERSE EFFECTS	NURSING IMPLICATIONS
amoxicillin (Amoxil, Polymox, Trimox, Wymox)	PO—250 mg–500 mg q8h For gonorrhea—single dose of 3 g	To treat infections caused by susceptible organisms	See penicillin G potassium.	See penicillin G potassium.
amoxicillin + potassium clavulanate (Augmentin)	PO—250 mg–500 mg q8h	To treat otic, respiratory, skin, and urinary tract infections caused by β-lactamase-producing organisms	See penicillin G potassium.	See penicillin G potassium.
ampicillin (Polycillin, Omnipen)	PO—250 mg–500 mg q6h IM, IV—250 mg–3 g q6h	See oxacillin.	See penicillin G potassium.	See penicillin G potassium.
carbenicillin (Geocillin, Geopen, Pyopen)	PO—1–2 tablet qid IM—1 g–2 g q6h IV—4 g–40 g qd in divided doses or continuously	To treat acute and chronic infections of the upper and lower urinary tract and asymptomatic bacteriuria and prostatitis due to susceptible organisms	See penicillin G potassium.	See penicillin G potassium.
dicloxacillin (Dycill, Dynapen, Pathocil)	PO—125 mg–500 mg q6h	See oxacillin.	See penicillin G potassium.	See penicillin G potassium.
methicillin (Staphcillin)	IM—1 g q4–6h IV—1 g q6h	To treat infections caused by penicillinase-producing staphylococci; to treat suspected staphylococcal infection	See penicillin G potassium, *plus:* oral and rectal moniliasis, glossitis, or stomatitis	See penicillin G potassium.
mezlocillin (Mezlin)	IM—6 g–8 g/day in divided doses IV—12 g–24 g/day in divided doses q4h	To treat serious infections caused by susceptible strains of specific organisms in intra-abdominal infections, urinary tract infections, gynecologic infections, septicemia, lower respiratory tract infections, skin infections, bone and joint infections, and gonococcal infections.	See penicillin G potassium.	See penicillin G potassium.
nafcillin (Unipen)	PO—250 mg–1 g q4–6h IM—500 mg q4–6h IV—500 mg–1 g q4h	See oxacillin.	See penicillin G potassium.	See penicillin G potassium.
oxacillin (Bactocill, Prostaphlin)	PO—500 mg–1 g q4–6h IM, IV—250 mg–1 g q4–6h	To treat mild to moderate upper respiratory tract and localized skin and soft tissue infections due to susceptible organisms.	See penicillin G potassium.	See penicillin G potassium.

(continued on page 60)

TABLE 7-1   (continued)

DRUG	ROUTE AND DOSAGE RANGE	USE	ADVERSE EFFECTS	NURSING IMPLICATIONS
penicillin G benzathine (Bicillin Long-Acting)	IM—600,000 U–2.4 million U qd	See penicillin G potassium.	See penicillin G potassium.	See penicillin G potassium, *plus:* Give only deep IM injection.
penicillin G procaine (Wycillin, Crysticillin, Duracillin)	IM—300,000 U–4.8 million U qd	See penicillin G potassium.	See penicillin G potassium, *plus:* mental disturbances, weakness, seizures, fear of impending death (symptoms of procaine toxicity)	See penicillin G potassium, *plus:* Evaluate any change in mental status. Take seizure precautions. Must be given deep IM in upper outer quadrant of the buttock.
penicillin V potassium (Pen-Vee-K, V-Cillin-K, Veetids)	PO—125 mg–500 mg (200,000 U–800,000 U) q6–8h	See penicillin G potassium.	See penicillin G potassium.	See penicillin G potassium.
piperacillin (Pipracil)	IM—2 g–8 g/day in single or divided doses	See mezlocillin.	See penicillin G potassium.	See penicillin G potassium.
ticarcillin (Ticar)	IM—50 mg–100 mg/kg/day in divided doses; (maximum of 2 g per injection) IV—150 mg–300 mg/kg/day in divided doses q3–6h	To treat bacterial septicemia, skin and soft tissue infections, acute and chronic respiratory tract infections, intra-abdominal infections, and infections of the female pelvis and genital tract	See penicillin G potassium.	See penicillin G potassium.
CEPHALOSPORINS				
cephalothin (Keflin, Seffin)	IM, IV—500 mg–2 g q4–6h	To treat infections of the respiratory tract, skin and soft tissue, bone, GU tract, prostate, and middle ear that are due to susceptible organisms; to treat GI infections, endocarditis, septicemia, and meningtis	*CNS:* headache, dizziness, fatigue *GI:* nausea, vomiting, diarrhea, abdominal pain, liver dysfunction, glossitis *Skin:* rash, itch (especially genital and anal) *Others:* edema, anaphylaxis, vaginal infections, blood disorders, pain on IM injection, kidney damage if given with aminoglycosides	Cephalothin may cause false-positive results if testing urine for sugar with Clinitest (use Tes-Tape). A careful drug history must be obtained, since those with penicillin allergy may also be allergic to cephalosporins. Observe skin for any signs of sensitivity. Watch for superimposed infections. Assist with activities as necessary. Blood tests should be done at regular intervals.
cefaclor (Ceclor)	PO—250 mg–500 mg q8h (to a maximum 4 g/day in severe infections)	See cephradine.	See cephalothin.	See cephalothin.
cefadroxil monohydrate (Duricef, Ultracef)	PO—500 mg–1 g bid	To treat urinary tract infections or skin and skin structure infections caused by susceptible organisms	See cephalothin.	See cephalothin.

(continued on page 61)

TABLE 7-1 (continued)

DRUG	ROUTE AND DOSAGE RANGE	USE	ADVERSE EFFECTS	NURSING IMPLICATIONS
cefamandole (Mandol)	IM, IV—500 mg–2 g q4–8h	To treat serious infections caused by susceptible organisms in the lower respiratory tract, urinary tract, peritonitis, septicemia, skin and related structures, bone and joints; to treat pelvic inflammatory disease	See cephalothin.	See cephalothin.
cefazolin (Ancef, Kefzol)	IM, IV—250 mg–1 g q6–12h (to a maximum 12 g/24 h if life-threatening infection) Prophylactic treatment—0.5 g–1 g ½ to 1 hr before; at intervals during; and q6–8h postoperative	See cephalothin, *plus:* To treat biliary tract infections and use as prophylactic treatment pre-, intra-, and postoperatively to reduce the incidence of infections	See cephalothin, *plus:* pain at injection site with possibility of phlebitis	See cephalothin, *plus:* Give injection into a large muscle mass. Watch for redness, swelling, pain, or warmth at the injection site.
cefonicid (Monocid)	IM, IV—1 g–2 g once daily	To treat infections caused by susceptible organisms	See cephalothin.	See cephalothin.
cefoperazone (Cefobid)	IM, IV—2 g–12 g/day in equally divided doses q6–12h	To treat infections caused by susceptible organisms	See cephalothin.	See cephalothin.
cefuranide (Precef)	IM, IV—0.5 g–1 g q12h	See cefonicid.	See cephalothin.	See cephalothin.
cefotaxime (Claforan)	IM—1 g–2 g q6–12h IV—2 g–12 g in divided doses	See cephalothin, *plus:* CNS infections	See cephalothin.	See cephalothin.
cefoxitin (Mefoxin)	IM, IV—0.5 g–2 g q4–8h For prophylaxis—2 g ½–1 hr before surgical incision; then 2 g q6h for 24–72 hr	To treat serious lower respiratory, GU intraabdominal, gynecologic, bone and joint, skin and skin structure infections; to treat septicemia; for prophylactic treatment pre-, intra-, and postoperatively	See cephalothin.	See cephalothin.
ceftizoxime (Cefizox)	IM, IV—1 g–12 g/day in divided doses q8–12h	See cefonicid.	See cephalothin.	See cephalothin.
cefuroxime (Zinacef)	IM, IV—750 mg–3 g q8h	See cefonicid.	See cephalothin.	See cephalothin.
cephalexin (Keflex)	PO—1 g–4 g qd in divided doses	See cephalothin.	See cephalothin.	See cephalothin.
cephapirin (Cefadyl)	IM, IV—500 mg–1 g q4–6 h (to a maximum of 12 g/day in serious cases)	To treat infections of the respiratory and urinary tracts, endocarditis, septicemia, and osteomyelitis that have been caused by susceptible organisms	See cephalothin.	See cephalothin.

(continued on page 62)

TABLE 7-1 (continued)

DRUG	ROUTE AND DOSAGE RANGE	USE	ADVERSE EFFECTS	NURSING IMPLICATIONS
cephradine (Anspor, Velosef)	PO—250 mg–1 g q6–12h	To treat respiratory tract, skin and skin structure, and urinary tract infections and otitis media caused by susceptible organisms	See cephalothin.	See cephalothin.
moxalactam (Moxam)	IM, IV—2 g–12 g/day in divided doses q8–12h for up to 14 days	To treat infections caused by susceptible strains of organisms, especially when resistant to other penicillins, cephalosporins, or aminoglycosides	*GI:* diarrhea, nausea, vomiting *Others:* blood abnormalities, pain at injection site, rash, fever, abnormal liver and renal function, anaphylaxis, superimposed infections	Observe for any signs of hypersensitivity. Blood tests should be done at regular intervals to assess liver and renal function. Monitor bleeding time if high-dose therapy is maintained for more than 3 days. Keep stool chart. Observe for any superimposed infection.

ANTITUBERCULAR DRUGS

DRUG	ROUTE AND DOSAGE RANGE	USE	ADVERSE EFFECTS	NURSING IMPLICATIONS
aminosalicyclic acid (PAS, Parasal)	PO—10 g–12 g qd in divided doses	To treat pulmonary and extra pulmonary tuberculosis	*GI:* nausea, vomiting, diarrhea, abdominal pain, hepatitis *Others:* fever, rashes, blood disorders, goiter, hypokalemia, acidosis, crystalluria	Used along with other antituberculotic medications, not alone. Check skin for rashes. Monitor temperature. Keep stool chart. Blood tests should be done at regular intervals. Watch neck for any increase in size. Keep urine neutral or alkaline. Encourage fluids to flush urinary system.
isoniazid (INH)	PO—5 mg/kg/day to a maximum of 300 mg/day as a single dose	To treat active tuberculosis; for preventive therapy for persons susceptible or recently exposed to TB	*CNS:* malaise, paresthesias in hands and feet (especially in alcoholics and diabetics) *GI:* anorexia, nausea, vomiting, epigastric distress, liver dysfunction, vitamin B_6 deficiency, pellagra *Others:* fever, rash, hyperglycemia, gynecomastia, SLE-like syndrome	Evaluate appetite. Assess fine motor movements and sensation in hands and feet. Tests for liver function should be done at regular intervals. Check skin for rash. Monitor temperature. Evaluate breast size. Watch for symptoms of vitamin deficiency. Therapy usually continues for a period of months to years.
ethambutol (Myambutol)	PO—15 mg–25 mg/kg qd as a single dose	To treat pulmonary tuberculosis	*CNS:* malaise, headache, dizziness, mental confusion, peripheral neuritis, optic neuritis causing decreased vision *GI:* anorexia, nausea, vomiting, abdominal pain *Skin:* rash or itch *Others:* fever, joint pains, anaphylaxis, increased uric acid levels	Evaluate appetite. Check skin for rash or itch. Monitor temperature. Assist with activity as necessary. Evaluate mental status. Evaluate sensation in periphery. Evaluate vision, particularly change in color perception. Uric acid levels should be checked at regular intervals.

(continued on page 63)

TABLE 7-1 (continued)

DRUG	ROUTE AND DOSAGE RANGE	USE	ADVERSE EFFECTS	NURSING IMPLICATIONS
rifampin (Rimactane, Rifadin)	PO—600 mg qd as a single dose	To treat pulmonary tuberculosis and carriers of meningococcal infection	*CNS:* headache, drowsiness, ataxia, mental confusion, visual disturbances, muscle weakness and pains *GI:* anorexia, nausea, vomiting, diarrhea, abdominal cramps, abnormal liver function *Skin:* rash, itch, hives, stomatitis *Other:* changes in menstruation, may cause body substances (urine, stool, saliva, sweat, tears, and sputum) to turn red-orange	Evaluate appetite. Keep stool chart. Assist with activity as necessary. Evaluate mental status. Check skin for rash, itch, hives. Evaluate visual acuity. Check mouth for sores. Warn female patient of possible changes in monthly menstruation cycle. Blood tests should be done at regular intervals to assess liver function. Give at least 1 hour before or 2 hours after meals to obtain optimum absorption. Warn patients about possible discoloration of body substances.

BROAD-SPECTRUM ANTI-INFECTIVES

Tetracyclines

DRUG	ROUTE AND DOSAGE RANGE	USE	ADVERSE EFFECTS	NURSING IMPLICATIONS
tetracycline HCl (Achromycin, Sumycin)	PO—1 g–4 g qd in 2–4 divided doses IM—250 mg as single daily dose or 300 mg in 2–3 divided doses IV—250 mg–500 mg q6–12h	To treat infections caused by susceptible organisms; to treat severe acne; if penicillins are contraindicated	*Cardiovascular:* possible thrombophlebitis after prolonged IV therapy *GI:* anorexia, nausea, vomiting, diarrhea, dysphagia, glossitis *Skin:* rash, hives, photosensitivity *Others:* superimposed infections, anaphylaxis, renal toxicity, blood disorders, permanent discoloration of the teeth if taken during times of tooth development, local irritation after IM injection	Give 1 hour before or 2 hours after meals to avoid conflict with foods and dairy products, which can decrease drug effect. All medications containing calcium, aluminum, iron, or magnesium should be avoided. Keep stool chart. Assess mouth for lesions. Evaluate swallowing. Check skin and perineal area for inflammation. Keep I&O to evaluate renal function. Blood tests should be done at regular intervals. Watch for superimposed infections. If necessary to give to children under 8 years old, have them drink liquid medication through a straw. IV must run slowly to avoid phlebitis. IM injection must be given deep into a large muscle.
oxytetracycline (Terramycin)	PO—1 g–4 g qd in 4 divided doses IM, IV—see tetracycline.	See tetracycline HCl.	See tetracycline HCl.	See tetracycline HCl.
demeclocycline (Declomycin)	PO—600 mg qd in divided doses	See tetracycline HCl.	See tetracycline HCl.	See tetracycline HCl.
doxycycline (Vibramycin)	PO—first day—100 mg q12h; then 100 mg/day IV—first day—200 mg; then 100 mg–200 mg/day	See tetracycline HCl.	See tetracycline HCl.	See tetracycline HCl. Doxycycline may be taken with food or milk.

(continued on page 64)

TABLE 7-1 (continued)

DRUG	ROUTE AND DOSAGE RANGE	USE	ADVERSE EFFECTS	NURSING IMPLICATIONS
minocycline (Minocin)	PO—initial dose—200 mg; then 100 mg q12h or 50 mg qid IV—100 mg–200 mg q12h	See tetracycline HCl	See tetracycline HCl, *plus:* vestibular disorders, ataxia, vertigo, nausea, and vomiting	See tetracycline HCl.
Erythromycin erythromycin (EES, E-Mycin, Eryc, Erythrocin, Ilosone, Ilotycin)	PO, IV—1 g–4 g qd in divided doses	To treat mild to moderately severe infections of the upper and lower respiratory tract, skin and soft tissues; as long-term preventive therapy for rheumatic fever when penicillin is not used; to treat intestinal amebiasis and venereal disease in persons allergic to penicillin; and to treat legionnaires' disease	*GI:* nausea, vomiting, diarrhea, abdominal cramps *Skin:* mild allergic reactions, such as rash and hives *Others:* superimposed infections, possibility of anaphylaxis	Give on an empty stomach (1 hr before or 2 hr after a meal). Keep stool chart. Watch for superimposed infections. Check skin for rash or itch. Monitor temperature.
erythromycin + sulfisoxazole (Pediazole)	PO—in equally divided doses qid for 10 days. Total daily dose calculated based on child's weight to a maximum of 6 g/day of sulfisoxazole	To treat acute otitis media in children that is caused by susceptible strains of *Hemophilus influenzae.*	See erythromycin and sulfisoxasole.	See erythromycin and sulfisoxasole.
Aminoglycosides amikacin (Amikin)	IM, IV—15 mg/kg (to a maximum of 1.5 g qd in 2–3 divided doses)	For short-term treatment of serious infections caused by susceptible gram-negative bacteria	*CNS:* headache, tremors, numbness, tingling, muscle paralysis, ototoxicity *GI:* nausea, vomiting *Others:* joint aches, anemia, rash, hypotension, fever, superimposed infections, nephrotoxicity	Evaluate joint and muscle function. Blood and urine tests should be done regularly to assess renal function. Monitor vital signs. Watch for superimposed infections. Evaluate hearing. Encourage fluid intake to keep urine dilute. Keep accurate I&O records. Check specific gravity. Check skin for rash, itching.
gentamicin (Garamycin)	IM, IV—3 mg–5 mg/kg/day in divided doses Topical Cream—1% Ointment—1% Solution—3 mg/ml Ophthalmic ointment	To treat serious infections caused by susceptible organisms	See amikacin, *plus:* confusion, visual disturbances, anorexia, weight loss	See amikacin, *plus:* Evaluate mental status and vision. Check weight periodically.
kanamycin (Kantrex)	PO—(Bowel prep) 1 g qh for 4 hr, then 1 g q6h for 36–72 hr (Hepatic coma) 8 g–12 g qd in divided doses IM—15 mg/kg/day in 2 equal doses (to a maximum of 1.5 g qd)	To eliminate bacteria in the intestines; to treat hepatic coma	Nausea, vomiting, diarrhea, possible nephrotoxicity and ototoxicity if given long term	See amikacin.

(continued on page 65)

TABLE 7-1 (continued)

DRUG	ROUTE AND DOSAGE RANGE	USE	ADVERSE EFFECTS	NURSING IMPLICATIONS
kanamycin (*continued*)	IV—not more than 15 mg/kg/day in 2–3 equal doses			
neomycin (Mycifradin Neobiotic)	PO—(Bowel prep) 40 mg/lb/day in 6 equally divided doses (Diarrhea) 50 mg/kg/day in divided doses (Hepatic coma) 4 g–12 g qd in divided doses	To eliminate intestinal bacteria; to treat diarrhea caused by *E. coli*; to treat hepatic coma	See kanamycin.	See kanamycin.
netilmicin (Netromycin)	IM, IV—3 mg–6.5 mg/kg/day in divided doses q8–12h	For short-term treatment of serious or life-threatening bacterial infections caused by susceptible organisms	*CNS:* vertigo, tinnitus, nystagmus, hearing loss, acute paralysis *GI:* nausea, vomiting *Others:* abnormal liver function, rash, itching, blood disorders, fever, apnea	See amikacin.
spectinomycin (Trobicin)	IM—2 g–4 g	Male—To treat acute gonorrheal urethritis and proctitis Female—To treat acute gonorrheal cervicitis and proctitis	Urticaria, fever, chills, dizziness, insomnia, decreased urine output, pain at injection site	Use a 20-gauge needle and give deep IM. Monitor temperature. Assess sleeping pattern. Check skin for itch. Keep accurate I&O records.
streptomycin sulfate	IM—1 g–4 g qd in divided doses	In combination with other drugs to treat all forms of tuberculotic infection; to treat serious nontuberculous infections after other less toxic drugs have been considered	See amikacin.	See amikacin.
tobramycin (Nebcin)	IM, IV—3 mg–5 mg/kg qd in divided doses given q6–8h	See gentamicin.	See amikacin.	See amikacin.
Other Broad-spectrum Anti-infectives				
bacitracin (Baciguent)	IM—(Infants only) 900 U–1000 U/kg qd in divided doses Topical—500 U/g	To treat infections caused by susceptible organisms; to treat staphylococcal pneumonia in infants	Nausea, vomiting, skin rashes, pain at the injection site, overgrowth of nonsusceptible organisms, nephrotoxicity	Observe skin for rash. Watch for superimposed infections. Maintain fluid intake and urinary output to avoid kidney toxicity.
chloramphenicol (Chloromycetin)	PO, IV—50 mg–100 mg/kg qd in divided doses Topical Cream—1% Ophthalmic solution—0.5% Ophthalmic ointment—1%	To treat serious infections caused by susceptible organisms; use in regimens for cystic fibrosis	*CNS:* headache, mild depression, mental confusion, optic and peripheral neuritis *GI:* nausea, vomiting, diarrhea, glossitis, stomatitis *Skin:* rash, hives *Others:* superimposed infections (including fungi), anaphylaxis, fatal blood disorders	Inspect mouth for irritations. Keep stool chart. Evaluate mental status. Note any visual difficulties. Check skin for rash or itch. Monitor temperature. Watch for superimposed infections. Blood tests should be done regularly. Chloramphenicol should never be used to treat minor infections.

(continued on page 66)

TABLE 7-1 (continued)

DRUG	ROUTE AND DOSAGE RANGE	USE	ADVERSE EFFECTS	NURSING IMPLICATIONS
clindamycin (Cleocin)	PO—150 mg–450 mg q6h IM, IV—600 mg–2700 mg qd in 2–4 divided doses (to a maximum of 4.8 g qd IV)	To treat serious infections caused by anaerobic bacteria after other less toxic drugs have been considered; to treat serious infections caused by susceptible streptococci, pneumococci, and staphylococci	*GI:* severe and persistent abdominal cramps, diarrhea, nausea, vomiting, blood and mucous in stools, esophagitis, jaundice, abnormal liver function *Skin:* rash, itching *Others:* superimposed infections (especially yeast), anaphylaxis, blood disorders	Keep a stool chart so changes in bowel frequency will be noted. Test stools for blood. Watch for superimposed infections. Check skin for rash. Monitor temperature. Blood tests should be done at regular intervals to assess liver function and blood components. Capsules should be taken with a full glass of water to avoid irritating the esophagus.
lincomycin (Lincocin)	PO—500 mg tid or qid IM—600 mg qd or bid IV—1.2 g–8 g qd in divided doses	To treat serious infections caused by susceptible organisms in patients who are allergic to penicillin; not used for minor bacterial or viral infections	See clindamycin, *plus:* tinnitus, vertigo, hypotension, cardiac arrest	See clindamycin, *plus:* No food or drink within 2 hours of drug will maximize the effect. Run IV infusions slowly.
nystatin + neomycin sulfate + gramicidin + triamcinolone (Mycolog)	Topical Cream—applied bid–tid and rubbed in Ointment—apply thin film bid–tid	To treat cutaneous candidiasis, superficial bacterial infections, conditions complicated by candidal and/or bacterial infections, infantile eczema, chronic lichen simplex, and pruritus ani or vulvae	Rare hypersensitivity, skin irritation, maceration of skin, loss of pigment, ototoxicity and nephrotoxicity, secondary infection	Observe skin for any irritation, color changes. Watch for secondary infections. Note any complaints of disturbed hearing. Keep I&O record. Check specific gravity of urine.
polymyxin B (Aerosporin)	IM—25,000 U–30,000 U/kg qd in divided doses IV—15,000 U–25,000 U/kg qd Intrathecal—50,000 U qd Topical—0.1%–0.25%	To treat acute infections of the urinary tract, meninges, bloodstream, and eye that are caused by susceptible organisms	*CNS:* dizziness, ataxia, paresthesias *Others:* drug fever, rash, nephrotoxicity, severe pain at injection sites, possible thrombophlebitis at IV injection sites, superimposed infections	Monitor temperature. Check skin for rash. Evaluate urinary output. Watch for signs of neurotoxicity. Give injections carefully. Observe for possible thrombophlebitis. Watch for superimposed infections.
polymyxin B + bacitracin + neomycin (Neosporin)	Topical—applied sparingly 2–5 times a day GU irrigant—as ordered	To topically treat localized infections or prevent infections in the following conditions: biopsy sites, vascular ulcers, decubitus ulcers, burns, dermabrasion, abrasions, cuts, lacerations, infected eczemas and dermatoses, skin grafts, and donor sites	See bacitracin, neomycin, and polymixin B.	See bacitracin, neomycin, and polymixin B.
vancomycin (Vancocin)	PO, IV—2 g qd in divided doses	To treat life-threatening diseases caused by infections that cannot be treated with other less toxic drugs	Nausea, chills, fever, anaphylaxis, rash, urticaria, ototoxicity and nephrotoxicity, pain and possible thrombophlebitis at injection site	Monitor temperature. Check for rash or itch. Evaluate hearing. Urine tests should be done at regular intervals to check for disorders in kidney. Run IV slowly and carefully.

the properties and actions of drugs in each of these categories.

Sulfonamides

Sulfonamides, commonly called sulfa drugs, were the first anti-infective agents to be used. Before penicillin was discovered they were the only drugs available to treat infections. Sulfa drugs are now useful in treating urinary tract infections, ulcerative colitis, and some forms of meningitis. They are also used topically to treat eye infections and prevent infections in patients with burns or rheumatic fever.

Sulfones have actions similar to those of the sulfonamides. They are effective in Hansen's disease (leprosy) and some skin diseases. These drugs are given for very long periods—months and years. Improvement may not begin until months after therapy has been started.

Most of the sulfonamides are absorbed from the gastrointestinal tract and excreted through the kidneys. However, if urine flow is below normal, crystals may form in the urine. If allowed to accumulate, these crystals can cause obstruction of urine flow and lead to renal shutdown or complete kidney failure. An uncommon, although potentially fatal adverse effect, called the Stevens-Johnson syndrome, is possible with sulfonamide therapy. It is a severe allergic reaction that begins with fever, cough, and muscular aches. Blisters or wheals appear on the skin, mucous membranes, and respiratory tract. Respiratory arrest and death can occur if the growth and expansion of the blisters cannot be checked.

Urinary tract antiseptics

The urinary antiseptics are drugs active in the urine against infectious organisms. They have little, if any, systemic effect. They are used chiefly in the treatment of urinary tract infections (infections of the kidney and bladder). Nalidixic acid (NegGram) and methenamine mandelate (Mandelamine) are prescribed in both acute and chronic urinary tract infections. Methenamine mandelate is effective only in acid urine, hence an acidifying agent, such as ascorbic acid (vitamin C) or ammonium chloride, also will be prescribed.

Penicillins and cephalosporins

Drugs belonging to the penicillin and cephalosporin groups are highly effective against certain gram-negative organisms and are widely used. Penicillin is a true antibiotic, being produced from the living *Penicillium* mold. Semisynthetic compounds, such as the newer penicillins and the cephalosporins, are also in wide use. These drugs, although also derived from *Penicillium* mold, have a chemical structure altered to make them effective in many situations in which the natural penicillins are not. Both the penicillins and cephalosporins are most effective when given parenterally, since gastric acids destroy most of them. They are excreted rapidly through the kidneys. Penicillins and cephalosporins also are widely used prophylactically, for example, before surgery or dental extractions.

The penicillins and cephalosporins are similar in structure, action, and adverse effects. Although mild allergic reactions are common, a serious life-threatening allergic reaction called *anaphylactic shock* may develop in some patients. This reaction is manifested within minutes of administration of the offending drug. The patient may go into circulatory collapse and must receive cardiopulmonary resuscitation (CPR) immediately. The larynx, pharynx, and bronchi may swell, threatening suffocation, and an emergency tracheostomy is necessary to save the patient's life. Early symptoms of anaphylaxis are pallor, a drop in blood pressure, increased perspiration, and severe dyspnea; these are followed by loss of consciousness.

Antitubercular drugs

Tuberculosis (TB) is an infection caused by the tubercle bacillus. There are two problems involved in the drug treatment of tuberculosis, and both are related to the fact that treatment takes 1 to 3 years. First, the drugs have toxic effects, and the longer they are given, the greater the likelihood of serious cumulative effects. The other problem is that the tubercle bacilli often, and quickly, become drug resistant. For these reasons, a combination of drugs is usually prescribed in order to intensify the therapy and delay drug resistance.

Prophylactic treatment is necessary for some persons who do not have the disease. This group includes anyone who has had a positive reaction to the TB test and has been in close contact with a person diagnosed as having TB and persons whose previously negative tests later become positive (if below the age of 20). Isoniazid is the preferred drug for prophylactic treatment. In active disease, streptomycin is highly effective but has a definite disadvantage in that it may cause hearing damage. Aminosalicylic acid (PAS, Parasol), although less effective against the bacillus, does raise the blood level of isoniazid, and it helps to retard resistance to both streptomycin and isoniazid. Current drug therapy usually includes isoniazid plus other drugs.

Broad-spectrum anti-infectives

Broad-spectrum anti-infectives are ordered when many different bacterial organisms have been identified by culture or when the organisms have not been identified. A mixed infection is one in which more than one pathogen is present. *Tetracyclines* are one group of broad-spectrum drugs. These drugs are useful in treating mixed bacterial infections, as well as in cholera, typhus, and Rocky Mountain spotted fever. Another use is in long-term treatment of acne.

All tetracyclines are easily absorbed from the stomach. The presence of food, milk, milk products, and some antacids will, however, inhibit absorption. Tetracyclines are usually ordered to be given orally, but many other forms are available—injectable solutions, ointments, powders, and vaginal tablets.

Erythromycins are another group of broad-spectrum anti-infectives. They are frequently prescribed for patients who are allergic to the penicillins. Diphtheria, amebiasis, and infections caused by group A β-hemolytic streptococci are sensitive to erythromycin.

Aminoglycosides are potent drugs used in bacterial infections. They are not absorbed well in the digestive tract and, for this reason, are usually given by IM injection. There are few topical preparations available.

Streptomycin has been used since 1944 when it was the major antitubercular drug. It is still used in combination therapy for TB. Penicillin and streptomycin are often combined in the treatment of subacute bacterial endocarditis. Neomycin sulfate (Mycifradin) is given orally to destroy intestinal bacteria in preparation for bowel surgery and (in combination with other antibacterial drugs) is applied topically to treat skin infections.

The most serious adverse effects of the aminoglycosides are ototoxicity and nephrotoxicity. Ototoxicity—damage to the eighth cranial nerve (auditory)—may cause permanent deafness, dizziness, and loss of balance. Nephrotoxicity—damage to the kidneys—causes nitrogen retention and proteinuria.

Polymyxins are broad-spectrum anti-infectives that are so potent and toxic that they are ordered only when other drugs have failed. Infections of the skin, mucous membranes, eye, and ear respond to the polymyxins. These drugs are not absorbed if taken orally; therefore they are given topically and parenterally. Also included in the category of miscellaneous anti-infectives are drugs, or combinations of drugs, that fit into none of the specific categories listed above.

NURSING IMPLICATIONS

All anti-infectives share some undesirable characteristics, and these need to be kept in mind if you are to administer the drugs safely. All anti-infectives have the potential for causing allergic (hypersensitivity) reactions. These may range from mild skin rash, urticaria, and itching to life-threatening anaphylactic shock, as described earlier in this chapter. Before any drug is given, if possible during the initial nursing assessment, you should discuss the patient's allergies with him. A patient who is allergic to penicillin, or for that matter to any drug or other substance, such as certain foods, dust, or pollen, is likely to be allergic to other medications. Observe the patient closely as he receives the first dose of the drug, since a serious reaction may develop within minutes. Be sure to observe the patient's skin for evidence of a rash or other eruption. You may have to ask the patient to remove his pajama top so you can observe his chest and back. Notify the nurse in charge immediately if you notice changes in skin color or appearance.

Another occurrence common to all anti-infective therapy is the growth of resistant organisms. Document the appearance of the infected site during the course of therapy to aid in assessing the drug's effectiveness. If you have responsibility for collecting specimens for cultures of the infected site, be sure to use the proper container and avoid contaminating the specimen.

In their battle with pathogenic organisms, the

anti-infectives destroy some nonpathogenic organisms as well. These harmless organisms are called the *normal flora*. They are essential to normal health and help protect the body against infection. Thus, when the normal flora of the mouth and digestive tract is destroyed, those areas are susceptible to superimposed infection (one infection imposed on another). Suspect superimposed infection if you notice or your patient complains of any of the following: mouth sores; patchy, dark fur on the tongue; diarrhea; perineal itching; discharge; or discomfort.

Bacteria that normally live in the intestine manufacture vitamin K, which is necessary for proper blood coagulation. Long-term therapy with anti-infectives can cause a deficiency of this vitamin and thus lead to prolonged bleeding. If you notice any bruises on the patient's skin, report and record them, because they may indicate bleeding under the skin.

Gastrointestinal disturbances, such as anorexia, nausea, vomiting, and diarrhea, sometimes occur with anti-infective drug therapy. The medication may have to be changed if they continue.

It is very important that anti-infectives be administered on time. Remember that if the blood level of the drug is not maintained at the required concentration, the drug will be less effective. If the patient is to leave the hospital with a prescription for an anti-infective, be sure to explain the importance of regular, around-the-clock dosing. If necessary, the patient should set an alarm clock so he is certain to get the nighttime or early morning dose. The person's own schedule should be accommodated, if possible. For example, a drug ordered to be given every 6 hours could be given at 10 AM–4 PM–10 PM–4 AM or 7 AM–1 PM–7 PM–1 AM. If the patient usually gets up around 7 AM and goes to bed after midnight, with the latter schedule he will not have to wake up in the middle of the night just to take his medication.

Another point to stress is that every pill must be taken. Many patients go home and take their pills until their symptoms clear or they feel better. If they stop taking the pills, they are likely to have a relapse or a reinfection. Anti-infectives must be taken for the entire time they are ordered.

With the sulfonamides and urinary tract antiseptics, it is essential that the patient's fluid intake and output be monitored. Since the formation of crystals and their accumulation in the kidney can cause serious damage, encourage your patient to drink at least 3000 cc of water every 24 hours. This will not only discourage formation of crystals but will also help flush the pathogens from the urinary tract. The presence of crystals will be noted on the urinalysis report. You can test for hematuria, which is often the result of kidney damage, by doing the dipstick test.

As was stated earlier, the absorption of some anti-infectives is inhibited by the presence of food, milk products, or antacids in the stomach. Thus, if these drugs are to be given, be sure you are aware of the stomach contents. In most cases, absorption will not be influenced if the drugs are given 1 hour before or 2 hours after meals.

If it is known that the drug will cause a change in the color of the urine, tell the patient about it before it happens. The sight of bright red or brown urine may cause unnecessary anxiety if it is not anticipated.

Some anti-infectives cause a false-positive result when the urine is checked for sugar with Clinitest tablets. This is especially true of the cephalosporins. You will need to use another method, such as Tes-Tape, to test your diabetic patient's urine if he is receiving these drugs.

Some anti-infectives may cause photosensitivity—the patient looks as though he has a severe sunburn. Caution patients to stay out of direct sunlight as much as possible and to wear protective clothing if they must go out into direct sunlight.

ANTIFUNGAL AGENTS

The second major group of anti-infectives are the drugs used to treat fungus (mycotic) infections (Table 7-2). Either yeasts or molds can cause fungus infections. The previously discussed superimposed infections owing to anti-infective therapy are often fungal in nature. Fungus infections can be either superficial or deep. If superficial, they are treated with specific topical agents. Deep infections must be treated systemically. Compared with the number of drugs used to treat bacterial infections, the number of antifungal agents is quite small. This is because fungi are immune to most drugs that are not extremely toxic.

Amphotericin B (Fungizone) is the only agent effective in deep, potentially fatal fungus infections. It is given intravenously. Nystatin (Mycostatin) is useful in topical fungus infections. It is available in creams, powders, ointments, and suppositories. It can also be given by mouth if the intestine is involved. A liquid preparation is available as a rinse for fungus infections of the tongue. Griseofulvin (Fulvicin, Grifulvin V) is the only an-

TABLE 7-2 ANTI-INFECTIVES (ANTIFUNGAL AGENTS)

DRUG	ROUTE AND DOSAGE RANGE	USE	ADVERSE EFFECTS	NURSING IMPLICATIONS
amphotericin B (Fungizone)	IV—0.25 mg–1 mg/ kg qd infused over 6 hr; 1.5/kg/day for alternate-day therapy Topical Cream—3% Lotion—3% Ointment—3% apply liberally q6–12h	To treat patients with progressive potentially fatal fungal infections; to treat skin and mucous membrane fungal infections	*CNS:* headache, malaise, generalized muscle and joint pains, vision and hearing losses, peripheral neuropathy *Cardiovascular:* cardiac arrhythmias, hypo- or hypertension *GI:* nausea, vomiting, diarrhea, anorexia *GU:* abnormal renal function, decreased urine output *Skin:* rash, itching, flushed skin *Others:* fever, weight loss, anemia and other blood disorders, anaphylaxis, irritation at injection site	Several months of therapy is usually necessary. Evaluate appetite. Keep stool chart. Check weight periodically. Monitor temperature, pulse, and blood pressure. Blood tests should be done at regular intervals. Check skin for rash or itch. Evaluate urinary output. Evaluate vision and hearing. Watch for tremors. Assess injection site. Give IV injections very slowly.
clotrimazole (Lotrimin, Mycelex, Gyne-Lotrimin, Mycelex-G)	Topical Cream—1% Solution—1% apply bid (morning and evening) Vaginal tablets—2 per day for 3 days Vaginal cream—daily for 7–14 days	For topical treatment of fungal infections caused by susceptible organisms	*Skin:* redness, stinging, blistering, peeling, edema, hives, itching, general skin irritation	Observe skin for reactions.
griseofulvin microsize (Fulvicin, Grifulvin V) ultramicrosize (Fulvicin P/G, Gris-Peg)	PO—(microsize) 500 mg in one daily dose or 1 g in divided doses (ultramicrosize) 250 mg in one daily dose or 500 mg qd in divided doses	To treat ringworm infections of the skin, hair, and nails caused by fungi	*CNS:* headache, fatigue, dizziness, insomnia, mental confusion *GI:* nausea, vomiting, diarrhea *Skin:* rash, hives, tissue swelling, photosensitivity *Other:* blood disorders	Check skin for rash or swelling. Keep stool chart. Assist with activity if necessary. Assess sleeping patterns. Evaluate mental status. Warn patient to avoid bright artificial or natural lights. Blood tests should be done at regular intervals.
ketoconazole (Nizoral)	PO—200 mg–400 mg qd	To treat systemic fungal infections	*CNS:* headache, dizziness, sleepiness *GI:* nausea, vomiting, diarrhea, abdominal pain *Others:* rash, chills, fever, jaundice, swelling of breasts, light sensitivity	Assess for gait instability and assist as necessary. Note level of alertness. Keep stool chart. Check skin for rash. Note any complaints of light sensitivity and if present avoid brightly lit areas. Monitor temperature. Warn about possible breast swelling (gynecomastia). Blood tests to monitor liver function should be done at regular intervals. Do not administer with antacids.

(continued on page 71)

TABLE 7-2 (continued)

DRUG	ROUTE AND DOSAGE RANGE	USE	ADVERSE EFFECTS	NURSING IMPLICATIONS
miconazole (Monistat)	IV—200 mg–3600 mg qd	To treat severe systemic fungal infections	*Cardiovascular:* tachycardia, arrhythmias (if infused too rapidly), phlebitis, changes in blood composition *GI:* anorexia, nausea, vomiting, diarrhea *Skin:* flushed skin, rash, itching *Other:* fever	Be sure infusion runs slowly. Take frequent apical pulses. Monitor temperature. Blood tests should be done at regular intervals. Evaluate appetite. Keep stool chart. Observe skin for color, rash, or itch.
miconazole nitrate (Monistat 7)	Topical Cream—2%; 1 applicatorful at hs for 7 days	To treat vulvovaginal candidiasis (moniliasis)	Vaginal burning, itch, irritation, generalized rash, hives, headache, pelvic cramps	Note complaints of vaginal irritation. Observe skin for rash, itch, or hives.
(Monistat-Derm)	Topical cream and lotion—2% bid Suppository 100 mg: 1 at hs × 7 days 200 mg: 1 at hs × 3 days			
nystatin (Mycostatin, Nilstat)	PO—Suspension— 400,000 U– 600,000 U qid; Tablets—500,000 U–1,000,000 U tid Topical Cream Lotion Powder Ointment	To treat candidal infections of the mouth, skin, and mucous membranes, especially the intestines and vulvovaginal area	Usually none; large doses may cause nausea and vomiting	When oral suspension is given, patients should be instructed to hold it in their mouth as long as possible before swallowing.

tifungal agent effective when given by mouth for the treatment of superficial fungus infections. It does not kill the fungus but prevents the spread of infection to other cells. Eventually, as the infected cells die, the infection clears.

NURSING IMPLICATIONS

Intravenous administration of antifungal agents can cause local inflammation as well as thrombophlebitis. They must be administered slowly and the site checked frequently for signs of tissue irritation.

If the patient will be sent home with instructions to apply a topical preparation daily, be sure he knows how to do this. Some drugs must be applied sparingly, some liberally; and the drug will not be fully effective unless it is correctly applied.

As with other anti-infectives, it is important to continue therapy even though the infection may appear to have cleared. A relapse may occur if treatment is not completed.

ANTIVIRAL AGENTS

A third major group of anti-infectives are those used to treat virus infections (Table 7-3). The treatment of viral infections is complicated for two reasons: First, the virus is a parasite, living within the cells of the host, so that a drug that destroys the virus will also destroy the host cells. Second, by the time symptoms are noticed, it is too late to alter the course of the disease. To date, the only truly effective treatment is prevention.

There are only a few antiviral drugs in common use. Amantadine (Symmetrel) is prophylactic against one type of influenza. It is toxic, however, and is given only to persons at high risk or during

TABLE 7-3 ANTI-INFECTIVES (ANTIVIRAL AGENTS)

DRUG	ROUTE AND DOSAGE RANGE	USE	ADVERSE EFFECTS	NURSING IMPLICATIONS
acyclovir (Zovirax)	PO—Initial dose: 200 mg q4h (5 times in 24 hr) × 10 days Chronic suppressive therapy: 200 mg 3–5 times a day for up to 6 months IV—15 mg/kg/day in 3 divided doses Topical Ointment— Apply q3h (6 times/day) × 7 days	To treat initial and recurrent episodes of mucosal, cutaneous, and genital herpes simplex infections	*CNS:* headache, dizziness, fatigue, insomnia, irritability, depression, with IV administration may cause seizures, cerebral edema, coma *GI:* nausea, vomiting, diarrhea, anorexia *Skin:* rash, acne, alopecia *Others:* edema, sore throat, muscle cramping, superficial thrombophlebitis, menstrual abnormalities	Counsel patient to avoid sexual intercourse when visible lesions are present. Be sure patient is aware that medication is not a cure. Advise patient to use finger cot when applying ointment to prevent spreading infection. Evaluate mental status. Keep stool chart. Note changes in appetite. Assess skin for any rash, hair loss, or acne eruptions. Note any swelling in extremities. Check legs for any redness, warmth, or swelling. Warn female patients of possible abnormalities in menstruation. Encourage fluid intake. Keep record of I&O.
amantadine HCl (Symmetrel)	PO—100 mg–400 mg qd in divided doses	To treat Parkinson's disease; to treat drug-induced extrapyramidal reactions, influenza A virus, and respiratory tract illness	*CNS:* headache, fatigue, dizziness, ataxia, anxiety, depression, confusion, psychosis, slurred speech, visual disturbances *Cardiovascular:* orthostatic hypotension, peripheral edema, congestive heart failure (CHF) *GI:* anorexia, nausea, vomiting, constipation, dry mouth *Others:* urinary retention, rash	Evaluate appetite. Keep stool chart. Assist with activity as necessary. Evaluate mental status. Keep accurate I&O records. Take orthostatic BP. Caution patient not to change position rapidly. Check extremities for edema. Check skin for rash. Evaluate clarity of speech. Evaluate vision.
idoxuridine (Stoxil, Herplex Liquifilm)	Topical Solution—0.1% gtt i OU qh while awake, q2h at night Ointment—5 mg/g; apply about q4h	To treat herpes simplex of the cornea	Pain, irritation, pruritus or edema of the eye and eyelids, photophobia, corneal defects, rare allergic reactions	Note any irritations in the eye and eyelids. Warn the patient to avoid brightly lit areas. Watch for allergic manifestations.
vidarabine (Vira-A, Ara-A)	IV—15 mg/kg qd Ophthalmic ointment—3%—apply a line (½ inch) 5 times day (at 3-hr intervals) into lower conjunctival sac	To treat herpes simplex virus conditions of the eye and herpes simplex encephalitis	*CNS:* malaise, weakness, ataxia, dizziness, hallucinations, psychosis, confusion *Cardiovascular:* thrombophlebitis (at IV infusion site), bone marrow depression *GI:* anorexia, nausea, vomiting, weight loss, GI bleeding, abnormal liver function *Others:* rash, itch, muscle tremor	Assess appetite. Check weight daily. Give antiemetics prn. Check insertion site of IV for any swelling or tenderness. Check skin for rash or itch. Test emesis and stools for blood. Assist with activities as necessary. Note any abnormal muscle movements. Evaluate mental status. Blood tests should be done at regular intervals to check on liver and bone marrow function.

an epidemic. Idoxuridine (Herplex liquifilm, Stoxil) is available as a solution or ointment to treat herpes simplex virus of the cornea. Herpes simplex encephalitis is treated with vidarabine (Ara-A, Vira-A). Immune serum globulin (gamma globulin) containing specific antibodies can be given to counteract specific viral antigens. It is valuable against measles, hepatitis, rabies, and poliomyelitis (see Chapter 9).

ANTIPARASITIC AGENTS

The final group of anti-infectives are those used to treat parasitic diseases (Table 7-4). Although infestation with protozoa, helminths (worms), and other parasites is uncommon in the United States, it is a major health problem in other countries, especially those with tropical climates. Overcrowded, unsanitary living conditions can accelerate the transmission of parasitic diseases. Therefore, although treatment with drugs is possible, the elimination of environmental conditions that favor

these diseases is also important. Of the diseases caused by protozoa, malaria is the most common. It infects humans through the bite of the *Anopheles* mosquito, which carries the causative organism.

Helminths are a more common cause of parasitic disease in the United States and worldwide. They are usually found in the gastrointestinal system, but can invade other tissues as well. *Cestodes* (tapeworms or flatworms) gain entrance to the body in improperly cooked or contaminated food. Pork that has not been thoroughly cooked is a good example. Drugs used to treat these infections are called *anthelmintics*. They are specific in their action, so it is important that the organism be properly identified before treatment is begun. Organisms may be found in stool, urine, sputum, blood, or tissue samples. It is possible for more than one type of worm to be present at the same time.

Pediculosis is an infestation of lice. It is usually diagnosed after the eggs (nits) are found in clothing or hair. The female itch mite, another parasite, burrows into the skin causing a condition called *scabies*. Areas of mite infestation appear scaly. Com-

TABLE 7-4 ANTI-INFECTIVES (ANTIPARASITIC AGENTS)

DRUG	ROUTE AND DOSAGE RANGE	USE	ADVERSE EFFECTS	NURSING IMPLICATIONS
chloroquine (Aralen)	IM—160 mg–800 mg (base) in the first 24 hr Acute attack PO—initial dose— 600 mg (base) then 300 mg at 6 hr, 24 hr, and 48 hr later For suppression— 300 mg (base) every week on exactly the same day (start 2 weeks prior to exposure and continue 6–8 weeks after leaving endemic area) Amebiasis—600 mg (base) daily for 2 days, then 300 mg (base) daily for 14–21 days	To treat acute attacks of malaria and extraintestinal amebiasis; to suppress malaria when exposure is expected	*CNS:* headache, psychic stimulation, visual disturbances *GI:* anorexia, nausea, vomiting, abdominal cramps, diarrhea *Skin:* skin disorders, itch	Give at mealtime to decrease gastric upset. Evaluate mental status. Evaluate appetite. Keep stool chart. Evaluate vision. Check skin for rash or itch. This medication must be taken exactly as ordered. Remind the patient not to skip a dose or change times. Suppressive therapy must continue for 6–8 weeks after leaving the endemic area.
lindane (Kwell, Scabene)	Topical Cream Lotion Shampoo	To treat infestation with scabies, lice, crab lice, and their eggs (nits)	Skin disorders or itching after treatment	Follow directions carefully. Be sure patient knows exactly how to apply the medication.

(continued on page 74)

TABLE 7-4 (continued)

DRUG	ROUTE AND DOSAGE RANGE	USE	ADVERSE EFFECTS	NURSING IMPLICATIONS
mebendazole (Vermox)	PO—1 tablet AM and PM × 3 days	To treat infestation with whipworm, pinworm, roundworm, and hookworm	Fever, abdominal pain, diarrhea	Keep stool chart. Monitor temperature. Encourage good personal hygiene to prevent future infestations or reinfestation.
metronidazole (Flagyl)	PO—(Amebic dysentary) 750 mg tid for 5–10 days (Trichomoniasis) 250 mg tid for 7 days or 2 g as single dose or two divided doses	To treat amebic dysentery; to treat patients with trichomoniasis and their sexual partners	*CNS:* dizziness, ataxia, seizures, paresthesias in the extremities, confusion, depression *GI:* anorexia, nausea, vomiting, diarrhea or constipation, abdominal cramps, metallic taste, furry tongue, stomatitis, dry mouth *Skin:* flushed skin, hives *GU:* difficult urination, cystitis *Others:* superimposed infections (especially *Candida* in the mouth and vagina), nasal congestion	Evaluate appetite. Keep stool chart. Assess mouth for irritation or infection. Watch for superimposed vaginal infections. Assist with activity as necessary. Note any tremors or unusual sensation in extremities. Evaluate mental status. Check skin for rash, itch, discoloration. Keep accurate I&O and evaluate voiding pattern and any complaints
piperazine salts (Antepar)	PO—Adult—3.5 g qd for 2 days Child—75 mg/kg (to a maximum of 3.5 g) as a single dose for 2 days	Anthelmintic to treat infections caused by roundworms and pinworms	*CNS:* headache, ataxia, muscle weakness, paresthesias, blurred vision, memory loss, EEG changes, convulsions *GI:* nausea, vomiting, diarrhea, abdominal cramps *Others:* hives, joint pains and redness, fever, cataracts	Keep stool chart. Check skin for irritations. Monitor temperature. Evaluate joint appearance and function. Assist with activity as necessary. Evaluate vision, memory. Encourage good hygiene to prevent future reinfestations.
primaquine	PO—3 tablets once a week, taken on the same day for 8 weeks or 1 tablet daily for 14 days	In combination with chloroquine for prevention of malaria	See chloroquine.	See chloroquine, *plus:* Tablets should be taken at least 1 day before entering the malaria zone.
pyrantel pamoate (Antiminth)	PO—11 mg (base) per kg to a maximum of 1 g	To treat common roundworm and pinworm infestations	*CNS:* headache, dizziness, drowsiness, insomnia *GI:* anorexia, nausea, vomiting, abdominal cramps, diarrhea *Others:* rash, increased liver enzyme levels	Assist with activity as necessary. Evaluate appetite. Assess sleep pattern. Keep stool chart. Check skin for rash. Blood levels of liver enzymes should be checked periodically.
pyrimethamine (Daraprim)	PO—25 mg once a week or 50 mg–75 mg qd	To prevent malaria; to treat toxoplasmosis	Anemia, glossitis, and CNS stimulation (with large doses)	When used to treat toxoplasmosis, this drug must be accompanied by a sulfonamide drug.
pyrvinium pamoate (Povan)	PO—Single dose—5 mg/kg; may repeat in 2–3 weeks	Anthelmintic to treat pinworm infestation	Nausea, vomiting, abdominal cramps, photosensitivity, allergic reactions, turns stools bright red	The solution stains most materials, therefore be careful not to spill it. Warn patient about change in stool color (bright red). If patient should vomit, the emesis will be red and will stain. Avoid brightly lit areas. Check for allergic skin reactions.

monly affected are the wrists, axillae, breasts, waist, buttocks, and the area between the fingers. Pediculosis and scabies are seen most often in persons who live in crowded conditions and who fail to practice personal hygiene. Infestation spreads rapidly from person to person in household, classroom, or hospital ward.

Drugs used to treat pediculosis are called *pediculicides*, and those to eliminate scabies, *scabicides*. These drugs can easily control infestation, and usually only one or two applications are needed. Reinfestation is the main problem. Thus, while the person is taking medication, all his personal belongings, clothes, and linens must be laundered and sterilized to destroy all eggs or mature parasites.

Gamma benzene hexachloride, now called lindane (Kwell), is useful in both scabies and pediculosis. The first application usually kills the mature parasites but not the eggs. A second application 6 to 7 days later destroys eggs and any remaining mature parasites. This drug is available as a cream, lotion, or shampoo. It can cause extensive skin and mucous membrane irritation and should be applied carefully, according to directions. Crotamiton (Eurax) is specifically for scabies. It is less toxic than lindane and is applied topically as a cream.

Amebic dysentery is caused by an intestinal parasite. It is also called *intestinal amebiasis*. It occurs worldwide, in all climates. In conditions of poor sanitation, the presence of diarrhea and parasites in the stool usually indicates amebiasis. In the United States, most affected persons are seen in institutions for the very young or the elderly.

NURSING IMPLICATIONS

All antiparasitics must be taken as ordered. Oral preparations must not be skipped or taken at times other than as ordered. The dose may need to be repeated at specific intervals, either daily or weekly. Instructions for topical administration must be followed carefully, since some of these drugs must be applied in a specific manner. Drugs in liquid form must be diluted in a specific manner. Instructions as to how and when to remove the preparation also must be explained to the patient. Epigastric distress is a common problem with antiparasitics taken internally. This can be lessened by taking the medication at mealtime. If alcohol is taken along with antimalarial drugs, the patient may have a reaction similar to a reaction from disulfiram (Antabuse); therefore, you should warn your patients about this.

Sanitary conditions in the patient's environment should be evaluated to assess the possibility of reinfestation. Occasionally, it may be possible to effect improvements in housing or food preparation. Patient teaching should include an explanation about the transmission of these diseases. The importance of thorough handwashing, especially after going to the bathroom, should be stressed. Also warn your patient to watch for symptoms of reinfestation, such as anal itching or any change in stool color, frequency, or consistency.

PRACTICE PROBLEMS—ANTI-INFECTIVES

1. The order reads: gentamicin (Garamycin) 50 mg IV in 150 ml D$_5$W. Gentamicin comes 40 mg/ml. How many milliliters would be added to the D$_5$W?

$$\frac{D}{H} \times A = G$$

$$\frac{5\emptyset \text{ mg}}{4\emptyset \text{ mg}} \times 1 \text{ ml} = G$$

$$\frac{5}{4} \times 1 \text{ ml} = \frac{5}{4} \text{ ml} = 1\frac{1}{4} \text{ ml} = 1.25 \text{ ml}$$

Thus, 1.25 ml of gentamicin (Garamycin) is added to 150 ml D$_5$W.

2. Sulfisoxazole (Gantrisin) syrup 1 g PO qid is ordered. The syrup contains 500 mg/5 ml. How much would be given?

$$\frac{D}{H} \times A = G$$

(remember: 1 g = 1000 mg)

$$\frac{100\cancel{0} \text{ m}\cancel{g}}{50\cancel{0} \text{ m}\cancel{g}} \times 5 \text{ ml} = G$$

$$\frac{2 \cancel{10}}{1 \cancel{5}} \times 5 \text{ ml} = \frac{2 \times 5 \text{ ml}}{1} = 10 \text{ ml}$$

Thus, 10 ml of sulfisoxazole (Gantrisin) is given.

Work the following problems:
1. The order reads: penicillin G 200,000 U IM q6h.
   The label reads: penicillin G 250,000 U/5 ml.
   How much penicillin G would you give?

2. The physician orders cephalothin (Keflin) 1 g IM q6h.

Cephalothin comes 2 g /5 ml. How much would be given?

3. The order reads: tetracycline syrup 500 mg PO q4h.
   The label reads: tetracycline 125 mg/5 ml.
   How much syrup would be given?

4. The order reads: cefoxitin (Mefoxin) 1.5 g IV q6h in 50 ml D_5W.
   The label reads: 2 g cefoxitin/6 ml.
   How many milliliters will be added to the IV solution?

Answers are given on p. 283.

CHAPTER 8
Dermatologic drugs

The largest organ in the human body is the skin. Dermatology is a specialized branch of medicine that deals with the diagnosis and treatment of diseases of the skin. Since it is not possible to list every dermatologic preparation in this text an outline of drug categories will be presented, along with representative examples of the important ones. Some drugs, for example the corticosteroids, which are discussed in other chapters, are also useful in treating skin disease. In these cases the dermatologic use is described in the present chapter, while the drug action is described in Chapter 34.

Skin diseases often give rise to an inflammatory response, with swelling, redness, and pain. Blisters, hives, wheals, or pustules may form, and their rupture is followed by the appearance of crusts, scaling, and scabs. Besides being inflamed, the skin may become scaly (mild as in dandruff or severe as in psoriasis) or corns, calluses, warts, or moles may appear. The skin is also subject to tumor formation.

Although absorption through the skin is poor (it is naturally waterproof), various substances can pass through the sweat glands and sebaceous glands to the underlying tissues. Absorption is increased if the skin is softened by water or perspiration, if the skin surface is broken, or if its outer layer is thin. Fat-soluble drugs are absorbed more rapidly than water-soluble drugs.

Dermatologic preparations (Table 8-1) have one of two basic actions: they either cause skin irritation or prevent or lessen it. The purpose of causing irritation is to hasten the sloughing of outer layers of skin cells, which are then replaced by new, healthy cells. Keratolytics and depilatories are used for this purpose. Topical corticosteroids, soothing medications, and protectives help lessen inflammatory skin reactions.

DRUGS THAT CAUSE SKIN IRRITATION (IRRITANTS)

Keratolytics are substances that dissolve the outer layer, or keratin, of the skin. Mild keratolytics are also called stimulants. Strong concentrations of stimulants may destroy tissues and cause inflammatory reactions. Salicylic acid, resorcinol, and various tar substances are examples of keratolytics. *Depilatories* are keratolytic agents incorporated in a cream or a lotion that remove hair by destroying the hair shaft. Most of them cause some local irritation (reddening) of the surrounding skin. The strongest irritant substances are the caustic chemicals, such as glacial acetic acid, liquid phenol, and silver nitrate. They are used to destroy overgrown skin tissue such as warts and granulomatous tissue.

DRUGS THAT PREVENT OR LESSEN SKIN IRRITATION

Topical preparations of the *corticosteroid drugs* are widely used in the treatment of skin disorders (see Chapter 34). In addition to their anti-inflammatory

(*Text continues on p. 80.*)

TABLE 8-1 DERMATOLOGIC DRUGS

DRUG	ROUTE AND DOSAGE RANGE	USE	ADVERSE EFFECTS	NURSING IMPLICATIONS
salicylic acid	Topical Shampoo—1%–6% Gels—1%–6% Soaps—1%–6% Scrubs—1%–6% Plaster—4%	To cleanse skin with acne or oily conditions; to remove excess keratin in skin diseases, such as ichthyosis and psoriasis	Skin irritation and dryness	Do not use on or near the eyes or other mucous membranes.
coal tar	Topical Gel—5% Shampoo—0.5%–1% Emulsion—300 mg/ml Ointment Cream	To treat eczema, psoriasis, and other skin diseases responsive to tar	Stains clothing, unpleasant odor, possibility of allergic reactions and photosensitivity Shampoo may temporarily discolor blond, tinted, or bleached hair	Do not use on inflamed or broken skin. Apply at night (areas treated with tar must be shielded from sunlight). When the emulsion is used in a bath, be sure the water is lukewarm, not hot. Tar is often used in combination with ultraviolet radiation therapy.
vitamins A & D	Topical Ointment	To treat diaper rash, chafed skin, minor burns and abrasions; to help prevent dry skin	None	
zinc oxide	Topical Paste Powder Ointment	To treat diaper rash, minor burns, sunburn, and skin irritations from urine or other wound drainage; sunscreen	Possible folliculitis and maceration of the skin	Do not apply repeatedly to hairy areas. Do not cover with occlusive dressings. Apply sparingly.
boric acid	Topical Ointment 5%–10% Solution 1.9%–2%	To treat otitis media; as a mouthwash and bladder or vaginal irrigant; to paint the throat; as a heated soak for ulcers, boils, and carbuncles	None usually, but if absorbed systemically: *CNS:* headache, restlessness, hyperthermia, weakness, delirium, coma *GI:* anorexia, nausea, vomiting, diarrhea *Other:* skin lesions	Apply only to unbroken skin (avoiding systemic absorption). Evaluate appetite. Check skin for lesions. Monitor temperature. Evaluate mental status.
aluminum acetate (Burow's solution)	Topical Lotion—10% Solution	To relieve the itching and weeping of poison ivy, oak, and sumac; to alleviate the itching of insect bites and other minor skin irritations	Occasional skin irritation	Check skin for any irritation. If lesions are weeping, cover with gauze rather than an occlusive dressing. Do not get medication near the eyes.
hydrogen peroxide	Topical Solution—3% (usually diluted with an equal volume of water)	To cleanse wounds, as a disinfecting gargle and as a deodorizing mouthwash	Oral mucosal irritation, bubbling action on contact with organic matter from wounds	Heat, sunlight, and reactive organic matter will cause solution to become unstable. Check the lining of the mouth for any irritation.
benzalkonium chloride (Zephiran)	Topical—solution, tincture, spray, 1:750 Concentrate—12.5%, 17%, 50% Vaginal gel	Antiseptic for the skin, mucous membranes, and wounds; to prep surgeons' hands and arms	Hypersensitivity (rare)	Use proper dilutions according to use and directions.

(continued on page 79)

TABLE 8-1 (continued)

DRUG	ROUTE AND DOSAGE RANGE	USE	ADVERSE EFFECTS	NURSING IMPLICATIONS
thimerosal (Merthiolate)	Topical Solution Powder Ointment Cream Tincture	Topical antiseptic and a preservative	Rashes	Observe skin for any rash.
gentian violet	Topical—Solution—1% Vaginal tablets—1–2 qd	Anthelmintic for pinworms; to treat vulvovaginal candidal infections	Purple stools, may cause purple staining on clothes	Tablets must be swallowed whole, not chewed, and followed by a glass of water. Warn the patient about the change in stool color. Apply carefully to avoid staining.
tolnaftate (Aftate, Tinactin)	Topical Cream—1% Solution—1% Powder—1% Gel—1%	To treat superficial fungus infections of the skin	Mild irritation, rare sensitivity reactions	Use sparingly and massage in gently until it has disappeared. Watch for any manifestations of skin reaction.

TOPICAL CORTICOSTEROIDS

DRUG	ROUTE AND DOSAGE RANGE	USE	ADVERSE EFFECTS	NURSING IMPLICATIONS
betamethasone valerate (Valisone)	Topical Cream—0.1% Lotion—0.1% Ointment—0.1% Apply tid to qid	To relieve the inflammatory manifestations of acute contact dermatitis	*Skin:* burning sensation, itching, irritation, abnormal hair growth, dry skin, folliculitis, acne, lightening of skin color, skin atrophy, secondary infections, striae, miliaria	Do not use under occlusive dressings or when infection is present. Observe skin for signs of reaction. Evaluate hair growth. Warn patient of possible changes in skin color, acne, or dryness. Watch for secondary infections.
flurandrenolide (Cordran)	Topical Tape—4 mcg/sq cm; change q12h Cream—0.025%–0.05% Ointment—0.025%–0.05% Lotion—0.05% Apply bid to tid	To relieve the inflammatory manifestations of corticosteroid-responsive skin diseases	See betamethasone, *plus:* allergic contact dermatitis and perioral dermatitis	See betamethasone, *plus:* Flurandrenalide may be used under occlusive dressings.
fluocinolone (Synalar, Fluonid)	Topical Cream—0.01% and 0.025% Ointment—0.025% Solution—0.01% Apply sparingly and rub in well tid to qid	See flurandrenolide.	See flurandrenolide.	See flurandrenolide.
fluocinonide (Lidex, Topsyn)	Topical Cream—0.05% Ointment—0.05% Gel—0.05% Apply small amount to affected area and gently massage tid to qid	See flurandrenolide.	See flurandrenolide.	See flurandrenolide.

(continued on page 80)

TABLE 8-1 (continued)

DRUG	ROUTE AND DOSAGE RANGE	USE	ADVERSE EFFECTS	NURSING IMPLICATIONS
iodochlorhydroxyquin + hydrocortisone (Vioform-Hydrocortisone)	Topical Cream Lotion Ointment Apply a thin layer to affected parts 3–4 times daily	To treat dermatitis, eczema, pyoderma, acne, urticaria, neurodermatitis, lichen simplex chronicus, anogenital pruritus, folliculitis, bacterial and fungal dermatoses, candidiasis, and intertrigo	Especially under occlusive dressings: *Skin:* rash, hypersensitivity reactions, burning, itching, dryness, folliculitis, increased hair growth, acne, lightening of skin color, maceration, atrophy, striae *Others:* mouth sores, secondary infections	Observe skin carefully for changes that signal adverse effect. Inspect the mouth at regular intervals. Watch for superimposed infections.
triamcinolone acetonide (Kenalog, Aristocort)	Topical Cream—0.025%, 0.1%, 0.5% Ointment— 0.025%, 0.1%, 0.5% Lotion—0.025%, 0.1% Spray Apply tid to qid	See flurandrenolide.	See flurandrenolide.	See flurandrenolide, *plus:* Cream should be rubbed in gently until it disappears.

action, the topical corticosteroids cause local vasoconstriction, relieve redness and itching, and retard skin cell growth. They are most effective in ointment form, but are available as creams, lotions, and sprays as well. The usual adverse effects of corticosteroids, including cushingoid appearance and symptoms, rarely occur with topical applications.

Many medications are applied to the skin for their soothing effect. *Emollients* are fat- or oil-based substances that help keep the skin moist and soft. Other agents may be mixed into an emollient and then applied to the skin. Examples of emollients are glycerin, lanolin, vitamin A and vitamin D ointment, petrolatum, cold cream, rosewater ointment, and zinc oxide. Lotions and other solutions are also soothing. Powders such as cornstarch and talc soothe irritated skin and relieve pruritus (itching). Soothing baths can be made by adding bran, starch, gelatin, or oatmeal to the bath water. *Protectives* are soothing substances that cool the skin and coat it with a light film. They prevent drying and protect irritated areas from air, light, and dust particles.

A diluted solution of hydrogen peroxide is commonly used as a cleanser. It helps to clean wounds by removing mucus, foreign particles, and dead tissue. It is also useful for cleaning mucus and tissue from instruments used during tracheostomy care and other procedures.

Some skin infections (impetigo, eczema, and cellulitis) are caused by bacteria. They are best treated with systemic anti-infectives, although topical combinations of drugs are also used. Fungal infections of the skin, such as athlete's foot, may be treated by topical or systemic drugs.

NURSING IMPLICATIONS

Drugs applied topically usually are not associated with the widespread or serious adverse effects of drugs taken by mouth or administered parenterally. There is, however, the danger of allergic reactions. Question the patient about any possible allergies. Patients having a history of allergies should be cautioned not to change medications without consulting their physician, because this practice may lead to other allergies.

Persons with fair complexions do not tolerate topical medications as well as dark-skinned persons. You may want to remind the patient about this. Topical agents are more potent when an occlusive dressing, such as plastic wrap, is applied over them. When using this method, watch the patient for systemic reactions, especially when using corticosteroids. Many dermatologic preparations stain skin and clothing. Protect unaffected areas on the patient and your own skin and clothing when applying these preparations. Follow directions as to whether the agent is to be applied thickly or lightly, as this will influence the drug's effectiveness. It is also important to know whether to wash the area between applications or let the medication build up. Strong irritant drugs must be applied carefully only to affected areas, since they will cause destruction of healthy tissues as well. Use a medicine dropper or special applicator when administering these medications.

CHAPTER 9
Serums and vaccines

Immunity to disease can be either natural or acquired. A person with natural immunity is born with the ability to resist certain infections. A person may acquire immunity by having the particular disease once or simply by being exposed to the organisms that cause the disease. In either case, the body's defenses produce protein substances called *antibodies* that fight off the disease-producing organisms, and there are certain antibodies that are specific against certain diseases. Even after the last pathogen has been killed, cells retain the ability to produce the same antibodies should other pathogens of the same strain reappear. It is the antibodies that confer immunity to a disease. *Active acquired immunity* is when the antibodies are produced by activity of the person's own cells. In some cases, infectious organisms, or *antigens*, are purposely injected into the body to induce the cells to produce antibodies. They may be a living, dead, or attenuated (weakened) form of virus, bacteria, or foreign protein. Substances of this type are called *vaccines*. They may also be substances produced by the infectious organism, in which case they are called *toxins*. A weakened toxin is called a *toxoid*. *Antitoxins* are substances manufactured by the body in response to the presence of toxins (as antibodies are formed in response to antigens).

Passive acquired immunity occurs when the blood serum of a human or animal that has active acquired immunity is administered to a person so he can borrow the antibodies to fight infectious organisms in his own body. Antibodies can also be borrowed by the transfer of blood serum from a human with natural immunity to the disease. This type of immunity is called passive, because the recipient's body does not actively produce the antibodies but makes good use of donated antibodies. It is also a temporary immunity, since once the antibodies have been used up the person is again susceptible to the disease.

Immune human serum globulin, or gamma globulin, contains antibodies against many diseases. It is given by IM injection to prevent rubeola (measles), rubella (German measles), pertussis (whooping cough), poliomyelitis, viral hepatitis, and repeated bacterial infections. Occasionally the disease is not totally prevented, but its symptoms and severity are reduced. Rh_0 (D) immune human globulin (RhoGam) is given to prevent the formation of antibodies in an Rh-negative mother when her child is Rh positive or the woman has aborted an Rh-negative fetus.

Antitoxic serums can come from human or animal sources. They are used to prevent botulism, tetanus (lockjaw), and diphtheria. When routine immunization is done, vaccines are given to produce active rather than passive immunity. It may take weeks before antibodies are produced, but they will continue to circulate in the blood for years. Booster injections of vaccine are sometimes necessary to keep the level of antibodies up to effective levels. Vaccines are given to protect against many infections, including cholera, influenza, measles, mumps, pneumonia, rabies, pertussis, polio-

TABLE 9-1 SERUMS AND VACCINES

DRUG	ROUTE AND DOSAGE RANGE	USE	ADVERSE EFFECTS	NURSING IMPLICATIONS
immune human serum globulin (Gamma Globulin, Gamimune, Sandoglobulin)	IM—0.2 ml–1.3 ml/kg Hepatitis A—0.02 ml–0.05 ml/kg Hepatitis B—0.06 ml/kg Measles—0.2 ml/kg IV—100 mg–300 mg/kg	For protection against hepatitis A (infectious hepatitis), measles (rubeola), German measles (rubella); to treat antibody-deficient diseases, immunodeficiency syndrome, idiopathic thrombocytopenic purpura	Local irritation after injection (pain, redness, muscle stiffness), possible anaphylaxis, sharp decrease in blood pressure	Observe injection site for irritation. Monitor temperature and BP closely. Check skin for rash. Refrigerate the serum. Have antidote (epinephrine) ready.
$RH_0(D)$ immune human globulin (RhoGam, Gamulin-Rh, HypRho-D)	IM—1 vial (give within 72 hours of birth or removal of the products of conception)	To prevent Rh incompatibility reactions in the Rh-negative mother who gives birth to a Rh-positive infant; given to a Rh-negative woman who has an abortion, miscarriage, or ectopic pregnancy	Possible increase in temperature, muscle aches, and lethargy	Monitor temperature. Warn patient of possible lethargy.
tetanus immune human globulin (TIG, Hu-Tet, Hyper-Tet)	IM—250 U–6000 U	For immediate passive immunization against tetanus; to treat clinical tetanus	See immune human serum globulin.	See immune human serum globulin.
diphtheria and tetanus toxoids and pertussis vaccine, combined (DPT)	IM—for 2 months to 26 years—0.5 ml every month for 3 months; then a booster 1 year after 3rd dose	For active immunization against diphtheria, tetanus, and pertussis	Local soreness and redness, irritability, loss of appetite, vomiting, temperature elevation	Note inflammation at injection site. Assess appetite. Monitor temperature.
Influenza virus vaccine	IM—0.5 ml	To induce active immunization against influenza	Local reactions (redness, tenderness, stinging), malaise, backache, headache, fever	Note reactions at injection site. Monitor temperature. Refrigerate vaccine.
rubella virus vaccine	SC, IM—0.5 ml	Promotes immunity to German measles in children from 1 yr of age to puberty	Transient muscle and joint pains and swelling, rash, fever, cough, pain at injection site, anaphylaxis (rare)	Note complaints of muscle aches and pains. Note any joint swelling. Monitor temperature. Check injection site for any reactions. Refrigerate vaccine.
measles, mumps, rubella virus (M-M-R-II)	SC—1 vial	For simultaneous immunization against measles, mumps, and German measles in children 15 months of age to puberty	See rubella vaccine, *plus:* swollen salivary glands, blood disorders	See rubella vaccine, *plus:* Blood tests should be done and the results checked. Note swelling of neck.
poliovirus vaccine (Sabin, Orimune Trivalent)	PO—2 doses 8 weeks apart; 3rd dose 8–12 months after 2nd dose	To provide immunity to poliomyelitis	Paralytic disease (rare)	Poliovirus vaccine may be mixed with water, syrup, or milk or absorbed on bread, cake, or a sugar cube. Keep vaccine refrigerated.

(continued on page 85)

TABLE 9-1 (continued)

DRUG	ROUTE AND DOSAGE RANGE	USE	ADVERSE EFFECTS	NURSING IMPLICATIONS
hepatitis B immune globulin (H-BIG, Hep-B-Gammagee, Hyperhep)	IM—0.06 ml/kg as soon after exposure as possible; repeat 28–30 days after exposure	For postexposure prophylaxis following parenteral exposure, mucous membrane contact, or oral ingestion of hepatitis B antigen-positive materials	Anaphylaxis, local pain and tenderness at injection site, urticaria, angioedema	Use buttock or deltoid area for injection. Monitor BP and other vital signs. Observe skin for flushing, urticaria, pruritus. Do not give IV.
pneumococcal vaccine (Pneumovax, Pnu-Immune)	IM, SC—0.5 ml; revaccinate after 3 yr	For immunization against pneumococcal disease in all persons age 2 yr or older in whom there is increased risk of morbidity and mortality from pneumococcal pneumonia; to treat chronic heart disease, pulmonary, renal, or hepatic disease, diabetes mellitus, in persons over age 50 yr	Local erythema and soreness at injection site, low-grade fever, local swelling, anaphylaxis	Monitor BP and other vital signs. Be alert for signs of anaphylaxis. Inject into deltoid muscle on lateral midthigh.

myelitis, smallpox, tuberculosis, typhoid, typhus, and yellow fever. Many of these are available in combination, such as the DPT (diphtheria, pertussis, and tetanus), and are commonly given to young children. Although routine vaccination for smallpox and typhoid is no longer required, the vaccines are available for international travelers. Additional information on serums and vaccines is provided in Table 9-1.

NURSING IMPLICATIONS

Prevention of many childhood diseases has been accomplished largely through the results of early vaccination programs. Nurses in contact with the parents of young children, for example on pediatric units, have an excellent opportunity to discuss immunization programs. Without continued attention to prevention, diseases that once killed or crippled thousands of children have the potential to do so again.

Vaccines should not be given to persons already taking anti-inflammatory or antineoplastic agents. These drugs can reduce the effectiveness of the vaccination and lead to serious illness. Mumps or measles vaccine may cause invalid results on tuberculosis tests. Virus vaccines given to patients undergoing x-ray treatment may cause death owing to cumulative adverse effects.

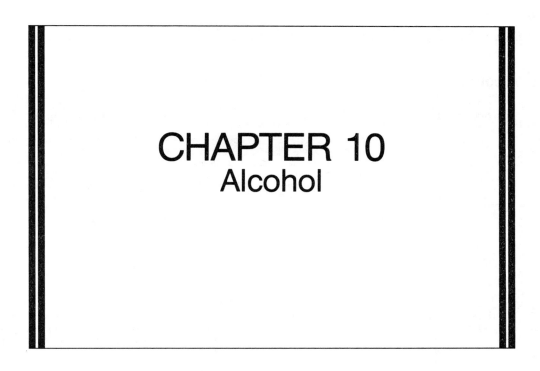

CHAPTER 10
Alcohol

In the early days of medicine alcohol was thought to cure most diseases. The alcohol used today is usually ethyl, or grain, alcohol, although there are other types. Alcohol's action in the body may be either local or systemic. As a local preparation, alcohol may function as an anti-infective, an irritant, or a cooling agent. The systemic effects of alcohol, aside from those associated with abuse, lead to its use as a vasodilator and an appetite stimulant. It also is used as a solvent and a medicinal preservative (see Table 10-1).

LOCAL EFFECT

Ethyl or grain alcohol, also called ethanol, or simply alcohol, is usually a 70% solution. Isopropyl alcohol, another form of alcohol, is used full strength. Doses and concentrations ordered will depend on use.

As a cleansing agent, alcohol destroys surface microorganisms. The mechanical action of applying the alcohol also helps to remove organisms. Alcohol is commonly used to cleanse the area around wounds and to prepare the skin for introduction of the SC, IM, or IV injection.

The irritating effect on the skin is taken advantage of in prevention of decubitus ulcers. When rubbed into a pressure area, the alcohol dries and hardens the outer layer of skin, so it is less likely to break down. As an astringent, alcohol helps de-crease inflammation and stop minor bleeding. This is due to its vasoconstrictive action.

Alcohol injected into subcutaneous tissue, where there are nerve endings, can destroy the nerves. This produces analgesia in the area and is called *nerve block*. Its effects last until the nerve regenerates, which can take up to 3 years.

Alcohol evaporates quickly, causing an immediate drop in skin temperature. Thus, in a patient with a high fever, an alcohol sponge bath is often given to take advantage of this cooling effect.

SYSTEMIC EFFECT

Alcohol in the systemic circulation acts like a general anesthetic. It has a depressing effect on the central nervous system. What may appear to be stimulation is simply the depression of all learned inhibitions. Alcohol causes the peripheral blood vessels to dilate, which promotes loss of body heat. Urine flow and gastric and salivary secretions are all increased. The pulse rate speeds up. Visual acuity and reaction time become impaired. There may be changes in judgment and self-control, as well as increasing drowsiness.

Because of its vasodilating effect, alcohol is sometimes prescribed for patients suffering from peripheral vascular disease and problems with blood circulation to the heart. It also helps stimulate the appetite, not only by increasing digestive

TABLE 10-1 ALCOHOL

DRUG	ROUTE AND DOSAGE RANGE	USE	ADVERSE EFFECTS	NURSING IMPLICATIONS
alcohol	PO—ethyl alcohol (Ethanol)—70%–99% Topical—isopropyl alcohol (full strength)	Sedative, analgesic, hypnotic, anti-infective, astringent, cooling agent, solvent, preservative, vasodilator, appetizer, digestant, and skin toughener (in the prevention of decubitus ulcers)	*Local effects:* skin irritation, vasoconstriction, decrease in skin temperature *Systemic effects:* drowsiness, decreased visual acuity, reaction time, and judgment, increased salivary and GI secretions, vasodilation, increased urine flow, increased pulse (may lead to severe CNS depression)	Observe skin after topical application. Caution patients not to engage in dangerous activities after ingesting alcohol. Monitor vital signs and urinary output. Evaluate level of consciousness.
disulfiram (Antabuse)	PO—initial dose—up to 500 mg qd for 1–2 weeks Maintenance—125 mg–500 mg qd	To help in the management of the chronic alcoholic patient who wants to remain sober	*CNS:* optic neuritis, peripheral neuritis, polyneuritis, drowsiness, possible psychotic reactions *Skin:* rashes, acne *Others:* metallic taste, impotence *Disulfiram reaction (disulfiram plus alcohol):* *CNS:* fainting, weakness, vertigo, blurred vision, confusion, uneasiness *Cardiovascular:* throbbing in the head and neck, chest pain, palpitations, tachycardia, hypotension *GI:* nausea, severe vomiting, thirst *Others:* flushing, increased perspiration, hyperventilation, dyspnea. (Severe reactions can lead to death.)	Never give unless the patient has full knowledge of what will happen when he takes alcohol while receiving this drug. Warn the patient to check ingredients of foods and other drugs to avoid all alcohol. Reactions with alcohol may occur up to 2 weeks after taking disulfiram (reaction lasts as long as there is alcohol in the bloodstream). Encourage patients to wear a Medic-Alert tag stating they are receiving disulfiram. Stress that it is important to take the drug daily. Check skin for rash or changes in color. Monitor vital signs and level of consciousness. Evaluate visual acuity. Warn male patient that he may experience impotence as a result of the medication.

secretions but also by relieving anxiety and tension that often interfere with proper eating habits. Older patients who have difficulty with other drugs for sleep sometimes receive an order for alcohol in the evening to make them drowsy. In this way alcohol is used as a hypnotic drug.

ALCOHOL AS A SOLVENT

Ethyl alcohol is also used as a solvent in many medicines because it has the ability to lower surface tension and promote easy mixing of substances.

Spirits are concentrated alcoholic solutions. *Elixirs* are sweetened alcoholic solutions. *Fluid extracts* and *tinctures* are other medicinal substances that make use of alcohol as a solvent.

ALCOHOL ABUSE

Overingestion, or abuse, of alcohol (alcoholism) can be either acute or chronic. In *acute* alcoholism the patient may be comatose. Death can result if coma persists or respiratory infection is a complication. *Chronic* alcoholism is a much more common state.

It may result in cirrhosis of the liver, gastrointestinal and kidney inflammation, and damage to the heart muscle.

The person who wants to stop drinking can often be helped to do so. Psychological support groups, such as Alcoholics Anonymous (AA), help to rehabilitate the alcoholic. Disulfiram (Antabuse) is a specific drug for the treatment of the chronic alcoholic who really wants to stop drinking (see Table 10-1). A person regularly taking disulfiram finds that ingesting even a small amount of alcohol produces extremely unpleasant reactions. His skin turns bright red, the blood pressure falls, and he feels dizzy, faint, weak, and nauseated. He may vomit violently. He has a pounding headache, and he may complain of chest pains, dyspnea, and heart palpitations. The prospect of such reactions is often sufficient to keep the alcoholic from taking a drink.

CHAPTER 11
Analgesics and anesthetics

ANALGESICS

Analgesics are drugs used to relieve pain. They do this without causing loss of consciousness or reflex activity. When we deal with persons in pain, it is necessary to keep in mind that each person will experience pain in his own way. Many physical and psychological factors combine to form the total "pain experience." Emotional factors are especially important to consider as patients voice their complaints of pain.

The various analgesics work in different ways (see Table 11-1). Some analgesics induce chemical changes in the body. Others cause changes in mood, so the patient no longer focuses on the pain. Still others cause sedation, so the patient is less alert and, therefore, less aware of the painful stimulus.

Narcotic analgesics

The narcotic analgesics are further broken down into naturally occurring substances (opium, morphine, codeine) and synthetic, or man-made, preparations. Opium contains over 20 active ingredients, or alkaloids. Two of the most important ones are morphine (10%) and codeine (0.5%).

Sometimes the word *opiate* is used to refer to the entire group of narcotic analgesics. An opiate is any natural or synthetic drug that has a pharmacologic action similar to that of morphine. These drugs are used chiefly to relieve severe pain. Because all narcotic analgesics can cause physical and psychological dependence, they are usually given

only when other analgesics are ineffective (see Chapter 2). Unfortunately, there are no agents yet known that are as effective against severe pain, yet not potentially addicting.

The danger of addiction, however, should not be a reason to withhold a narcotic if it is being used to relieve temporary, severe pain. Narcotics given over a period of a few days will not cause addiction. In any case, the smallest dose that is effective should be given.

When given to a patient already in severe pain, the opiate seems to effect a change in his emotional response to pain. In other words, he still feels the pain, but he is not very concerned about it. If given before the patient experiences severe pain, the blocking effect seems to be increased and he may not experience the pain. Patients who benefit most from this early administration of medication are those who have had recent surgery or are in the terminal stage of a painful illness.

In addition to their desired effect of analgesia, the narcotic analgesics have many adverse effects. They affect consciousness and mood in various ways. Some patients become restless, excited, and euphoric, while others seem drowsy, calm, and mentally unclear. Narcotics depress the cough center in the brain. The pupils are constricted. The respiratory center in the brain is depressed, and both rate and depth of respirations are decreased. This can lead to respiratory arrest in severe cases of narcotic overdose. Gastrointestinal disturbances

(*Text continues on p. 96.*)

TABLE 11-1 ANALGESICS

DRUG	ROUTE AND DOSAGE RANGE	USE	ADVERSE EFFECTS	NURSING IMPLICATIONS
NARCOTICS				
Natural morphine	PO—5 mg–20 mg (or more) q4h SC, IM—10 mg–15 mg q4h prn IV—10 mg–15 mg diluted in 5 ml NS and injected slowly PR—5-, 10-, 20- mg suppositories	To relieve severe pain; preanesthetic agent	CNS: excitement, depression of CNS functions, physical and psychological dependence ANS: pupil constriction, increased smooth muscle tone (bladder, biliary tract, ureters) Respiratory: respiratory rate decrease GI: nausea, vomiting, constipation	Morphine is more effective against a dull, continuous pain than pains of a sharp, intermittent nature. Monitor respiratory rate (withhold medication if rate is less than 12 per minute) and BP. Keep record of I&O. Keep stool chart. Watch for signs of dependence.
codeine	PO, SC, IM—15 mg–60 mg q3–4h	To relieve moderate to severe pain; antitussive to relieve cough	See morphine.	See morphine, plus: Codeine has about ⅙ the analgesic effect of morphine.
Synthetic butorphanol (Stadol)	IM, IV—1 mg–4 mg q3–4h	To relieve moderate to severe pain	CNS: sedation, dizziness, vertigo, headache, nervousness, depression, restlessness, crying, euphoria, hostility, confusion, unusual dreams, hallucinations, numbness, tingling, feeling of faintness or unreality, physical and psychological dependence Cardiovascular: hyper- or hypotension, brady- or tachycardia Respiratory: decreased respiratory rate, dyspnea, asthma GI: nausea, vomiting, cramps, upset stomach, bitter taste in mouth Skin: itching, rash, burning sensation, flushing, sweating/clammy feeling Others: speech impairment, urinary urgency, blurred vision, dry mouth	Evaluate for change in mental status. Evaluate any complaints of unusual sensations. Assess BP and pulse. Evaluate respiratory rate and character. Assist with activity, as needed. Caution patient not to engage in any potentially dangerous activity. Check skin for rash and color. Evaluate speech and visual acuity. Note any problems with urination. Watch for signs of dependence.
dihydrocodeine + aspirin + caffeine (Synalgos-DC)	PO—1–2 capsules q4h prn	To relieve moderate to moderately severe pain	CNS: physical and psychological dependence, tolerance (if used repeatedly), impairment of judgment/physical ability, lightheadedness, dizziness, drowsiness, sedation GI: nausea, vomiting, constipation Skin: rash, itching	Note any change in alertness, judgment, or coordination. Caution patient to avoid potentially dangerous activities. Keep stool chart. Check skin for rash.

(continued on page 93)

TABLE 11-1 (continued)

DRUG	ROUTE AND DOSAGE RANGE	USE	ADVERSE EFFECTS	NURSING IMPLICATIONS
hydromorphone (Dilaudid)	PO—2 mg–4 mg q4–6h prn IM, SC—2 mg–4 mg q4–6h prn PR—3-mg suppository	To relieve moderate to severe pain	*CNS:* dizziness, drowsiness, lethargy, anxiety, fear, mood changes, mental clouding, increased CSF pressure, physical and psychological dependence, tolerance *ANS:* pupil constriction, urinary retention *GI:* nausea, vomiting, constipation *Others:* respiratory depression, hyperglycemia	Warn patients not to engage in dangerous activities. Evaluate mental status and behavioral changes. Monitor respiratory rate (withhold medication if rate is less than 12 per minute) and BP. Check urine for sugar and acetone. Keep stool chart. Keep record of I&O. Watch for signs of dependence or tolerance.
meperidine (Demerol)	PO, IM, SC—50 mg–150 mg q3–4h prn IV—1 mg–10 mg/ml diluted; slow IV	To relieve moderate to severe pain; a preoperative medication; to support general anesthesia and obstetric analgesia	*CNS:* dizziness, lightheadedness, sedation, mood changes, headache, weakness, tremors, muscle incoordination, disorientation, visual disturbances, hallucinations, syncope, physical and psychological dependence. *ANS:* sweating, dry mouth, constipation, biliary spasm, urinary retention *Cardiovascular:* tachy- or bradycardia, palpitations, hypotension *Respiratory:* respiratory depression *GI:* nausea, vomiting *Skin:* flushed face, skin rashes *Others:* pain and possible phlebitis after injection	Caution patients not to attempt activities that are dangerous or require alertness. Evaluate mental status and mood. Note any muscle weakness or abnormal movements. Check skin color. Evaluate vision. Keep stool chart. Monitor vital signs, especially respirations and pulse. Note any rash. Watch for local irritation at injection sites. Watch for signs of dependence.
methadone (Dolophine)	PO, SC, IM—2.5 mg–10 mg q3–4h prn	To relieve moderate to severe pain; to treat narcotic addiction in detoxification or maintenance programs	See meperidine.	See meperidine, *plus:* Detoxification should not exceed 21 days.
nalbuphine (Nubain)	SC, IM, IV—10 mg–160 mg/day (20 mg is maximum single dose)	To relieve moderate to severe pain; for preoperative analgesia, a supplement to surgical anesthesia, and obstetric analgesia during labor	See butorphanol.	See butorphanol.
oxycodone + aspirin (Percodan)	PO—1–2 tablets q6h prn	To relieve moderate to moderately severe pain	See meperidine.	See meperidine.

(continued on page 94)

TABLE 11-1 (continued)

DRUG	ROUTE AND DOSAGE RANGE	USE	ADVERSE EFFECTS	NURSING IMPLICATIONS
oxycodone + acetaminophen (Percocet, Tylox)	PO—1–2 tablets or capsules q4–6h	To relieve moderate to moderately severe pain	See meperidine and acetaminophen.	See meperidine and acetaminophen.
pentazocine (Talwin)	PO—50 mg–100 mg q3–4h prn IM, SC, IV—30 mg–60 mg q3–4h	See oxycodone.	See meperidine. CNS, ANS, allergic, cardiac, and respiratory problems are rare.	See meperidine.
pentazocine + naloxone (Talwin NX)	PO—1–2 tablets q3–4h prn (maximum 12 tablets per 24 hr)	See oxycodone.	See pentazocine.	See pentazocine. Note: Talwin NX tablets contain a narcotic antagonist, naloxone, to eliminate the abuse potential of pentazocine.
propoxyphene HCl (Darvon)	PO—32 mg–65 mg q4h prn (to a maximum of 390 mg/day)	To relieve mild to moderate pain	(Rarely) *CNS:* dizziness, sedation, headache, light-headedness, weakness, euphoria, mood changes, visual changes, possible physical and psychological dependence *GI:* nausea, vomiting, abdominal pain, constipation, liver dysfunction *Other:* rash	Caution patients to avoid dangerous activities. Keep stool chart. Observe skin for rash. Evaluate mental status. Evaluate vision. Blood tests should be done regularly to monitor liver function. Watch for signs of dependence. Encourage patients to limit alcohol intake.
propoxyphene HCl + aspirin + caffeine (Darvon compound)	PO—1 capsule q4h prn	To relieve mild to moderate pain, either when pain is present alone or accompanied by fever	See propoxyphene HCl and aspirin.	See propoxyphene HCl and aspirin.
propoxyphene napsylate + acetaminophen (Darvocet-N)	PO—100 mg q4h prn	To relieve mild to moderate pain and reduce fever	See propoxyphene HCl and acetaminophen.	See propoxyphene HCl and acetaminophen.

NARCOTIC ANTAGONIST

DRUG	ROUTE AND DOSAGE RANGE	USE	ADVERSE EFFECTS	NURSING IMPLICATIONS
naloxone (Narcan)	IM, SC, IV—0.1 mg–0.4 mg for 2–3 doses at 2–3 minute intervals	To reverse respiratory depression due to narcotics and opium overdosage; to reverse overdosage with propoxyphene and pentazocine	Nausea, vomiting, sweating, tachycardia, hypertension, tremor, excitement (if no narcotic is present in the patient there will be no adverse effects)	Monitor vital signs. Watch for abnormal muscle movements. Evaluate mental status and level of consciousness.

NON-NARCOTICS

DRUG	ROUTE AND DOSAGE RANGE	USE	ADVERSE EFFECTS	NURSING IMPLICATIONS
aspirin (Empirin)	PO—325 mg–650 mg q4h prn (up to 12 tablets per day) Higher doses for arthritis and acute rheumatic fever PR—Suppository strength from 65 mg–1.2 g	For relief of headache, painful discomfort and fever of colds and flu, and muscular aches and pains; for temporary relief of joint pains, toothache, nerve pain, and menstrual cramps	Nausea, vomiting, gastric irritation, tinnitus, dizziness (large doses may cause decreased clotting time)	Give with meals or milk to decrease gastric irritation. Drink plenty of water when taking the pills. Check for GI bleeding by testing all vomitus, stool for blood. Patients taking high doses should have their clotting time checked regularly.

(continued on page 95)

TABLE 11-1 (continued)

DRUG	ROUTE AND DOSAGE RANGE	USE	ADVERSE EFFECTS	NURSING IMPLICATIONS
aspirin + magnesium-aluminum hydroxide (Ascriptin)	PO—2–3 tablets qid	To relieve pain in headache, neuralgia, minor injuries, and dysmenorrhea; to relieve pain and reduce fever in colds and influenza; to relieve pain and reduce inflammation in arthritis and other rheumatic diseases	See aspirin and magnesium-aluminum hydroxide (Maalox).	See aspirin and magnesium-aluminum hydroxide.
acetaminophen (Tylenol, Phenaphen)	PO—325 mg–650 mg q4–6h prn (up to 12 tablets per day)	See aspirin.	Sensitivity (rare)	This drug is often used when aspirin causes adverse effects in the patient.
chlorzoxazone + acetaminophen (Parafon Forte)	PO—2 tablets qid	With rest and physical therapy to relieve discomfort associated with acute painful musculoskeletal conditions	(Rarely) *CNS:* drowsiness, dizziness, malaise, overstimulation *GI:* nausea, vomiting, GI disturbances *Skin:* rash, allergic reactions *Other:* discolors urine	Caution patients to avoid dangerous activities. Evaluate mental status. Keep stool chart. Check skin for rash. Warn patient about possible change in urine color.
aspirin + caffeine + orphenadrine citrate (Norgesic)	PO—1–2 tablets tid to qid	To relieve mild to moderate pain caused by acute musculoskeletal disorders	*CNS:* weakness, headache, dizziness, drowsiness, confusion (especially in the elderly) *ANS:* dry mouth, blurred vision, dilated pupils, increased intraocular pressure *Cardiovascular:* tachycardia, palpitations *GU:* urinary hesitancy or urinary retention *GI:* nausea, vomiting, constipation *Skin:* (rare) itching and rash	Assist with activities as necessary. Evaluate mental status. Assess visual acuity. Encourage fluids or hard candy if mouth is excessively dry. Monitor apical pulse at regular intervals. Evaluate voiding pattern. Keep record of I&O. Keep stool chart. Observe skin for rash.
meprobamate + aspirin (Equagesic)	PO—1–2 tablets tid to qid	To treat pain accompanied by tension or anxiety in patients with musculoskeletal disease or tension headache	*CNS:* dizziness, drowsiness, ataxia, visual disturbances *GI:* nausea, vomiting, gastric distress *Others:* allergic reactions, physical or psychological dependence	Assist with activities as necessary. Assess visual acuity. Observe for allergic reactions. Watch for signs of dependence. Warn patient that his tolerance for alcohol may be reduced.
butalbital + aspirin + caffeine (Fiorinal)	PO—1–2 tablets or cap q4h (to a maximum of 6 qd)	To relieve tension (muscle contraction) headache	*CNS:* drowsiness, dizziness, light-headedness *GI:* nausea, vomiting, flatulence *Other:* physical or psychological dependence	Assist with activities as necessary. Watch for signs of dependence.
phenazopyridine (Pyridium)	PO—200 mg tid	To relieve the pain, burning, frequency, urgency, and other discomforts associated with lower urinary tract irritations	GI disturbances, turns urine bright red-orange	Give with meals to avoid GI upset. Warn the patient to expect his urine to be bright red-orange.

include anorexia, nausea, vomiting, decreased intestinal secretions, biliary spasms, and constipation. Urine output may drop. The skin may become flushed and warm, while body temperature may drop. The blood pressure may become unstable as the patient changes position (postural hypotension). Allergic reactions, such as rash, urticaria (hives), and itching, may also occur.

Natural opium products. Morphine was first extracted from opium in the 19th century. It is the standard by which other analgesics are judged, since none of the newer analgesics is more effective in relieving severe pain. Morphine seems most effective when it is used to relieve constant, dull pain as compared to intermittent, sharp pain. Any type of pain will be alleviated, however, as the dosage of morphine is increased. In addition to relieving severe pain, morphine is also frequently used as premedication before surgery. It relieves apprehension, thus allowing smoother induction of general anesthesia.

Codeine is another naturally occurring analgesic derived from opium. Although it is much less potent than morphine, it is also less likely to cause respiratory problems or constipation. It has little or no effect on the pupil in low doses and is less likely to lower the level of consciousness. Codeine also appears to be less habit forming than morphine. For this reason, it is usually given to suppress cough, although morphine is as effective for the purpose.

Synthetic derivatives of morphine. Some synthetic narcotic analgesics are less depressing to both the respiratory center and to the level of consciousness. Their effect on the pupil is minimal. Like the natural opiates, however, they cause a decrease in the urinary output, cause constipation, and potentially are addicting.

Meperidine (Demerol) is only slightly more potent than codeine. Its usual use is as a substitute for morphine in the treatment of severe pain. Meperidine is less likely to cause nausea, vomiting, and constipation than morphine, but occasionally it does cause hypotension and tachycardia. It does not affect the pupils or cough center. Like morphine, meperidine is often used as a preanesthetic agent.

Hydromorphone (Dilaudid) is more than twice as potent as morphine, although its duration of action is shorter.

Methadone (Dolophine) is very similar to morphine although it produces less sedation and euphoria. It is used primarily as an analgesic but also to treat withdrawal symptoms in patients dependent on opiate drugs, such as heroin.

Pentazocine (Talwin) is classified as a narcotic or non-narcotic, depending on the source of information. The reason for this discrepancy may be that when given orally, pentazocine is no more potent than codeine and has a low potential for dependence. When injected, however, it is similar to morphine in its ability to control severe pain. It has been abused by addicts and does give rise to a withdrawal syndrome when discontinued abruptly.

Another widely used narcotic analgesic is propoxyphene (Darvon). It is similar to codeine, although not as potent. It does not suppress cough but is effective in treating mild to moderate pain. Headache, dizziness, rash, gastrointestinal upset, and sedation are associated problems. Overdose can lead to respiratory depression, convulsions, and coma. The abuse of this drug has recently been recognized. There is evidence of tolerance, as well as both physical and psychological dependence after repeated use.

NURSING IMPLICATIONS (NARCOTIC ANALGESICS)

All narcotics must be kept in a locked cabinet and counted and signed for as used; the administration equipment should be disposed of properly as stipulated in the federal regulations. Because the opiates depress respirations, as well as decrease patient responsiveness and alertness, they should not be given to patients with head injuries and those who have had brain surgery. Anyone suffering from a convulsive disorder or alcoholism should receive these drugs only under careful supervision. Patients who have had chest or abdominal surgery usually need to cough to avoid the accumulation of mucus in their lungs. For this reason narcotic analgesics, which depress the cough center, are not given. If an elderly patient needs relief from severe pain, a narcotic analgesic may be ordered, but the dose should be low.

Before a narcotic is given, it is the nurse's responsibility to count the patient's respirations. If the respiratory rate is below 12 per minute the narcotic should be withheld and the doctor notified. As soon as pain becomes less severe, a non-narcotic analgesic should be substituted for the opiate to reduce the danger of drug dependence.

When you give the patient his pain medication, tell him it is a pain medication. Anxiety may make the medication less effective. Some patients are afraid or unwilling to ask what is in the shot or pill. Warn the patient not to get out of bed quickly, sit up in bed, or change position quickly because of the possibility of postural hypotension and fainting. Blood pressure should be taken in both supine and upright positions to see if this is a problem. Encourage the patient to cough and take deep breaths, because pulmonary stasis can lead to complications in the hospitalized patient. Do not forget to check back on your patient about 30 minutes after you give the narcotic analgesic. Observe his general appearance, as well as his vital signs, including depth of respirations. A pale, moist complexion and rapid weak pulse may be signs of overmedication. Lastly, ask the patient whether the medication has eased his pain.

All antidepressants increase the analgesic action of narcotics. Patients receiving diuretics or antihypertensive drugs may have episodes of postural hypotension. There can also be a dangerous buildup of adverse effects when narcotics are given to patients already receiving other central nervous system depressants, such as alcohol, barbiturates, general anesthetics, hypnotics, sedatives, or muscle relaxants. If severe, the combined effect can lead to respiratory depression, coma, and death.

Narcotic antagonists

This group of drugs, also called the anti-narcotics, is used in the management of narcotic overdose and in treatment of opiate dependence. In patients who have been given too much opiate, these drugs will cause an immediate increase in respiratory rate.

NURSING IMPLICATIONS (NARCOTIC ANTAGONISTS)

Drugs such as butorphanol and nalbuphine have both narcotic analgesic and narcotic antagonist action. In other words, they provide analgesia and have a lower potential for causing drug dependence and respiratory depression. Narcotic-dependent patients should *not* receive this type of analgesic because it can cause withdrawal reactions (abdominal cramps, nausea and vomiting, runny nose, tearing, anxiety and restlessness, and fever).

Non-narcotic analgesics

Non-narcotic analgesics are either salicylates, such as aspirin, or nonsalicylates, such as phenol derivatives. They are nonaddicting. While their major use is as analgesics, they may also be antipyretic (fever reducing).

Salicylates. In 1899 the Bayer Company produced acetylsalicylic acid, commonly called aspirin. It is a good analgesic for mild to moderate pain and is more effective in relieving bone and muscle pain than visceral pain or severe pain due to trauma. In the doses prescribed for pain relief, aspirin does not produce mental changes, euphoria, sleepiness, or drug dependence, as the opiates do.

Aspirin is helpful in reducing inflammation. In large doses (5 g/day) it promotes the secretion of uric acid into the urine. Other properties of aspirin are discussed in later chapters.

Aspirin is very irritating, not only to skin but also to mucous membranes. In the gastrointestinal tract it can cause nausea, vomiting, and ulceration of tissues, with bloody stools. Large doses may prolong bleeding time, as well as lower the blood sugar level. There have been occasional hypersensitivity reactions, which have led to respiratory difficulty and death.

Nonsalicylates. Acetaminophen (Tylenol) and phenacetin (Acetophenetidin) have analgesic effects similar to aspirin but do not usually cause gastric irritation or respiratory problems. They relieve pain of moderate intensity and are used to treat patients who cannot take aspirin because of extreme gastrointestinal disturbance or allergy.

Acetaminophen is given alone, while phenacetin is usually combined with aspirin and caffeine in a tablet called APC. Both acetaminophen and phenacetin are given by mouth. Although adverse effects are rare, prolonged use may lead to kidney, blood, and bone marrow disorders. There have also been rare hypersensitivity reactions in the form of rashes, urticaria, and gastrointestinal distur-bances.

NURSING IMPLICATIONS (NON-NARCOTIC ANALGESICS)

Gastric irritation can often be avoided if irritating drugs are given along with food or milk. Buffered forms of aspirin, such as aspirin plus magnesium-aluminum hydroxide (Ascriptin), or enteric-coated tablets will also decrease the possibility of gastro-intestinal upset. Stools should be examined for the presence of blood, a sign of gastrointestinal bleed-ing. The prothrombin time should be checked for evidence of increased bleeding time in a patient re-ceiving large doses of aspirin over long periods of time.

Aspirin should not be given to patients with vi-tamin K deficiency, bleeding disorders, or ulcers or to patients on anticoagulant therapy. Aspirin should not be used by persons scheduled for operations, since prolonged bleeding could lead to serious complications. Diabetics taking aspirin regularly should have periodic checks of blood sugar levels. With large doses of aspirin, the dose of oral hypo-glycemics and insulin may need to be changed.

When taken in prescribed doses, aspirin usually causes no ill effects. However, if by self-medication, a person greatly increases the dose, toxicity may develop. Salicylism is a form of mild poisoning, which is first noticed as hearing and visual distur-bances, dizziness, and increased sweating. Nau-sea, vomiting, and diarrhea may also occur. A more serious form of salicylism may be seen in children who mistake aspirin for candy. The clinical features proceed to drowsiness, fever, mental confusion, and increased respiratory and pulse rate. There is no specific antidote, and treatment is symptomatic.

ANESTHETICS

Anesthetics are drugs that cause a loss of sensation (see Table 11-2). They may be either *general* or *local* in action. A general anesthetic causes loss of con-sciousness, as well as loss of sensation throughout the body. *Preanesthetic* agents are drugs given to prepare the patient for general anesthesia and the operative experience. Local anesthetics are admin-istered to a specific area, which then loses sensa-tion. A local anesthetic does not affect the level of consciousness. The action of most anesthetics is re-versible; that is, once the drug leaves the body, sen-sation returns.

General anesthetics

The general anesthetics are used to achieve sur-gical anesthesia, the state in which surgery may be done. These drugs, given by inhalation or in-travenous injection, induce sleep, analgesia, and muscle relaxation, and certain reflexes are tem-porarily abolished. Unless you are a nurse-anes-thetist you will not administer these drugs, but you need to understand their action so you can deal with their effects.

One thing to keep in mind is that patients do not recover from general anesthesia at predictable rates. Regardless of which general anesthetic has been used, you need to be observant of the patient for the development of nausea, vomiting, hypoven-tilation, and a drop in blood pressure. Oliguria (se-verely diminished urine excretion) and intestinal distention are also potential problems.

Preanesthetic agents.   On the day of surgery, most patients receive drugs that help prepare them, both physically and psychologically, for the experience of surgery. These preanesthetic agents (often called *premedication*) help to calm the pa-tient. Anxiety in a preoperative patient is to be expected, but it can interfere with smooth admin-istration of the general anesthetic. A relaxed pa-tient may also require less of the anesthetic. Pre-anesthetic agents include narcotic analgesics, anticholinergics, barbiturates, skeletal muscle re-laxants, sedative-hypnotics, antianxiety agents (tranquilizers), and specialized agents. Once the patient has received the medication, he will appear calm and perhaps even uninterested in what is hap-pening around him. Other effects will vary accord-ing to which drug has been administered.

Local anesthetics

Local anesthetics decrease sensation in a particular area. They may be rubbed into the skin as oint-ments or creams, sprayed on in aerosol form, in-jected into the skin and subcutaneous layers, or injected into the spinal canal to produce more extensive anesthesia. The area recovers sensation

TABLE 11-2 ANESTHETICS

DRUG	ROUTE AND DOSAGE RANGE	USE	ADVERSE EFFECTS	NURSING IMPLICATIONS
GENERAL ANESTHETICS				
enflurane (Ethrane)	Inhalation—dose is individualized	To induce and maintain general anesthesia, to provide analgesia for vaginal delivery, and to supplement other anesthetic agents during delivery by cesarean section.	Unusual motor activity and/or seizures, hypotension, respiratory depression, malignant hyperthermia, decreased intellectual function for 2–3 days following use.	Monitor vital signs. Note any unusual muscle activity. Evaluate changes in mental status.
halothane (Fluothane)	Inhalation—dose is individualized	General anesthetic for operative procedures	Liver damage, cardiac arrhythmias, hypotension, fever, chills, nausea, vomiting, malignant hyperthermia	Keep emesis basin at hand. Monitor vital signs closely. Take apical pulses. Evaluate level of consciousness.
thiopental (Pentothal)	IV—individualized	General anesthetic for short (less than 15 minute) surgical procedures; to supplement other general anesthetics	*CNS:* prolonged sedation and recovery *Cardiovascular:* arrhythmias *Respiratory:* respiratory depression, sneezing, coughing, bronchospasm, laryngospasm *Others:* shivering, hypersensitivity reactions	See halothane, *plus:* Be alert for signs of respiratory distress. Check skin for rash or other sensitivity reactions.
methohexital (Brevital)	IV—individualized	See thiopental.	*CNS:* muscle twitching, headache, delirium *ANS:* salivation *Cardiovascular:* circulatory depression, thrombophlebitis *Respiratory:* respiratory depression, laryngospasm, bronchospasm, hiccoughs *GI:* nausea, vomiting *Others:* pain at injection site, acute allergic reactions	See halothane, *plus:* Note any abnormal muscle movements. Check skin for any reactions. Watch for signs of thrombophlebitis. Evaluate mental status and level of consciousness. Be alert for signs of respiratory distress.
ketamine (Ketalar)	IV, IM—individualized	General anesthetic for diagnostic and surgical procedures that do not require skeletal muscle relaxation; to supplement other general anesthetics	*CNS:* diplopia, nystagmus, increased intraocular pressure *Cardiovascular:* increased pulse, hypertension, arrhythmias, rapid breathing *GI:* anorexia, nausea, vomiting *Others:* pain at injection site, rash, emergence reaction (pleasant, dreamlike states, vivid hallucinations, delirium, confusion, irrational behavior)	Emergence reactions may last from a few hours to 24 hours (no lasting effects). To reduce the occurrence of emergence reactions reduce verbal, tactile and visual stimulation of the patient during the recovery period. Evaluate mental status. Monitor vital signs closely. Evaluate vision. Check skin for rash. Evaluate appetite.

(continued on page 100)

TABLE 11-2 (continued)

DRUG	ROUTE AND DOSAGE RANGE	USE	ADVERSE EFFECTS	NURSING IMPLICATIONS
PREANESTHETIC AGENTS				
droperidol (Inapsine)	IM, IV—individualized	Preoperative medication to produce tranquilization and reduce the incidence of nausea and vomiting in surgical and diagnostic procedures; helps in maintaining general and regional anesthesia	*CNS:* postoperative drowsiness, extrapyramidal symptoms, restlessness, hyperactivity, anxiety, dizziness, chills, sweating *Cardiovascular:* mild to moderate hypotension, tachycardia *Other:* respiratory muscle rigidity	Evaluate mental status. Note any unusual muscle movements. Assist with activities as necessary. Monitor BP, pulse, and temperature. Evaluate rate, rhythm, and ease of respirations. Always have emergency resuscitation equipment and a narcotic antagonist nearby.
droperidol + fentanyl citrate (Innovar)	IM, IV—individualized	To aid in producing tranquility and decreasing anxiety and pain	See droperidol, *plus:* *CNS:* drug dependence, postoperative delirium and confusion, muscle twitching, blurred vision *Cardiovascular:* mild to moderate hypertension, bradycardia *Respiratory:* respiratory depression, apnea, laryngospasm, bronchospasm *GI:* nausea, vomiting	See droperidol, *plus:* Watch for signs of drug dependence. Assess visual acuity.
LOCAL ANESTHETICS				
bupivacaine (Marcaine, Sensorcaine)	0.25%–0.75% solution for injection	See procaine.	Usually none	See procaine.
chloroprocaine (Nesacaine)	1%–3% solution for injection	See procaine.	Usually none	See procaine.
cocaine	Topical—solution— 1%–2%	For local anesthesia of the ear, nose, throat, rectum, and vagina	*CNS:* euphoria, excitement, restlessness, tremors, pupil dilation, possibility of physical and psychological dependence *GI:* nausea, vomiting, abdominal pain *Others:* hypersensitivity reactions, perforated nasal septum, changes in cornea, fever, chills, increased BP and pulse, arrhythmias	Check skin for any signs of rash. Assess mental status. Monitor vital signs. Be alert to changes in the eye and nose. Watch for signs of dependence.
dibucaine (Nupercainal)	PR—2.5-mg suppository Topical Cream—0.5% Ointment—1% Spray—0.25%	Local anesthetic for relief of painful hemorrhoids, sunburn, minor burns, cuts, scratches, or nonpoisonous insect bites	Occasionally, irritation at the site of application	Do not use on or near the eyes. Avoid prolonged use. Check site for irritation.

(continued on page 101)

TABLE 11-2 (continued)

DRUG	ROUTE AND DOSAGE RANGE	USE	ADVERSE EFFECTS	NURSING IMPLICATIONS
lidocaine (Xylocaine)	PR—100-mg suppository (patient should not receive more than 5 in 24 hr) Topical Jelly—(20 mg/ml)—2% Ointment—2.5%–5% Solution—4%–10% Solution for injection: 0.5%–5%	To produce local anesthesia by infiltrating techniques; to relieve pain and discomfort of oral, anorectal, and urethral conditions; minor pains, burns, itching	*CNS:* dizziness, nervousness, tremors, drowsiness, convulsions, blurred vision *Cardiovascular:* hypotension, bradycardia *Other:* allergic skin reactions	Evaluate mental status. Monitor vital signs, especially pulse and BP. Note any unusual muscle movements or rash. Assist patient with activities as necessary.
procaine (Novocain)	Solution for injection—0.25%–10%	Local anesthetic, especially in nerve block	Usually none	

quickly once the local anesthetic is removed or wears off. One of the oldest local anesthetics is cocaine, a substance made from the leaves of a South American shrub. Synthetic local anesthetics are now preferred to cocaine.

Serious adverse effects, such as overstimulation and central nervous system depression or cardiovascular collapse, may occur if local anesthetics reach the bloodstream and travel to the brain or heart muscle. This usually happens as a result of the drug being injected into or too near a blood vessel. Early manifestations of a toxic reaction are nausea, vomiting, increased pulse, hypotension, pale skin, and dyspnea. Convulsions may follow.

NURSING IMPLICATIONS

It is important to give preanesthetic medications on time because the anesthesiologist has carefully planned for maximum effect to occur at a specific time. Be sure to explain to the patient what effects may be noticed (dry mouth, change in mood, etc.) before you give the drugs, since he may not be able to understand what you say once they have taken effect. Patients may be unsteady on their feet and should not be allowed out of bed after receiving their premedication, so be sure they have been to the bathroom, called their family, shaved, and so on first. Always put the bedrails up after giving these drugs—a confused patient may fall trying to climb out of bed.

Some general anesthetics cause hallucinations or nightmares as the drug effects wear off. The patient may become delirious and irrational. This behavior may go on for up to 24 hours. Remember that the patient needs to be reassured and protected from harming himself and others. Intellectual function may be impaired for 2 to 3 days following use of some general anesthetics. Patients and their families should be made aware of this fact.

When the patient is returned to his room from either the operating room or the recovery room, his vital signs must be taken at frequent intervals. His temperature and the condition of the operative site need to be observed. It is best to position the patient either on his side or with his head turned to the side to avoid the possibility of secretions falling back into the lungs and being aspirated while the gag reflex is absent.

PRACTICE PROBLEMS—ANALGESICS AND ANESTHETICS

1. The order reads: morphine sulfate 6 mg q4h prn incisional pain.
The label reads: morphine sulfate 10 mg/ml. How much morphine sulfate will be given for pain?

$$\frac{D}{H} \times A = G$$

$$\frac{3 \ \cancel{6} \ \cancel{mg}}{5 \ \cancel{10} \ \cancel{mg}} \times 1 \ ml = G$$

$$\frac{3}{5} \times 1 \ ml = \frac{3}{5} \ ml = 0.6 \ ml$$

Thus, 0.6 ml of morphine sulfate will be given for pain.

2. "Codeine 45 mg PO q4h prn pain" is ordered for the patient who has pain in the left shoulder. Codeine 30 mg/tablet is available. How many tablets would be given?

$$\frac{D}{H} = G$$

$$\frac{3 \ \cancel{45} \ \cancel{mg}}{2 \ \cancel{30} \ \cancel{mg}} = 1\frac{1}{2}$$

Thus, $1\frac{1}{2}$ tablets of codeine are given.

3. The order reads: ASA gr X × PO q4h prn headache.

The label reads: ASA 325 mg/5 gr tablet. How much ASA will be given?

$$325 \ mg = gr \ V$$

$$\frac{D}{H} = G$$

$$\frac{\cancel{gr} \ \cancel{10} \ 2}{\cancel{gr} \ \cancel{5} \ 1} = 2 \ tablets$$

Thus, 2 tablets of ASA will be given.

Work the following problems:
1. The order reads: hydromorphone (Dilaudid) 4 mg PO q4h prn severe pain.
The label reads: hydromorphone 2 mg/tablet. How many tablets will be given?

2. The physician orders pentazocine (Talwin) 45 mg IM q4h prn pain in the left leg. Available is pentazocine 30 mg/ml. How many milliliters will be given?

3. The order reads: phenazopyridine (Pyridium) 200 mg PO tid.
The label reads: phenazopyridine 100 mg/tablet.
How many tablets will you give?

Answers are given on p. 283.

PART 3
Drugs used to help meet patients' needs for activity, exercise, rest, and sleep

CHAPTER 12
Stimulant drugs

A stimulant is a drug that stimulates the central nervous system (CNS). Some drugs in this class are also called *analeptics*. Their use in recent years has declined due to their lack of specific action and potential for abuse. Stimulants are divided into four groups: (1) convulsants, (2) respiratory stimulants, (3) xanthines, and (4) amphetamines (see Table 12-1).

Convulsants cause convulsions or seizures. They are occasionally used in the treatment of psychiatric disorders but more commonly to aid in the diagnosis of epilepsy. *Respiratory stimulants* are administered when, because of the presence of respiratory disease or overdose with barbiturates, alcohol or anesthesia, the patient is suffering from respiratory insufficiency (see Chapter 23). The *xanthines* comprise caffeine, theophylline, and theobromine. These drugs are mild stimulants that increase alertness, relieve drowsiness and fatigue, improve memory, and promote quicker judgment and reaction time. Of the three, caffeine is the most frequently used. It is found in coffee and tea, as well as in various medications. Amphetamines are a group of drugs sharing similar chemical composition and action. They are CNS stimulants used to treat narcolepsy (recurrent attacks of an uncontrollable desire to sleep), hyperactive behavior disorders (especially in children), and obesity. Amphetamines increase alertness, promote euphoria, and affect behavior. Persons receiving these drugs tend to talk excessively and to behave in an excited manner. There may be an increase in perspiration and pupillary dilation. Tolerance and psychological dependence may develop if these drugs are used for long periods. Overdose can cause convulsions, coma, and death.

Methylphenidate (Ritalin) is similar to the amphetamines, but it is not used to treat obesity. It is the drug of choice in the treatment of minimal brain dysfunction in children. Children with this problem (also called hyperkinetic behavior) are excessively active, easily distracted, and often the cause of classroom disruptions. The drug is mildly sedating so that behavioral excesses tend to be diminished. Methylphenidate appears to bring about improved motor ability, mood, and mental function, but the use of this drug in children is controversial.

NURSING IMPLICATIONS

Stimulants used for convulsant or respiratory effect are usually given for short-term therapy. When stimulants, such as the amphetamines, are given for a period of days, however, personal health and safety are threatened. A person using amphetamines tends to severely limit his food intake and get little sleep. The outcome may be exhaustion, confusion, and disorientation. Repeated use can also lead to tolerance and dependence.

If stimulants are given as an aid to diagnosis of epilepsy, be sure the proper seizure precautions

TABLE 12-1 STIMULANT DRUGS

DRUG	ROUTE AND DOSAGE RANGE	USE	ADVERSE EFFECTS	NURSING IMPLICATIONS
diethylpropion (Tenuate, Tepanil, Tepanil Ten-Tab, Tenuate Dospan)	PO—1 (25-mg tablet) tid 1 hr āc and mid evening, if desired; 1 (75-mg controlled-release tablet) qd in mid morning	To treat exogenous obesity as a short-term (few weeks) adjunct in a regimen of weight reduction based on limited calories	*CNS:* nervousness, restlessness, dizziness, insomnia, anxiety, euphoria, depression, tremor, dyskinesias, mydriasis, drowsiness, malaise, headache, psychotic episodes, increased seizures in the epileptic, tolerance *Cardiovascular:* palpitations, tachycardia, hypertension, precordial pain, arrhythmias *Endocrine:* impotence, changes in sexual drive and desire, gynecomastia, irregular menses *GI:* dry mouth, unpleasant taste, nausea, vomiting, diarrhea or constipation, abdominal discomfort *GU:* dysuria, polyuria *Skin:* hives, rash, bruised areas, redness, increased perspiration *Others:* bone marrow depression, dyspnea, hair loss, muscle pain	Evaluate mental status. Assist with activities if necessary. Note any abnormal muscle movements. Note pupil size. Observe for signs of drug dependence and tolerance. Be alert and prepared for seizures in the patient who has a tendency toward seizures. Monitor apical pulse and blood pressure. Note rate and rhythm of respirations. Warn patient of possible changes in sexual function or drive. Warn patient about possible breast and menstrual changes. Keep a stool chart. Record I&O and note changes in output. Observe skin for change in color, moisture, and any allergic reactions. Blood tests should be done at regular intervals. Warn patient and look for hair loss. Check weight daily.
phentermine (Fastin, Ionamin)	PO—15 mg–30 mg capsule qd before breakfast or 10–14 hr before bedtime	See diethylpropion.	*CNS:* restlessness, dizziness, insomnia, euphoria, depression, tremor, headache, psychotic episodes, drug dependence *Cardiovascular:* palpitations, tachycardia, hypertension *Endocrine:* impotence, changes in libido *GI:* dry mouth, unpleasant taste, diarrhea or constipation, other GI upset *Skin:* hives	Evaluate mental status. Note any unusual muscle movements. Watch for signs of dependence. Monitor apical pulse and BP. Warn patient about possible changes in sexual function and desire. Keep a stool chart. Observe skin for any reaction. Check weight daily.
methylphenidate (Ritalin, Ritalin-SR)	PO—10 mg–60 mg qd in one or divided doses	To treat minimal brain dysfunction in children, narcolepsy, mild depression, and apathetic or withdrawn senile behavior	*CNS:* nervousness, insomnia, dizziness, headache, muscle weakness, drowsiness, possible psychological dependence, tolerance *Cardiovascular:* palpitations, tachy- or bradycardia, hypo- or hypertension, angina, arrhythmias *GI:* anorexia, nausea, vomiting, abdominal pain, weight loss *Others:* rash, fever, joint pains	If insomnia is a problem, do not give after 6 PM. Observe skin for any rash. Monitor vital signs. Assist with activity as necessary. Evaluate mental status. Check weight daily. Watch for dependence.

(continued on page 107)

TABLE 12-1 (continued)

DRUG	ROUTE AND DOSAGE RANGE	USE	ADVERSE EFFECTS	NURSING IMPLICATIONS
dextroamphet-amine (Dexedrine)	PO—2.5 mg–60 mg qd in divided doses	To treat exogenous obesity, narcolepsy, minimal brain dysfunction in children	*CNS:* agitation, restlessness, dizziness, insomnia, headache, mental changes, muscle tremors, physical and psychological dependence *Cardiovascular:* palpitations, tachycardia, increased BP *Endocrine:* impotence, changes in libido *GI:* anorexia, diarrhea or constipation, weight loss, unpleasant taste, dry mouth *Other:* hives	Potential for abuse of this drug is high. Watch for dependence. Do not give these drugs in late evening, because they will interfere with sleep. Caution patients against performing any dangerous activities. Warn the patient about possible change in sexual desire or function. Keep stool chart. Check weight daily. Monitor vital signs. Check skin for rash or itch. Evaluate mental status. Note any abnormal muscle movements.
methamphet-amine (Desoxyn)	PO—5 mg–25 mg qd	To treat exogenous obesity and minimal brain dysfunction in children	See amphetamine.	See amphetamine.

have been taken; an oral airway, oxygen, and suction equipment should be nearby. The patient should be positioned in a safe environment so he will not be injured should he have a generalized seizure.

Hyperactivity is common with respiratory stimulants. More than one person should be available to deal with an excited patient who may thrash about. When prescribed for psychiatric disorders, the dose range of stimulants is wide. It is necessary, therefore, to observe the patient carefully and document his response to the drug so that the dosage may be corrected for optimum effect.

Amphetamines should not be given after approximately 4:00 PM, so as not to interfere with sleep. After amphetamines are discontinued, a tranquilizer or barbiturate may be necessary to combat the restlessness and nervousness that may interfere with sleep. A period of severe mental depression may follow discontinuation of amphetamines, so you must beware of the potential for suicide.

PRACTICE PROBLEMS—STIMULANT DRUGS

1. The order reads: dextroamphetamine (Dexedrine) 7.5 mg PO tid.
   The label reads: dextroamphetamine 5 mg/tablet.
   How many tablets would be given?

   $$\frac{D}{H} = G$$

   $$\frac{7.5 \text{ mg}}{5 \text{ mg}} = 1\frac{1}{2} \text{ tablet}$$

   Thus, you would give $1\frac{1}{2}$ tablets.

Work the following problems:
1. The physician orders 15 mg dextroamphetamine (Dexedrine) elixir daily. The pharmacy sends dextroamphetamine elixir containing 5 mg/ml. How many milliliters would you give?

2. Your patient is depressed. The physician orders methylphenidate (Ritalin) 25 mg PO q6h prn depression. The methylphenidate comes 10 mg/tablet. How many tablets would you give?

Answers are given on p. 283.

CHAPTER 13
Anti-inflammatory, antirheumatic, and uricosuric drugs

Normal physical activity and exercise are possible only if the musculoskeletal system is functioning normally. Disorders such as arthritis, bursitis, degenerative joint disease, gout, and muscle strains and sprains create limitations to normal movement. Drugs used to treat these conditions fall into several categories. Drugs with analgesic effect relieve pain (see Chapter 11). *Anti-inflammatory* agents decrease the swelling, redness, heat, and loss of function of affected parts. Fever is reduced by antipyretic drugs. *Uricosuric* drugs promote urinary excretion of uric acid, which can cause inflammatory disease. *Antirheumatic* drugs relieve symptoms of bone and joint diseases, owing to their anti-inflammatory action.

Anti-inflammatory drugs are discussed elsewhere in the text as well as in this chapter because they are used to treat many conditions. This chapter discusses their use in the treatment of musculoskeletal diseases. Antirheumatic and uricosuric drugs are prescribed specifically for musculoskeletal disorders. Gout and rheumatism are often seen in patients with an alteration in musculoskeletal function. Thus, discussion of anti-inflammatory, antirheumatic, and uricosuric drugs is devoted to these two problems.

Gout is a metabolic disorder in which uric acid accumulates in various joints. Attacks of pain and swelling in certain joints (most often the big toe, ankle, knee, elbow) are characteristic. If left untreated, gout can lead to serious joint, kidney, and blood vessel disease. The drugs used in treatment aim either to relieve pain and inflammation or to increase uric acid elimination, and some combine these actions. Salicylates, corticosteroids, uricosuric drugs, and specific anti-inflammatory agents are widely used.

Salicylates have analgesic, anti-inflammatory, and antipyretic effects. They are uricosuric if given in doses of 5 g to 6 g/day (see Chapter 11). *Corticosteroids* are commonly used to treat gout and other musculoskeletal disorders because of their potent anti-inflammatory action. They can be given orally or parenterally. Often they are injected directly into affected joints.

Specific *anti-inflammatory* drugs include phenylbutazone (Butazolidin), colchicine, and indomethacin (Indocin). They are potent drugs that relieve pain, as well as reduce inflammation. However, because of serious adverse effects, they are used only if there has been no improvement with other less toxic drugs.

Uricosuric drugs promote elimination of uric acid in the urine, thereby decreasing the buildup that causes gout attacks. Allopurinol (Zyloprim) also decreases uric acid in the body, but by a different action. It blocks the formation of uric acid. Although not technically uricosuric, it does produce the same end result.

Rheumatism is a term that refers to any of the approximately 75 rheumatic diseases, such as rheumatic arthritis, gouty arthritis, connective tissue disorders, rheumatic fever, degenerative joint

(*Text continues on p. 114.*)

TABLE 13-1 ANTI-INFLAMMATORY, ANTIRHEUMATIC, AND URICOSURIC DRUGS

DRUG	ROUTE AND DOSAGE RANGE	USE	ADVERSE EFFECTS	NURSING IMPLICATIONS
ANTI-INFLAMMATORY DRUGS				
phenylbutazone (Butazolidin)	PO—First week—300 mg–600 mg/day in 3 to 4 divided doses maintenance—100 mg–400 mg qd	To relieve pain, fever, and swelling in gout, rheumatoid arthritis, rheumatoid spondylitis, osteoarthritis, psoriatic arthritis, acute superficial thrombophlebitis, painful shoulder	*CNS:* eye and optic nerve damage, increased thyroid activity, agitation, mental confusion, lethargy *Cardiovascular:* edema, myocarditis, hypertension *GI:* ulceration with perforation and hemorrhage, salivary gland enlargement, gastritis, epigastric pain, nausea, vomiting, diarrhea, abdominal distention, hepatitis *Others:* blood disorders, electrolyte imbalances, skin lesions, Stevens-Johnson syndrome, possible anaphylaxis, kidney stones and kidney failure, hyperglycemia	Warn patients to take the drug exactly as ordered and to report any adverse reaction to the doctor at once. Test vomitus and stool for blood. Keep stool chart. Check weight daily. Blood tests should be done at regular intervals (usually every 1–2 weeks) Assess skin for any rash, wheals, or other lesions that may be signs of allergic reactions. Record I&O accurately. Monitor BP. Evaluate hearing and vision. Evaluate mental status. Assist with activity if necessary. Caution patients not to engage in dangerous activities. Severe toxic reactions are especially likely in the elderly patient.
colchicine	PO—Initial dose—0.6 mg–1.2 mg; then 0.6 mg–1.2 mg q1–2h; then 0.5 mg–0.6 mg bid to once a week IV—Initial dose—1 mg–3 mg; then 0.6 mg q6–12h prn (to a maximum of 4 mg/24 hr)	To treat gout	Abdominal pain, nausea, vomiting, diarrhea (long-term use may lead to blood disorders, peripheral neuritis, and hair loss)	Keep stool chart. Be sure blood tests are done regularly (with long-term use).
indomethacin (Indocin, Indocin-SR)	PO—25 mg–75 mg bid or tid (to a maximum of 200 mg qd) PR—50 mg bid–tid	To treat acute gouty arthritis; to treat moderate to severe rheumatoid arthritis, ankylosing spondylitis, and osteoarthritis of the large joints	*CNS:* headache, dizziness, sedation, depression, tinnitus *GI:* nausea, vomiting, epigastric pain, diarrhea or constipation *Other:* visual disturbances	Always give with food, immediately after a meal, or with antacids to reduce gastric upset. Evaluate mental status. Keep stool chart. Assist with activities if necessary. Caution patient not to engage in dangerous activities. Warn patient to avoid aspirin while taking this medication. Assess visual acuity.

(continued on page 111)

TABLE 13-1 (continued)

DRUG	ROUTE AND DOSAGE RANGE	USE	ADVERSE EFFECTS	NURSING IMPLICATIONS
ANTIRHEUMATIC DRUGS				
aurothioglucose (Solganal)	IM—Initial dose—10 mg; 2nd and 3rd—25 mg; 4th and following doses—50 mg Give at weekly intervals until cumulative dose is 0.8 g–1 g	In combination with other drugs to treat arthritis	*CNS:* headache, fainting, dizziness, weakness *GI:* metallic taste, GI upset, diarrhea, abdominal cramps, stomatitis, jaundice *GU:* albuminuria, hematuria *Skin:* dermatitis, hair loss, flushing, rash, itch *Others:* upper respiratory tract inflammations, blood disorders, possibility of severe toxic reactions and anaphylaxis, eye disorders	This is a very expensive drug preparation. Keep stool chart. A specimen for urinalysis must be taken before each injection. Assess skin for any lesions. Instruct the patient in careful oral hygiene practices. Caution patient not to engage in dangerous activities. Complete blood testing should be done every 2 weeks. Rash may be worsened by sunlight.
gold sodium thiomalate (Myochrysine)	IM—Initial dose—10 mg; 2nd dose—25 mg; 3rd and following doses—25 mg–50 mg Given at weekly intervals until cumulative dose is 1 g	See aurothioglucose.	See aurothioglucose.	See aurothioglucose.
fenoprofen (Nalfon)	PO—300 mg–600 mg qid	To relieve signs and symptoms of rheumatoid arthritis and osteoarthritis	*CNS:* headache, drowsiness, dizziness, nervousness, tremor, insomnia, confusion, tinnitus, weakness, blurred vision, decreased hearing *Cardiovascular:* palpitations, tachycardia, peripheral edema *GI:* indigestion, abdominal pain, nausea, vomiting, diarrhea, constipation, anorexia, GI bleeding, gas, dry mouth *Skin:* rash, itching, hives, increased perspiration *Others:* anemia, difficult urination	Evaluate mental status. Assess sleeping pattern. Note any tremor. Assess visual acuity and hearing. Monitor apical pulse. Check weight daily. Note any edema. Evaluate appetite Keep stool chart. Test stool and emesis for blood. Observe skin for rash, hives, and itching. Note increased perspiration. Keep record of I&O. Note any difficulty with urination. Give medication 30 minutes before or 2 hours after meals unless GI upset occurs, in which case it may be given with meals or milk.

(continued on page 112)

TABLE 13-1 (continued)

DRUG	ROUTE AND DOSAGE RANGE	USE	ADVERSE EFFECTS	NURSING IMPLICATIONS
ibuprofen (Motrin, Rufen)	PO—300 mg–600 mg tid or qid	To relieve the signs and symptoms of rheumatoid arthritis and osteoarthritis	*CNS:* headache, dizziness, nervousness, tinnitus, visual changes, depression, insomnia *GI:* nausea, vomiting, epigastric pain, diarrhea or constipation, bleeding, bloating, anorexia *Skin:* rash, hives, itching *Others:* increased BP, fluid retention, blood disorders	Give with meals or milk to decrease GI upset. Test all stool and vomitus samples for presence of blood. Keep stool chart. Evaluate mental status. Evaluate hearing and visual acuity. Assess skin for lesions. Monitor BP. Keep accurate I&O records. Blood tests should be done at regular intervals.
meclofenamate (Meclomen)	PO—200 mg–400 mg qd in 3 to 4 divided doses	To relieve signs and symptoms of acute and chronic rheumatoid arthritis and osteoarthritis (not used as initial treatment)	*CNS:* headache, tinnitus, dizziness *GI:* nausea, vomiting, anorexia, gas, constipation, diarrhea, bleeding, ulcers, abdominal pain, stomatitis *Skin:* rash, itching, hives *Other:* edema	Assess hearing. Assist with activity as necessary. Assess appetite. Keep stool chart. Test all stool and vomitus samples for the presence of blood. Observe skin for rash, hives, or itching. Check weight daily. Note any edema. Take medication with meals, milk, or an antacid to decrease GI upset.
naproxen (Anaprox, Naprosyn)	PO—500 mg–1000 mg qd in 2 divided doses, one morning, one evening	To relieve the signs and symptoms of rheumatoid arthritis; to relieve mild to moderate pain and primary dysmenorrhea	*CNS:* headache, drowsiness, dizziness, vertigo, inability to concentrate, depression, tinnitus, visual disturbances *GI:* heartburn, nausea, abdominal pain, indigestion, stomatitis, diarrhea or constipation, vomiting, bleeding *Skin:* rash, itch, sweating, ecchymosis *Others:* edema, dyspnea, palpitations	Question the patient about indigestion. Inspect mouth and skin for lesions. Test all stool and vomitus samples for the presence of blood. Keep stool chart. Assist with activities as necessary. Caution the patient not to engage in dangerous activities. Evaluate mental status. Evaluate hearing and visual acuity. Note any edema. Monitor vital signs and I&O.
piroxicam (Feldene)	PO—20 mg qd (single dose)	In acute or long-term treatment to relieve signs and symptoms of osteoarthritis and rheumatoid arthritis	See naproxen, *plus:* *CNS:* insomnia, malaise, nervousness. *Others:* anorexia, Stevens-Johnson syndrome, colic, decreased hemoglobin, hematocrit and other blood changes, altered liver function, weight gain or loss, swollen eyes	Caution patient not to engage in dangerous activities. Note any behavioral changes. Keep stool chart. Evaluate appetite and any complaints of GI discomfort. Check weight daily. Assess skin for rash or unusual color. Test all stool and vomitus samples for the presence of blood. Monitor I&O.

(continued on page 113)

TABLE 13-1 (continued)

DRUG	ROUTE AND DOSAGE RANGE	USE	ADVERSE EFFECTS	NURSING IMPLICATIONS
piroxicam (*continued*)				Blood tests should be done at regular intervals. Patients on coumarin-type anticoagulants need to be observed closely due to possible drug interactions. Full effect of therapy may not be evident for 2 weeks or more.
sulindac (Clinoril)	PO—150 mg–200 mg bid	To treat rheumatoid arthritis, osteoarthritis, ankylosing spondylitis, acute shoulder pain, acute gouty arthritis	*CNS:* dizziness, headache, nervousness, vertigo, tinnitus *GI:* GI upset, diarrhea, or constipation, flatulence, anorexia, bleeding, stomatitis, abdominal cramps *Others:* rash or itch, edema	Give with food to decrease stomach upset and GI irritation. Test vomitus and stool samples for the presence of blood. Keep stool chart. Inspect mouth and skin for lesions. Assist patient with activities as necessary. Caution patient about engaging in dangerous activities.
tolmetin (Tolectin, Tolectin DS)	PO—600 mg–2000 mg qd in 3–4 divided doses (including one dose on arising and one at hs)	See ibuprofen.	See ibuprofen, *plus:* chest pain, anaphylaxis	See ibuprofen, *plus:* Note any complaints of chest discomfort. Avoid aspirin.

URICOSURIC DRUGS

DRUG	ROUTE AND DOSAGE RANGE	USE	ADVERSE EFFECTS	NURSING IMPLICATIONS
probenecid (Benemid)	PO—0.25 g–0.5 g bid (may increase by 0.5 g every 4 weeks to a maximum of 2 g qd)	To treat hyperuricemia associated with gout and gouty arthritis	*CNS:* headache, dizziness *GI:* nausea, vomiting, sore gums *Others:* urinary frequency, hypersensitivity reactions (rash, fever, anaphylaxis), flushing, anemia	Encourage the patient to increase fluid intake (total 2–3 liters/day). Urine should be kept alkaline. Give with food, milk, or antacids to decrease the GI upset. Keep accurate record of I&O. Assess skin for any lesions. Monitor temperature. Avoid aspirin.
sulfinpyrazone (Anturane)	PO—200 mg–800 mg qd in 2 divided doses	To treat chronic and intermittent gouty arthritis	GI upset, rash, and blood disorders	Give with food, milk, or antacids. Encourage fluids to keep the urine output high. Keep accurate record of I&O. Assess skin for rash. Blood tests should be done at regular intervals.
allopurinol (Lopurin, Zyloprim)	PO—200 mg–800 mg qd	To treat gout, primary or secondary uric acid nephropathy, recurrent uric acid stone formations; preventive drug for uric acid accumulation in patients with diseases or treatment that cause increased uric acid levels	*CNS:* drowsiness, peripheral neuritis *GI:* nausea, vomiting, diarrhea, abdominal pain *Skin:* rash, alopecia *Others:* Stevens-Johnson syndrome, vasculitis, blood disorders, cataracts	Watch for skin lesions. Push PO fluids and maintain a neutral, preferably alkaline urine. Keep accurate record of I&O. Take medication with meals to lessen GI upset. Warn patients to stop taking the drug at the first sign of a rash. Blood tests should be done at regular intervals. Evaluate visual acuity. Assist with activities as necessary.

disease, bursitis, and synovitis. In rheumatic disease the joints and associated structures become inflamed; in some types of arthritis, if the inflammation cannot be brought under control, there may be progressive changes in the joint until finally the joint is destroyed. The result is pain, stiffness, and limited motion. The principles of management in all these diseases are similar to those for rheumatic arthritis. Antirheumatic drugs used are the salicylates, corticosteroids, gold salts, antimalarials, and various specific agents.

Salicylates taken regularly in high doses are very effective in treating rheumatic disease but may not be sufficient to relieve especially acute inflammations. Corticosteroids are likewise effective in treating rheumatism, but long-term use leads to many undesirable consequences (see Chapter 34). Treatment with injections of gold salts is called *chrysotherapy.* Aurothioglucose (Solganal) and sodium thiomalate (Myochrysine) are gold salts effective in active rheumatic arthritis. Antimalarial drugs, such as chloroquine (Aralen) and hydroxychloroquine (Plaquenil), are sometimes used to treat arthritis patients (see Chapter 7). These are ordered when other less toxic drugs have not brought about improvement.

Anti-inflammatory drugs, such as colchicine, phenylbutazone, probenecid, and sulfinpyrazone, are effective in both gout and rheumatism. Ibuprofen (Motrin) is useful in chronic rheumatic arthritis and osteoarthritis. New nonsteroidal anti-inflammatory agents, such as naproxen (Naprosyn) and sulindac (Clinoril), have been introduced as alternatives to salicylates in the long-term treatment of rheumatic arthritis. They offer the advantages of prolonged action and fewer gastrointestinal disturbances.

Specific information on these types of drugs is given in Table 13-1.

NURSING IMPLICATIONS

Uricosuric agents are most effective when the urine is kept alkaline. For this reason, sodium bicarbonate is often given along with the uricosuric drug. It is also very important that patients receiving drugs be encouraged to drink large amounts of fluid to flush the urinary system, so that accumulation of uric acid crystals is avoided.

PRACTICE PROBLEMS—ANTI-INFLAMMATORY, ANTIRHEUMATIC, AND URICOSURIC DRUGS

1. The physician orders 10 mg aurothioglucose (Solganal) IM for the first day of therapy. The drug comes 50 mg/ml. How much would be given?

$$\frac{D}{H} \times A = G$$

$$\frac{1}{5} \frac{\cancel{10} \text{ mg}}{\cancel{50} \text{ mg}} \times 1 \text{ ml} = G$$

$$\frac{1}{5} \times 1 \text{ ml} = \frac{1}{5} \text{ ml} = 0.2 \text{ ml}$$

Thus, 0.2 ml of aurothioglucose (Solganal) will be given the first day.

2. The order reads: phenylbutazone (Butazolidin) 200 mg tid.

The label reads: 100 mg phenylbutazone/tablet. How much would you give?

$$\frac{D}{H} = G$$

$$\frac{2 \cancel{200} \text{ mg}}{1 \cancel{100} \text{ mg}} = 2 \text{ tablets}$$

Two tablets of phenylbutazone (Butazolidin) would be given.

Work the following problems:
1. Ibuprofen (Motrin) 450 mg PO tid is ordered. The pharmacy sends 300-mg tablets. How many tablets would you give?

2. The order reads: colchicine 1.2 mg PO bid. The label reads: colchicine 0.6 mg/tablet. How many tablets would you give?

3. The physician orders naproxen (Naprosyn) 250 mg PO bid. Available are 250-mg tablets. What quantity would you give?

4. The order reads allopurinol (Zyloprim) 400 mg PO bid. Allopurinol is dispensed in 100-mg tablets. How much medication would you give?

5. The order reads: gold sodium thiomalate (Myochrysine) 25 mg IM once a week. Gold sodium thiomalate comes 10 mg/ml. How much medication must be given?

Answers are given on p. 283.

CHAPTER 14
Skeletal muscle relaxants and antiparkinsonian drugs

Body movement, produced by skeletal muscles, is usually under voluntary control. Movement is initiated when the muscle is stimulated by cortical motor nerves passing through the spinal cord and connecting with the muscle fibers in any body part. The place where the motor nerve fiber and the skeletal muscle fiber meet is called the *myoneural junction*. At this point the neurohormone acetylcholine is produced. This substance enables the nerve impulse to travel from the motor nerve fiber to the muscle (motor) fiber.* A muscle so stimulated becomes tense and shortened—it *contracts*. Contraction continues as long as impulses continue across the myoneural junction. When no impulse is present, the skeletal muscle fibers are not stimulated—they are relaxed and they lengthen. Normally even a relaxed muscle is not completely limp because of the *tone* present in healthy muscle tissue. Sometimes it may happen that there is a loss of muscle tone, and the muscles become limp or *flaccid*.

Muscle fibers that are inflamed, traumatized, or diseased tend to contract in an abrupt involuntary movement known as *spasm*. Spasms can severely limit a person's ability to care for himself and to get adequate exercise. Cerebral palsy, multiple sclerosis, and spinal cord injuries are examples of problems involving spasticity. Many drugs given for other reasons also help relax muscles. Local, spinal, and general anesthetics have this

characteristic, as do barbiturates in large doses and other depressants (see Chapter 15). In this chapter we discuss drugs given specifically to relax muscles.

SKELETAL MUSCLE RELAXANTS

There are two general groups of skeletal muscle relaxants (see Table 14-1). In one group are the drugs that act on the central nervous system—the brain and the spinal cord. Drugs in the second group affect the peripheral areas, specifically the myoneural junctions of muscle fibers.

Centrally acting skeletal muscle relaxants

The centrally acting skeletal muscle relaxant drugs reduce muscle spasms in specific areas and also have a sedative effect. They are often combined with other drugs and prescribed in connection with physical therapy for muscle strains and sprains; low back problems; dislocated, fractured, or herniated disks; arthritis; and other inflammatory joint disease. Neurologic diseases also benefit from therapy with these drugs. Among these diseases are cerebral palsy, multiple sclerosis, amyotrophic lateral sclerosis, and poliomyelitis. They are often useful during spinal operations and in treatment of tetanus. Carisoprodol (Rela, Soma), chlorphenesin carbamate (Maolate), and methocarbamol

(Text continues on p. 122.)

---

* A more detailed description of the transmission of impulse is provided in Chapter 18, under Cholinergic Drugs.

TABLE 14-1 SKELETAL MUSCLE RELAXANTS AND ANTIPARKINSONIAN DRUGS

DRUG	ROUTE AND DOSAGE RANGE	USE	ADVERSE EFFECTS	NURSING IMPLICATIONS
SKELETAL MUSCLE RELAXANTS				
baclofen (Lioresal)	PO—5 mg–20 mg tid or qid	To alleviate the signs and symptoms of spasticity resulting from multiple sclerosis and spinal cord injuries	*CNS:* drowsiness, dizziness, weakness, fatigue, headache, confusion, insomnia, mental confusion, muscle pain and tremors, ataxia, rigidity, paresthesias, tinnitus, slurred speech, blurred vision, pupil changes, seizures, diplopia *Cardiovascular:* hypotension, chest pain, palpitations *GI:* nausea, constipation, dry mouth, weight gain *GU:* urinary frequency *Others:* rash, itching, increased perspiration, nasal congestion, ankle edema	Patients should be warned to avoid dangerous activities. Evaluate mental status and level of consciousness. Note any abnormal muscle movements or posturing. Assist with activities as necessary. Evaluate hearing, speech, and visual acuity. Keep stool chart. Record I&O. Check skin for rash, itching, and increased perspiration. Check weight daily. Monitor BP.
carisoprodol (Rela, Soma)	PO—350 mg qid	In combination with other therapies to relieve discomfort associated with acute painful musculoskeletal conditions	*CNS:* drowsiness, dizziness, ataxia, tremor, irritability, agitation, headache, depression, syncope, insomnia, possible psychological dependence, weakness *Cardiovascular:* hypotension, tachycardia *GI:* nausea, vomiting, epigastric distress *Skin:* rash, itching, flushing *Others:* asthmatic episodes, fever, anaphylaxis, hiccoughs	Watch for signs of dependence. Warn patients to avoid dangerous activities. Evaluate mental status. Monitor vital signs. Note any abnormal muscle movements. Check skin for rash or itching. Assist with activites as necessary. Give with meals or milk to decrease GI upset.
cyclobenzaprine (Flexeril)	PO—30 mg–60 mg qd in divided doses (should not be given for longer than 2 to 3 weeks)	Used along with physical therapy and rest to relieve muscle spasm associated with acute, painful musculoskeletal conditions	*CNS:* drowsiness, dizziness, ataxia, weakness, fatigue, nervousness, depression, hallucinations, euphoria, disorientation, confusion, headache, paresthesias, insomnia, blurred vision, tremors *Cardiovascular:* tachycardia *Respiratory:* dyspnea *GI:* dry mouth, abdominal pain, indigestion, coated tongue, unpleasant taste in mouth, nausea, constipation	Caution patient to avoid dangerous acts. Assist with activity as necessary. Evaluate mental status. Note any complaints of unusual sensations. Assess sleep patterns. Assess visual acuity. Note any unusual muscle tremors. Monitor apical pulse. Note quality and rate of respirations. Note any complaints of GI discomfort. Keep stool chart. Record I&O and watch voiding pattern.

(continued on page 119)

TABLE 14-1 (continued)

DRUG	ROUTE AND DOSAGE RANGE	USE	ADVERSE EFFECTS	NURSING IMPLICATIONS
cyclobenzaprine (*continued*)			*GU:* urinary retention, decreased bladder tone *Skin:* increased perspiration, rash, hives *Others:* edema of face and tongue, myalgias, *plus:* see tricyclic antidepressants.	Observe skin for increased moisture, rash, or hives, *plus:* See tricyclic antidepressants (Chapter 6).
diazepam (Valium)	PO—2 mg–10 mg qd–qid IM, IV—2 mg–20 mg q3–4h	To relieve tension and anxiety; to treat acute alcohol withdrawal; to decrease anxiety, stress, and memory of endoscopic procedures; to relieve skeletal muscle spasms; to treat status epilepticus; premedication for surgery	*CNS:* drowsiness, fatigue, ataxia, confusion, depression, headache, slurred speech, syncope, tremor, vertigo, blurred or double vision, possible psychological dependence *Cardiovascular:* venous thrombosis and phlebitis at injection site, hypotension, bradycardia *GI:* nausea, constipation *GU:* incontinence, urinary retention *Others:* rash, itch, changes in libido, hiccoughs, paradoxical reactions	Warn patients to avoid dangerous activities. Check injection site for any redness, swelling, or heat. Evaluate mental status. Assist with activities as necessary. Assess speech and visual acuity. Keep stool chart. Record I&O. Note any tremors. Warn patient of possible change in sexual desire. Monitor vital signs. Check skin for rash or itching. Watch for signs of physical and psychological dependence.
methocarbamol (Robaxin)	PO—4 g–8 g qd in divided doses IM, IV—1 g–3 g qd in divided doses	See carisoprodol.	*CNS:* dizziness, drowsiness, vertigo, syncope, blurred vision, headache *Cardiovascular:* hypotension, bradycardia, thrombophlebitis and tissue sloughing at injection site *GI:* GI upset, metallic taste *Others:* allergic skin reactions, conjunctivitis, nasal congestion, fever, anaphylaxis	Assist with activity if necessary. Warn patient to avoid dangerous activities. Monitor vital signs. Check skin for rash. Evaluate vision. Give with food to decrease GI upset. Inspect injection site.
pancuronium (Pavulon)	IV—individualized dose	In conjunction with general anesthesia to produce skeletal muscle relaxation and in the management of patients on mechanical respirators	Slightly increased pulse, increased salivation, transient rash, respiratory depression may lead to apnea	Monitor pulse. Evaluate and remove secretions as necessary. Observe skin for rash. Note rate and depth of respirations.
succinylcholine (Anectine)	IV—individualized dose	In conjunction with general anesthesia to produce skeletal muscle relaxation and to reduce the intensity of muscle contractions in seizures	See pancuronium, *plus:* hypo- or hypertension, brady- or tachycardia, cardiac arrhythmias, increased intraocular pressure	See pancuronium, *plus:* Monitor BP.

(continued on page 120)

TABLE 14-1 (continued)

DRUG	ROUTE AND DOSAGE RANGE	USE	ADVERSE EFFECTS	NURSING IMPLICATIONS
dantrolene (Dantrium)	PO—25 mg–100 mg qd–qid IV—1 mg/kg (maximum of 10 mg/kg)	To control muscle spasticity from spinal cord injuries, stroke, cerebral palsy, multiple sclerosis, or malignant hyperthermia	*CNS:* drowsiness, malaise, dizziness, visual, taste and speech disturbances, headache, seizures, insomnia, mental changes *Cardiovascular:* tachycardia, changes in BP *GI:* diarrhea or constipation, bleeding, anorexia, dysphagia, abdominal cramps, liver disease *GU:* difficult urination and erection, urinary frequency, incontinence, nocturia, retention *Skin:* abnormal hair growth, acne, rash, sweating *Others:* muscle aches, fever, chills, feeling of suffocation, increased tearing	Patients should avoid dangerous activities and be assisted with activity as necessary. Keep stool chart. Test all vomitus and stool samples for the presence of blood. Assess vision, taste, and speech. Monitor vital signs. Evaluate mental status. Warn male patients that erection may be difficult. Keep I&O records to evaluate urinary output, incontinence, and nocturia. Check skin for rash or abnormal hair growth and acne. Baseline liver function tests should be done at the beginning of therapy and repeated at regular intervals.

ANTIDOTES FOR NEUROMUSCULAR BLOCKERS

DRUG	ROUTE AND DOSAGE RANGE	USE	ADVERSE EFFECTS	NURSING IMPLICATIONS
neostigmine (Prostigmin)	PO—15 mg–375 mg qd SC, IM, IV—0.25 mg–2 mg q4–6h or prn	To prevent and treat postoperative distention and urinary retention; to control symptoms of myasthenia gravis and myasthenic crisis; for a diagnostic test for myasthenia gravis	*CNS:* muscle cramps and weakness, tremors *ANS:* increased saliva, bronchial secretions and perspiration, miosis *GI:* nausea, vomiting, diarrhea, abdominal cramps	Assess for increase in secretions and remove as necessary. Keep stool chart. Note pupil size. Note any abnormal muscle movements or complaints of weakness. Medication must be given at exact times as ordered. Tell patients to keep a record of daily condition (periods of weakness vs periods of increased activity) to aid in optimal dosage schedules.
edrophonium (Tensilon)	IM, IV—1 mg–10 mg	To diagnose myasthenia gravis; in combination with other drugs to treat myasthenia gravis and in myasthenic crisis; antagonist to curariform drugs	*CNS:* difficult speech and swallowing, convulsions, muscle weakness *ANS:* increased tearing, increased GI and respiratory secretions, urinary frequency, increased perspiration *Cardiovascular:* hypotension, cardiac arrhythmias *GI:* nausea, vomiting, diarrhea, abdominal cramps *Others:* visual changes, respiratory paralysis, incontinence	Assess for increase in secretions (GI, perspiration, sputum). Evaluate visual acuity. Note any difficulty swallowing or speaking. Monitor vital signs. Keep stool chart. Record I&O, noting frequency of urination. Note any cramps or muscle weakness.

(continued on page 121)

TABLE 14-1 (continued)

DRUG	ROUTE AND DOSAGE RANGE	USE	ADVERSE EFFECTS	NURSING IMPLICATIONS
ANTIPARKINSONIAN DRUGS				
benztropine (Cogentin)	PO, IM, IV—0.5 mg–6 mg qd in one dose or divided doses	To treat all forms of parkinsonism and to control extrapyramidal symptoms (except tardive dyskinesias) due to drugs	Dry mouth, blurred vision, nausea, vomiting, nervousness, constipation, numb fingers, lethargy, depression, allergic rashes	Offer fluids or hard candy to aid dry mouth. Assess vision. Keep stool chart. Evaluate mental status. Check skin for rash.
bromocriptine mesylate (Parlodel)	PO—1.25 mg–2.5 mg qd–tid with meals. In treatment of Parkinson's disease dosage may be titrated to achieve optimal therapeutic response by increasing 2.5 mg every 2–4 weeks to a maximum of 100 mg/day	To treat signs and symptoms of idiopathic or postencephalitic Parkinson's disease; for short-term treatment of amenorrhea/galactorrhea and female infertility associated with low levels of prolactin; to prevent lactation following childbirth or abortion	*CNS:* headache, dizziness, ataxia, vertigo, hallucinations, confusion, drowsiness, "on-off" phenomenon, visual disturbances, fatigue, insomnia, depression, anxiety *Cardiovascular:* shortness of breath, orthostatic hypotension, ankle and/or foot edema *GI:* anorexia, dysphagia, nausea, vomiting, constipation, abdominal discomfort or cramping, diarrhea *Others:* nasal congestion, abnormal involuntary movements, forced closure of the eyes (blepharospasm), mottled skin, rash, urinary incontinence or retention, ergotism, elevated liver function test results	Note instability of gait or unusual muscle movements. Assist with activities as necessary. Evaluate mental status. Assess visual acuity. Evaluate character/rate of respirations. Monitor BP closely; warn patient to change position slowly. Check for ankle/limb edema. Keep accurate record of I&O. Keep stool chart. Observe skin for any rash or unusual color. Blood tests to evaluate liver function should be done at regular intervals.
levodopa (Dopar, Larodopa)	PO—up to 8 g qd in divided doses	To treat Parkinson's disease and other forms of parkinsonism	*CNS:* involuntary muscle movements, difficulty starting and stopping movements, ataxia, mental changes, headache, dizziness, weakness, insomnia, nightmares, hallucinations, agitation, anxiety *Cardiovascular:* arrhythmias, palpitations, orthostatic hypotension, hypertension *GI:* bleeding, anorexia, nausea, vomiting, dry mouth, dysphagia, abdominal pain *Others:* urinary retention, blood disorders	Note any unusual muscle movements. Monitor vital signs. Warn patient to change positions slowly to avoid fainting. Evaluate mental status, sleeping, and dreaming. Test stool and vomitus samples for the presence of blood. Record I&O. Blood tests should be done at regular intervals. Assist with activity as necessary.

(continued on page 122)

TABLE 14-1 (continued)

DRUG	ROUTE AND DOSAGE RANGE	USE	ADVERSE EFFECTS	NURSING IMPLICATIONS
levodopa + carbidopa (Sinemet)	PO—mg carbidopa/ mg levodopa (10/ 100, 25/100, 25/ 250), 1 to 6 tablets qd (Highly individ- ualized as to inter- vals between doses)	To treat Parkinson's disease	See levodopa.	See levodopa, *plus:* Use of Sinemet enables dos- ages of levodopa to be de- creased, thereby decreas- ing the incidence of adverse effects from levo- dopa.
trihexyphenidyl (Artane, Tremin)	PO—1 mg–15 mg qd in divided doses	See benztropine.	*CNS:* drowsiness, dizzi- ness, nervousness, headache, mental changes, blurred vi- sion, increased intra- ocular pressure *GI:* dry mouth, constipa- tion, nausea, vomiting *Others:* rash, urinary re- tention, tachycardia	See benztropine, *plus:* Assist with activity as neces- sary. Monitor pulse. Record I&O.

(Robaxin) are among the drugs in this group. Bac-lofen (Lioresal) is particularly helpful in the treat-ment of spasticity owing to multiple sclerosis and spinal cord injuries. Diazepam (Valium), discussed in Chapter 6 as a minor tranquilizer, is also widely prescribed as a skeletal muscle relaxant, especially for the treatment of muscle spasms and back strain.

Peripherally acting skeletal muscle relaxants

Members of this group of skeletal muscle relaxants act directly at the myoneural junctions in the af-fected area. Since they block the impulses that travel from nerve to muscle, they are called *neu-romuscular blocking agents.* They are much more potent than the centrally acting drugs and are ca-pable of inducing relaxation to the point that the muscles become paralyzed. These drugs have no an-algesic or sedative effect, as have the centrally act-ing skeletal muscle relaxants. Their chief uses are during surgery, to relax muscles so insertion of an airway will be less risky and difficult and so less general anesthetic will be necessary; to decrease muscle contractions during electroconvulsive ther-apy (ECT); and to treat tetanus.

These drugs are not absorbed well from the gastrointestinal tract. They may be administered by intramuscular injection, but the intravenous route is faster and more predictable.

Curare, a natural substance long used by In-dians in South America to make poison-tipped darts, causes quick and complete relaxation of all muscles within 10 minutes of intravenous admin-istration. However, synthetic drugs with similar properties are now manufactured, for example, di-methyltubocurarine (Metubine Iodide), pancuron-ium (Pavulon), and succinylcholine (Anectine). Succinylcholine is considered the safest of these drugs. Its action is extremely rapid but short; re-laxation begins within 1 minute of intravenous ad-ministration, and it is effective for only 4 to 5 min-utes.

Dantrolene (Dantrium), another skeletal mus-cle relaxant, has a different action from the neu-romuscular blockers. It acts within the muscle fi-bers of the affected part rather than at the myoneural junctions, thereby decreasing muscle stiffness, reflex muscle contractions, and spasticity. Its chief use is in neurologic diseases where spas-ticity is a problem, such as cerebral palsy, multiple sclerosis, and spinal cord injuries.

ANTIPARKINSONIAN DRUGS

Parkinson's disease is a chronic, progressive neu-rologic disorder that results in disorders of body movement. The major symptoms are muscle rigid-ity, slowness of movement (bradykinesia), and tremor. These symptoms are thought to be due to decreased amounts of the chemical dopamine in the brain of the affected individual.

Several types of medications are given in an

effort to relieve the symptoms, which often interfere with the patient's ability to care for himself and get adequate exercise (see Table 14-1).

Anticholinergic drugs such as the belladonna alkaloids and the synthetic atropinelike drugs were the first drugs used to treat Parkinson's disease, and they are still useful. Newer synthetic anticholinergic drugs used are benztropine (Cogentin) and trihexyphenidyl (Artane).

Certain *antihistamine* drugs (see Chapter 26) such as diphenhydramine (Benadryl) and orphenadrine (Disipal) also have anticholinergic effects and may be used to treat Parkinson's disease.

Dopaminergic drugs contain substances that are converted to dopamine in the brain. Examples are levodopa (Dopar, Larodopa) and carbidopa plus levodopa (Sinemet). Although these drugs have many possible adverse effects, if they are ordered and monitored carefully they may relieve many symptoms.

Bromocriptine (Parlodel) is a new drug given to promote dopamine availability in the brain. It is usually ordered in combination with other drugs to treat Parkinson's disease. Amantadine (Symmetrel), a synthetic antiviral drug mentioned in Chapter 7, and propranolol (Inderal), a cardiac depressant also effective in decreasing tremor (see Chapter 31), may also be used in combination with other drugs to treat Parkinson's disease.

NURSING IMPLICATIONS

Because they have a sedative effect, the centrally acting skeletal muscle relaxants decrease alertness, which may pose a safety hazard. Persons receiving these medications should not operate dangerous machinery or perform activities that require alertness.

The peripherally acting skeletal muscle relaxants are very potent. They affect the respiratory muscles and may cause severe alterations in blood pressure and heart function as well. They are usually administered by a physician or in situations in which the patient can receive emergency care immediately. Respiratory paralysis is always possible. Resuscitation equipment, oxygen, and antidotes should be within reach.

The dose of drugs used to treat Parkinson's disease is carefully adjusted according to the severity of the patient's disease and his tolerance of adverse effects. It is essential that the patient be closely observed and observations be reported and recorded. Some patients experience orthostatic hypotension during the first few weeks of levodopa or bromocriptine treatment. You can explain that this is common and that it usually clears in a few weeks. Patients should be taught to get up from bed slowly and to progress from lying to sitting before standing. Wearing elastic stockings may help by preventing the blood from pooling in the legs. Explain that the blood pressure will be taken while they are lying, sitting, and standing, so that changes may be measured.

Long-term therapy with antiparkinsonian drugs may lead to adverse effects not seen in the initial treatment phase. Abnormal involuntary movements called *dyskinesias* may involve the eyelids, tongue, lips, face, neck, or extremities. In some cases the entire body may show abnormal posturing or writhing (choreiform) movements. There is no way to stop them except to decrease the dosage. Wearing-off of drug effect and loss of effect are also seen in some patients after years of treatment. An extremely upsetting adverse effect that may occur with any of the medications used to treat Parkinson's disease is a change in mental status, which can include memory problems, confusion, or hallucinations. Patients should inform their doctor as soon as any unusual movements, changes in response to medication, or changes in mental status occur.

PRACTICE PROBLEMS—SKELETAL MUSCLE RELAXANTS AND ANTIPARKINSONIAN DRUGS

1. The physician orders methocarbamol (Robaxin) 0.25 g IM qid. The vial of methocarbamol reads 100 mg/ml. How much should be given?

$$(0.25 \text{ g} = 250 \text{ mg})$$

$$\frac{D}{H} \times A = G$$

$$\frac{5}{2}\frac{\cancel{250} \text{ mg}}{\cancel{100} \text{ mg}} \times 1 \text{ ml} = G$$

$$\frac{5}{2} \times 1 \text{ ml} = 2\frac{1}{2} \text{ ml}$$

Thus, 2.5 ml of methocarbamol (Robaxin) will be given.

2. The order reads: dantrolene (Dantrium) 75 mg PO tid.
The label reads: 25 mg dantrolene/capsule. How much dantrolene would you give?

$$\frac{D}{H} = G$$

$$\frac{3\ \cancel{75} \text{ mg}}{1\ \cancel{25} \text{ mg}} = 3 \text{ capsules}$$

You will give 3 capsules of dantrolene (Dantrium).

Work the following problems:
1. Diazepam (Valium) 7.5 mg IM was ordered prn anxiety. The patient is very anxious and requests the medication. Diazepam is dispensed in ampules of 5 mg/ml. How much would you give?

2. The order reads: levodopa 2 g PO qid. Levodopa comes from the pharmacy in 500-mg capsules. How much would you give?

3. The order reads: cyclobenzaprine (Flexeril) 10 mg PO tid.
The label reads: cyclobenzaprine 10 mg/tablet. How much would you give?

Answers are given on p. 283.

CHAPTER 15
Sedatives and hypnotics

Sedatives and *hypnotics* are drugs that produce central nervous system depression resulting in sedation or sleep. Sedatives are usually given during the daytime and may make a person drowsy but do not bring sleep. They are given to calm and soothe a patient when anxiety is a problem. In some chronic diseases, such as hypertension, heart disease, and certain gastrointestinal disorders, anxiety may make the symptoms worse, and in these cases sedatives are given as long-term therapy. Sedatives are also prescribed for temporary relief of anxiety in the nervous or emotionally upset individual.

Drugs with hypnotic effect are given at bedtime to produce sleep. A good quality as well as quantity of sleep is necessary for optimal physical and psychological functioning. Persons who are deprived of sleep may become emotionally disturbed, as well as physically uncomfortable. Hypnotic drugs are given to avoid these problems in the patient whose sleeping habits have been altered by hospitalization, drugs, or disease. It is hoped that this induced sleep will be similar to normal sleep and the patient will wake up refreshed, with no side-effects.

CLASSIFICATION OF SEDATIVES AND HYPNOTICS

The drugs given for sedative or hypnotic effect are classified as either *barbiturate* or *non-barbiturate*

drugs (see Table 15-1). The distinction between sedative and hypnotic is often one of dose rather than drug. Small doses of a drug may have a sedative effect, while larger doses of the same drug will have a hypnotic effect.

The barbiturates are commonly called sleeping pills. They all depress the central nervous system and thus result in slower respiratory and heart rates and lower blood pressure and body temperature. A person may become tolerant to them and dependent on them. Barbiturates are classified according to their duration of action as long, intermediate, short, or ultra-short acting. They are used as anesthetic or preanesthetic agents (see Chapter 11), as anticonvulsants (see Chapter 36), in the treatment of psychosomatic disorders, delirium tremens, and other withdrawal states and to promote sedation and amnesia during labor and delivery. It is the variations in dose, specific drug, and route of administration that make barbiturates useful for inducing mild sedation to deep anesthesia.

The *non-barbiturates* differ from barbiturates in chemical makeup, but they also depress the central nervous system, are habit-forming, and may cause tolerance and dependence.

NURSING IMPLICATIONS

All barbiturates are general depressants, hence they depress the central nervous system, the respiratory

(Text continues on p. 128.)

TABLE 15-1 SEDATIVES AND HYPNOTICS

DRUG	ROUTE AND DOSAGE RANGE	USE	ADVERSE EFFECTS	NURSING IMPLICATIONS
BARBITURATES				
phenobarbital (Luminal)	PO—sedative—15 mg–30 mg bid to qid hypnotic—100 mg–300 mg at hs IM, SC, IV—100 mg–300 mg (to a maximum of 600 mg/24 hr)	To promote sleep and to treat conditions in which mild, relatively prolonged sedation is desired, such as hypertension, preoperative apprehension, GI disorders, anxiety, neuroses, and coronary artery disease; used along with other medications to treat epilepsy	*CNS:* drowsiness, paradoxical states (euphoria, excitement, hyperactivity, confusion), especially in elderly and children, drug hangover, possible physical and psychological dependence *Cardiovascular:* hypotension, shock *Skin:* skin reactions, photosensitivity *Others:* Stevens-Johnson syndrome, respiratory depression	Caution patients to avoid all dangerous activities in which alert behavior is a necessity. Watch for paradoxic reactions. Evaluate mental status. Monitor vital signs. Check skin for rash. Watch for signs of dependence. Give IM injections deep into a large muscle, never more than 5 ml at one site. IV injections must be given very slowly. If barbiturates are given to a patient with uncontrolled pain, they may cause excitement. Withdrawal from long-term barbiturate use must be gradual to avoid convulsions.
secobarbital (Seconal)	PO—100 mg–300 mg at hs IV—50 mg–250 mg IM—100 mg–200 mg PR—solution (5%); suppository (60 mg–200 mg) Dilute 5% solution to 1%–1.5% for rectal administration.	For insomnia; preoperative sedation; sedation in obstetrics, dentistry, and psychiatry; emergency control of certain acute convulsions	See phenobarbital.	See phenobarbital.
amobarbital (Amytal)	PO—65 mg–400 mg prn (to a maximum of 1 g qd) IM, IV—65 mg prn (to a maximum of 0.5 g qd)	See secobarbital.	See phenobarbital.	See phenobarbital.
pentobarbital (Nembutal)	PO—30 mg–100 mg at hs IM—150 mg–200 mg IV—100 mg–500 mg	See secobarbital.	See phenobarbital.	See phenobarbital.
sodium butabarbital (Butisol)	PO—sedative—15 mg–30 mg q6–8h hypnotic—50 mg–100 mg at hs	For sedation or to promote sleep	*CNS:* drowsiness, lethargy, hangover, physical and psychological dependence *Respiratory:* respiratory depression, apnea *Skin:* rash, hypersensitivity reactions *Other:* circulatory collapse	Evaluate mental status. Watch for signs of dependence. Monitor respiratory rate and BP. Observe skin for any reactions.

(continued on page 127)

TABLE 15-1 (continued)

DRUG	ROUTE AND DOSAGE RANGE	USE	ADVERSE EFFECTS	NURSING IMPLICATIONS
NON-BARBITURATES				
chloral hydrate (Noctec)	PO—sedative—250 mg tid hypnotic—500 mg–1 g at hs	For nocturnal sedation in all types of patients, especially the ill, young, and elderly; use as a preoperative medication	*CNS:* excitement, delirium, drowsiness, ataxia, staggering gait, lightheadedness, vertigo, dizziness, nightmares, malaise, mental confusion, hallucinations, tolerance, addiction, headache, hangover *GI:* gastric irritation, nausea, vomiting, gas, diarrhea, unpleasant taste *Skin:* reddened skin, rash, hives, itching *Others:* blood disorders, ketonuria	Capsules should be taken with a full glass of liquid. Evaluate mental status. Assist with activity as necessary. Observe for signs of tolerance or dependence. Keep stool chart. Observe skin for any allergic reaction. Check urine periodically for ketones. Blood tests should be done at regular intervals.
ethchlorvynol (Placidyl)	PO—500 mg–1000 mg at hs	To treat insomnia	*CNS:* dizziness, mild drug hangover, transient giddiness and ataxia, blurred vision, facial numbness, possible physical and psychological dependence *GI:* nausea, vomiting, GI upset, aftertaste *Others:* blood disorders, rash, itch, hypotension	Give with milk or an antacid to decrease GI upset. Caution patients to avoid dangerous activities. Monitor BP. Check skin for rash or itch. Evaluate mental status and behavior. Check blood tests at regular intervals. Watch for signs of dependence.
flurazepam (Dalmane)	PO—15 mg–30 mg at hs	To treat all types of insomnia	*CNS:* dizziness, drowsiness, lightheadedness, ataxia, disorientation, headache, nervousness, talkativeness, weakness, possible physical and psychological dependence *Cardiovascular:* palpitations, chest pains *GI:* GI upsets, diarrhea or constipation *Others:* GU complaints, joint pain	Caution patients to avoid dangerous activities such as driving or operating machinery. Assist patient with activity as necessary. Take medication with milk or an antacid to decrease GI upset. Keep stool chart. Evaluate mental status and behavior. Keep accurate I&O. Watch for signs of dependence. Monitor pulse. Caution the patient about possible combined effects of alcohol or other CNS depressant drugs with sleeping pills.

(continued on page 128)

TABLE 15-1 (continued)

DRUG	ROUTE AND DOSAGE RANGE	USE	ADVERSE EFFECTS	NURSING IMPLICATIONS
paraldehyde (Paral)	PO—5 ml–30 ml PR—10 ml–30 ml (mixed with NS or olive oil) IM—2 ml–10 ml (maximum 5 ml per site) IV—2 ml–10 ml (diluted)	As a sedative or hypnotic in delirium tremens, bromide psychosis, alcohol or morphine withdrawal or obstetrics	*Cardiovascular:* hypotension, brady- or tachycardia, palpitations *Respiratory:* nasal congestion, respiratory depression *GI:* dry mouth, nausea, vomiting, abdominal discomfort, jaundice *Others:* difficult voiding, pain on injection, chills, strong, offensive odor	Monitor vital signs. Evaluate voiding. If medication is given long-term, blood tests to evaluate liver function should be done. Injections should be into a large muscle. Be sure solution is colorless. Give liquid mixed in milk or iced fruit juices to mask the taste and odor. Patient's breath will have an offensive odor. Protect the medication from sunlight. Use a glass syringe for injections, as plastics will react with undiluted medication.
temazepam (Restoril)	PO—15 mg–30 mg at hs	To relieve insomnia associated with complaints of difficulty falling asleep, frequent nocturnal awakenings, and/or early morning awakening	*CNS:* drowsiness, dizziness, lethargy, confusion, euphoria, weakness, tremor, ataxia, lack of concentration, loss of equilibrium, falling, nystagmus, paradoxical reactions (excitement, stimulation, hyperactivity), physical and psychological dependence *Others:* anorexia, diarrhea, palpitations	See flurazepam.
triazolam (Halcion)	PO—0.125 mg–0.5 mg at hs	In short-term management of insomnia characterized by difficulty falling asleep, frequent nighttime awakenings, and/or early morning awakenings	*CNS:* drowsiness, dizziness, headache, nervousness, lightheadedness, ataxia or other incoordination, confusion, nightmares, euphoria, lethargy, depression *GI:* nausea, vomiting, diarrhea or constipation, loss of appetite *Others:* tachycardia, cramps/pain, visual disturbances, alteration in taste, dry mouth, rash	See flurazepam.

system, and the gastrointestinal system. Although the non-barbiturates have depressant effects, these are less likely to be generalized. Alcohol should never be taken with barbiturates or non-barbiturates because it, too, is a depressant, and the additive effect may be lethal.

Drug dependence, with slow development of tolerance, is possible with both the barbiturates and the non-barbiturates. These drugs are well known, easily obtained, and often abused. They are also commonly used with suicidal intent. The lethal dose is 15 to 20 times the therapeutic dose; thus, a single prescription, which contains many times the prescribed dose, is all the person needs to overdose. Sedative and hypnotic drugs should never be left at the patient's bedside. Any CNS depressant can cause poisoning if the dose is too high or if it is excreted too slowly. The symptoms of barbiturate poisoning progress from deep sleep to stupor to coma, with low blood pressure, a weak, slow pulse, and slow respirations. Death finally results from respiratory depression or sudden heart failure.

Most barbiturates cause depression, headache, nausea, and a sense of listlessness and lethargy the following day. This drug hangover can be prevented by giving a smaller dose or a different drug. Barbiturates given to a person in severe pain may cause restlessness, mental confusion, and delirium. In these cases, it is important to give an analgesic. Barbiturates are not analgesic—a patient unable to sleep because of pain will not be helped by a hypnotic.

Drugs that are given to help a hospitalized person sleep often disrupt his normal sleep patterns. When they are discontinued, increased dreaming and nightmares may occur.

The elderly patient taking a hypnotic may become confused and disoriented, so some precautions should be observed. Keep siderails up at night to prevent accidents. With sedatives there may be initial drowsiness and slowing of reflexes, so the person should be cautioned against performing potentially dangerous acts, such as driving a car or operating heavy machinery.

Barbiturates should be given by mouth whenever possible, although other routes are occasionally used. Some sedatives and hypnotics in liquid form, such as chloral hydrate and paraldehyde, have an extremely unpleasant taste; serve them cold and diluted with milk or juice to mask the taste. Knowing that hypnotic drugs may cause sleep disruptions, use discretion when following prn or sos orders for sleeping medications. They should not be given automatically at bedtime—assess the situation first. In your patient teaching, discuss ways to encourage sleep without the use of drugs. Simple measures such as emptying the bladder, reading for a short while, drinking a glass of warm milk, listening to soft music, or meditating may be enough to get the patient to fall sleep naturally. You may take a "sleep history"—ask your patient to describe his usual bedtime routine. Perhaps together you can find ways to modify it. Hypnotics should be administered only after other efforts to promote sleep have failed.

If the patient is taking sedatives or hypnotics regularly, be alert to the possibility of tolerance and dependence. A patient who complains that he cannot get to sleep without taking medication may be drug dependent. Suspect tolerance if the patient complains that one pill is no longer enough to produce sleep.

Sedatives and hypnotics should not be given along with narcotics or even within a short time of each other, unless there is a specific order to do so. Sedatives, hypnotics, and narcotics are all CNS depressants, and the combination of effects may lead to fatal respiratory and cardiac depression. Other CNS depressants, such as alcohol, anesthetics, tranquilizers, and antihistamines should also be avoided.

When some hypnotics are discontinued, a phenomenon known as "rebound insomnia" may occur. In such cases, insomnia on the night following discontinuance of sleeping medication may be even more severe than before treatment.

PRACTICE PROBLEMS—SEDATIVES AND HYPNOTICS

1. The order reads: flurazepam (Dalmane) 30 mg PO hs.
    The label reads: flurazepam 15 mg/capsule.
    How much flurazepam will you give the patient at bedtime?

    $$\frac{D}{H} = G$$

    $$\frac{2\ \cancel{30\ mg}}{1\ \cancel{15\ mg}} = G$$

    $$\frac{2}{1} = 2 \text{ capsules}$$

    You will give 2 capsules of flurazepam (Dalmane).

2. The physician orders pentobarbital (Nembutal) 75 mg IM hs prn sleeplessness. The patient is unable to sleep and asks for his medication. The

vial of pentobarbital reads 100 mg/2 ml. How much will you give?

$$\frac{D}{H} \times A = G$$

$$\frac{3}{4} \frac{75 \text{ mg}}{100 \text{ mg}} \times 2 \text{ ml} = G$$

$$\frac{3}{4} \times 2 \text{ ml} = \frac{6}{4} = 1\frac{1}{2} \text{ ml}$$

You will give $1\frac{1}{2}$ ml of pentobarbital (Nembutal).

Work the following problems:
1. The order reads: secobarbital (Seconal) 150 mg PO hs.

The label reads: secobarbital 50 mg/ml.
How much secobarbital will you administer at bedtime?

2. Chloral hydrate 1 g PO hs is ordered. It comes in 500-mg capsules. How many capsules will you give?

3. The order reads: phenobarbital elixir 30 mg PO bid.
The label reads: phenobarbital 20 mg/5 ml.
How much would you give?

Answers are given on p. 283.

PART 4
Drugs used to help meet patients' needs for intake and utilization of nutrients and the elimination of waste

CHAPTER 16
Vitamins, minerals, fluids, and electrolytes

VITAMINS

Vitamins are organic substances that are necessary for normal metabolism (Table 16-1). Only two vitamins—D and K— are produced in the body; the others must be obtained in food or vitamin supplements. Since only very small amounts of vitamins are needed, a balanced diet is adequate to provide daily needs. A person who is not properly nourished may have one or more vitamin deficiencies.

Two standards for vitamin intake have been adopted in the United States: minimal daily requirement (MDR) and recommended daily allowance (RDA). The minimal daily requirement is the amount of a vitamin that a person must receive to prevent symptoms of deficiency. The recommended daily allowance is a higher amount—sufficient amount to keep a normal, healthy person in good nutritional balance.

Vitamins are divided into two groups. The *fat-soluble* vitamins (A, D, E, and K) are stored in the liver and in adipose tissue. Deficiencies of these vitamins develop only after long periods of time or when there is some interference with absorption. The *water-soluble* vitamins (B complex and C) are not stored in the body, so a deficiency state may develop if they are not taken in for even short periods of time.

Vitamins are for the most part nontoxic, but allergic reactions may occur. For example, a large dose of thiamine (vitamin B_1) has been known to cause anaphylactic shock. A large dose of niacin may cause flushing of the face and neck and occasionally a drop in blood pressure. High doses of vitamin C may cause diarrhea. Vitamins are relatively free of undesirable effects, if taken properly in the normal diet or in a prescribed amount. It is best to stay within the RDA.

The only known diseases caused by vitamin overdose are hypervitaminosis D and hypervitaminosis A, and both develop when too much of that vitamin is ingested. In hypervitaminosis D the person becomes nauseated and anorexic. He complains of weight loss, nausea, vomiting, aches, stiffness, drowsiness, and weakness. Calcium moves out of the bones and into the bloodstream; from there it moves into the blood vessels, heart, or kidneys with damaging results. The signs and symptoms of hypervitaminosis A are swelling and tenderness of bone, dry, scaly skin lesions, anorexia, thinning hair, joint pains, and an enlarged liver and spleen. Normal growth and development in children are disrupted by an excess of either vitamin.

TABLE 16-1   VITAMINS

DRUG	ROUTE AND DOSAGE RANGE	USE	ADVERSE EFFECTS	NURSING IMPLICATIONS
vitamin A (Aquasol A)	PO and IM—(for severe deficiency) 100,000 IU qd for 3 days; then 50,000 IU qd for 2 weeks; then 10,000 to 20,000 IU qd for 2 months	To treat vitamin A deficiency	*With overdosage:* fatigue, malaise, lethargy, abdominal discomfort, anorexia, vomiting	Do not exceed prescribed dosage. Observe activity level. Note any GI discomfort.
calciferol or ergocalciferol (vitamin D)	PO—50,000 U– 1,000,000 U qd	To treat hypoparathyroidism and refractory rickets	Drowsiness, GI distress, renal failure, hypertension, increased levels of calcium and phosphorus in the blood, metastatic calcification	Evaluate mental status. Monitor BP. Check blood and urine regularly for levels of calcium. Record I&O, and note adequacy of output. Note any complaints of GI discomfort.
cyanocobalamin (vitamin B_{12}, Rubramin-PC)	PO—15 mcg qd for 1 month IM, SC (deep)—30 mcg qd for 5–10 days; then 100 mcg–200 mcg every month Schilling test—1000 mcg	To treat deficiency states; use in pregnancy, thyrotoxicosis, hemolytic anemia, hemorrhage, malignancy, hepatic and renal disease when requirements of vitamin B_{12} are increased; use as a Schilling test for pernicious anemia	Mild transient diarrhea, blood disorders, peripheral vascular thrombosis, itching, sensation of swelling in the entire body, pulmonary edema, CHF, anaphylaxis, death	Keep stool chart. Take regular blood tests. Observe for itching. Monitor respiratory rate and rhythm. Note complaints of swelling sensation.
thiamine (vitamin B_1)	PO—1 mg–50 mg qd in divided doses IM, IV—5 mg–100 mg tid	Use as a therapeutic and prophylactic nutritional supplement in stress, pregnancy and lactation, infections, burns, fractures, pre- and postoperative therapy, peptic ulcer, colitis, diabetes, alcoholism; use in special diets; to treat debilitated patients	Usually none; adverse effects may occur when vitamin preparations are given intravenously or in very large doses (allergic reactions, respiratory distress, vascular collapse)	Whenever possible, poor dietary habits should be corrected through patient education. Encourage the patient to take multivitamins to supplement his diet at home.
riboflavin (vitamin B_2)	PO—1 mg–30 mg qd in divided doses	To treat riboflavin deficiency, ariboflavinosis, and microcytic anemia	See thiamine.	See thiamine.
niacin (nicotinic acid)	PO—10 mg–500 mg qd in divided doses SC, IM—50 mg–100 mg up to 5 times/ day IV—25 mg–100 mg	To prevent niacin deficiency; to treat pellagra	*CNS:* headache, dizziness, visual changes *Cardiovascular:* hypotension, tachycardia *GI:* nausea, vomiting, bloating, flatulence, hunger pains, heartburn, diarrhea, liver damage *Skin:* flushing of the face and neck, burning, itching, and tingling skin, increased sebaceous secretions *Other:* blood disorders	Watch for adverse effects if doses over the average are given.

(continued on page 135)

TABLE 16-1 (continued)

DRUG	ROUTE AND DOSAGE RANGE	USE	ADVERSE EFFECTS	NURSING IMPLICATIONS
pyridoxine (vitamin B₆)	PO—2 mg–600 mg qd IM, SC, IV—10 mg–100 mg	To prevent and treat vitamin B₆ deficiency; to treat sideroblastic anemia associated with high iron concentration; to treat intractable seizures in infants	See thiamine.	See thiamine, *plus:* Medication must be protected from light.
ascorbic acid (vitamin C)	PO, IM, SC, IV—10 mg–500 mg qd To acidify urine: 4–12 g/day in divided doses	To prevent and treat scurvy; as a supplement in patients with GI disease, long-term parenteral nutrition, and chronic hemodialysis; after surgery to increase the rate of wound healing and as a urinary acidifier	Usually none; occasionally—nausea, vomiting, diarrhea, heartburn, abdominal cramps, fatigue, flushing, headache, insomnia, sleepiness	
phytonadione (vitamin K₁, Mephyton, Aqua-MEPHYTON)	PO, SC, IM—(coagulation disorders) 2.5 mg–50 mg, repeat after 6–8 hr if necessary; (newborn) 0.5 mg–2 mg	To treat coagulation disorders; use as preventive treatment in hemorrhagic disease of the newborn	Transient flushing, alterations in taste, dizziness, tachycardia, hypotension, profuse sweating, respiratory distress, pain at injection site, possible anaphylaxis	Protect medication from light at all times. Monitor vital signs. Assist with activity as necessary. Assess injection site.
menadione (vitamin K₃)	PO—5 mg–10 mg qd	To prevent and treat hypoprothrombinemia caused by vitamin K deficiency or drug therapy	Severe blood disorders and brain damage in infants, nausea, vomiting, headache, GI upset, hypersensitivity, allergic reactions	Observe skin for reactions. Blood tests should be done, especially in infants.
multivitamins	PO—1 qd	Use as a daily supplement	None	None

In the United States only mild forms of vitamin deficiency are generally seen, rather than the severe deficiency states of beriberi, rickets, scurvy, and pellagra. These diseases are seen in countries where poverty and lack of proper diet prevent people from getting enough vitamins. Patient teaching is a special need among persons whose vitamin intake is low. Those on restricted diets, whether by a physician's order or their own will, may need dietary instruction to alert them to the possibility of vitamin deficiency. Patients with gastrointestinal diseases that affect absorption of nutrients, alcoholics who generally eat poorly, pregnant or lactating women, and children all need extra vitamins.

There are many vitamin preparations available as nonprescription drugs. The thing to remember about vitamins is that any daily dose higher than the RDA is unnecessary and may be dangerous. High potency vitamins prescribed by a physician are called therapeutic vitamin formulations. Multivitamin capsules vary greatly in composition. The label should be read carefully to see that all the essential vitamins are present in amounts equal to the RDA. Remember that amounts greater than this are not needed and may increase the cost of the preparation.

Always check the date on the label; vitamins may lose their potency with time. Do not heat preparations containing water-soluble vitamins; they are destroyed by high temperatures. Vitamins are sometimes kept in dark containers to avoid the heat of the sun or of lights for this reason. Fat-soluble vitamins are not affected by heat.

MINERALS

Minerals are naturally occurring substances that are easily supplied in the diet. The most prominent minerals of the body are calcium (Ca), iron (Fe), iodine (I), potassium (K), sodium (Na), and phosphorus (P). Several others (chromium, cobalt, copper, fluorine, magnesium, molybdenum, selenium, and zinc), although important, are present in such tiny amounts that they are called trace elements. Minerals serve as regulators of some essential bodily functions. Calcium, magnesium, potassium, and sodium are *electrolytes* (substances capable of conducting electricity) that play extremely important parts in water balance, acid–base balance, and blood clotting. Other key functions controlled by minerals are transmission of nerve and muscle impulses and metabolism for energy production.

NURSING IMPLICATIONS

Iron preparations given by mouth can cause gastrointestinal disturbances and staining of the teeth. Giving iron along with meals lessens the likelihood of gastric distress. Iron absorption is also increased if orange juice or vitamin C is given at the same time. If a liquid iron preparation is ordered, be sure to suggest that the patient drink it through a straw, or place the drops on the back of the tongue to avoid staining the teeth. Intramuscular iron injections are very irritating to subcutaneous tissues.

Calcium and iron are the two minerals most frequently lacking in the diet. You can encourage your patients to eat foods that are good sources of these minerals, such as meat and milk. Women need about four times as much iron than men because of the loss of iron in menstrual blood.

FLUIDS AND ELECTROLYTES

Approximately 60% of body weight is water. Most of the water is found within the cells and is called intracellular fluid. It is absolutely essential for all metabolic reactions. Even slight alterations in fluid balance may adversely affect health. Fluids are taken into the body not only by ingesting fluids but also by eating foods that have a high water content. Fluid is lost in urine, perspiration, feces, tears, saliva, and exhaled air. Thirst is usually a good indicator of the need for fluids.

Electrolytes are necessary for normal health. An electrolyte is a substance that conducts electricity in a solution. The principal electrolytes are sodium (Na), potassium (K), calcium (Ca), magnesium (Mg), and chloride (Cl) (see Table 16-2). They are found in both the intracellular and the extracellular (outside the cell) fluid.

Fluids and electrolytes, like vitamins and minerals, are substances normally present in the body. When, for any reason, they are not present in the normal amount, drug therapy is needed. This type of treatment is called *replacement therapy*.

The quickest way to treat fluid and electrolyte disturbances is by intravenous replacement. Various solutions of water, electrolytes, and nutrients are administered alone or in combination. Replacement therapy with oral medications is another way to correct the imbalance, although it is slower and less efficient. Dehydration, electrolyte imbalance, acid–base imbalance, overhydration, and nutritional deficits, all of which are due to an inability to ingest, digest, or absorb nutrients normally, are treated by administering fluids and electrolytes. Severe nutritional deficits are sometimes treated by intravenous fluid therapy, known as *hyperalimentation* or *total parenteral nutrition (TPN)*. The solution administered for this purpose contains vitamins, minerals, glucose, and other nutrients, as well as sufficient calories so cellular functions can continue. Those who may benefit from such therapy are the severely malnourished, patients with extensive burns, and patients who have undergone extensive intestinal surgery.

Dehydration occurs when both fluid volume and sodium level are below normal.

Overhydration occurs when the internal fluid volume is abnormally high. Electrolyte solutions and other substances in the blood become too diluted.

Electrolyte imbalances usually accompany fluid imbalance. First, the fluid imbalance is corrected, then appropriate electrolyte solutions are administered.

Acid–base balance refers to the proportion of acid and base needed to keep blood and body fluids neutral. The relationship is measured in *p*H. A neutral *p*H (neither acid nor base) is 7.35 to 7.45. The reason this delicate balance is so important is that while the production of acids is an end result of metabolism, an alkaline fluid environment is required for essential cell activities. *Acidosis*, a *p*H less than 7.3, is a result of too much acid. It is treated by oral or intravenous administration of a base. *Alkalosis*, a *p*H greater than 7.5, is the opposite imbalance; there is too much base. In this

TABLE 16-2 ELECTROLYTES

DRUG	ROUTE AND DOSAGE RANGE	USE	ADVERSE EFFECTS	NURSING IMPLICATIONS
potassium (K-Lyte, K-Phos, K-Tab, Kaon, Kay-Ciel, Klorvess, Klotrix, Micro-K, Slow-K)	PO—20 mEq–100 mEq qd in divided doses	To prevent or treat hypokalemia; to treat cardiac arrhythmias due to digitalis toxicity	Nausea, vomiting, diarrhea, abdominal discomfort	Give with meals to decrease GI upset. Be sure to dilute liquid potassium preparations and dissolve powder and effervescent tablets in 3 to 4 ounces of iced water or cold fruit juice. Have the patient sip the medication slowly (over a 5- to 10-minute period). Different flavors are available in many preparations. Monitor electrolyte levels. Watch for signs and symptoms of hyperkalemia (paresthesias of the extremities, lethargy, confusion, flaccid paralysis, weak legs, hypotension, cardiac arrhythmias, heart block).
sodium polystyrene sulfonate (Kayexalate)	PO, PR—15 g–60 g qd	To treat hyperkalemia	Anorexia, nausea, vomiting, constipation, hypocalcemia, sodium retention, possible fecal impaction, diarrhea; may lead to severe hypokalemia	Monitor electrolyte levels closely. Keep stool chart. Watch for signs and symptoms of hypokalemia (irritability, confusion, mental slowness, ECG changes, severe muscle weakness).
sodium bicarbonate	PO—325 mg–650 mg prn (to a maximum of 8 g qd) IV—doses highly individualized	To treat metabolic acidosis; use for rapid relief from acid indigestion, heartburn, and sour stomach	Stomach distention, flatulence (gas), renal stones or crystals, sodium and water retention	Encourage patient to ambulate. Note urinalysis results. Monitor electrolytes. Check weight daily. Keep accurate record of I&O.

case, medications that raise the acid level are given.

Intravenous therapy

The solutions used to administer intravenous replacement therapy are grouped into three categories. *Isotonic* solutions (0.9% solution of NaCl) resemble normal blood plasma and are often called normal saline (NS) solutions. *Hypertonic* solutions are more concentrated than blood plasma. When these solutions are used, fluid leaves the blood cells and travels to the plasma and is also drawn from interstitial tissue into the bloodstream. *Hypotonic* solutions are less concentrated than blood plasma. When these solutions are used, fluid moves from the vascular compartment to the interstitial tissues.

Included in a written order for intravenous therapy are the name of the solution to be administered and the rate of administration. It is the responsibility of the nurse to determine the flow rate (in drops per minute) and regulate the flow. The flow is regulated by adjusting the roller clamp on the tubing (Fig. 16-1).

Intravenous infusion sets deliver either a macrodrip or a microdrip. A macrodrip delivers 10 to 20 drops/ml, depending on the manufacturer. The smaller microdrip (also called the minidrip, pedidrip, or Buretrol) delivers 60 drops/ml. *The drop per milliliter ratio is always printed on the package containing the infusion set.*

The formula for determining the drops per minute (gtt/min) is:

$$\frac{\text{total amount of solution} \times \text{drop factor}}{\text{minutes (hours} \times 60)}$$

$$= \text{drops/minute}$$

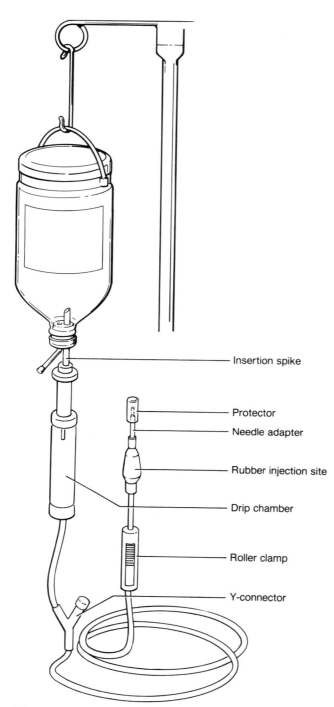

Figure 16-1. Intravenous tubing.

- Insertion spike
- Protector
- Needle adapter
- Rubber injection site
- Drip chamber
- Roller clamp
- Y-connector

COMMONLY USED INTRAVENOUS SOLUTIONS

Isotonic Solutions

0.9% sodium chloride (NS)
5% dextrose in water* (D_5W)
Lactated Ringer's solution (RL)

Hypertonic Solutions

5% dextrose with 0.9% sodium chloride (D_5NS)
5% dextrose with 0.45% sodium chloride ($D_5\frac{1}{2}NS$)
5% dextrose with 0.33% sodium chloride ($D_5\frac{1}{3}NS$)
10% dextrose in water ($D_{10}W$)

Hypotonic Solutions

0.45% sodium chloride ($\frac{1}{2}$ NS)

For example, the order reads: Run 3000 ml of $D_5 \frac{1}{3}$ NS over 24 hours. The administration set delivers 15 gtt/ml.

$$\frac{\text{total amount of solution} \times \text{drop factor}}{\text{hours} \times 60 \text{ minutes/hour}}$$
$$= \text{drops per minute}$$
$$\frac{3000 \text{ ml} \times 15 \text{ gtt/ml}}{24 \text{ hr} \times 60 \text{ min/hr}} = \text{gtt/min}$$
$$\frac{45,000 \text{ gtt}}{1440 \text{ min}} = 31.25 \text{ gtt/min} = 31$$

Thus, you will adjust the clamp so that 31 drops fall per minute.

With the microdrip infusion set, the drops per minute equal the milliliters per hour because the 60 gtt/ml cancels out the 60 min/hr. For example, if the order reads 50 ml D_5W qh and the set delivers 60 gtt/ml,

$$\frac{\text{total amount of solution} \times \text{drop factor}}{\text{hours} \times 60 \text{ minutes/hour}}$$
$$= \text{drops per minute}$$
$$\frac{50 \text{ ml} \times 60 \text{ gtt/ml}}{1 \text{ hr} \times 60 \text{ min/hr}} = 50 \text{ gtt/min}$$

* 5% dextrose in water contains 170 calories/liter.

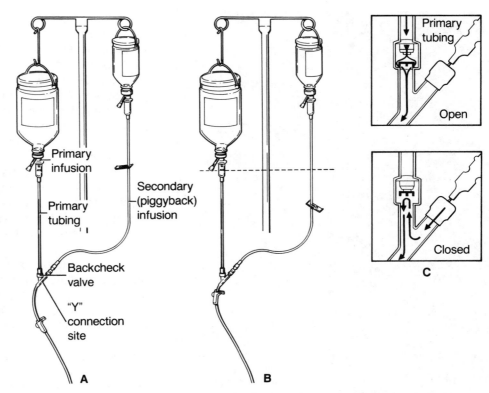

Figure 16-2. (A) The piggyback infusion setup. (B) The piggyback bottle is always hung higher than the primary infusion. (C) The valve in the primary tubing is closed while the secondary solution infuses. When the secondary solution is finished, the valve opens and the primary solution resumes its flow. (After Brunner LB, Suddarth DS: The Lippincott Manual of Nursing Practice, 3rd ed. Philadelphia, JB Lippincott, 1982)

Some intravenous medications are given "piggyback" with the main intravenous solution. This technique is used when one medication is given intermittently while the main intravenous solution is administered continuously. In this case when the second solution (the piggyback) is to be infused, the needle of the second tubing is inserted into the Y-site of the first line. The height of the primary bottle is adjusted so that it is lower than the piggyback solution. A valve in the primary tubing closes to stop the flow of the primary solution, allowing the other solution to flow. When the second solution is finished, the valve opens, allowing the primary solution to resume its flow (see Fig. 16-2).

Medication can also be administered through a volume-controlled administration set. These sets are called Buretrols, Solusets, Volutrols, or Peditrol sets. Directions for assembling and priming these sets are on each package. The set should be labeled with the name of the drug to be administered through it. If more than one drug is being given, there must be a separately labeled set for each drug.

When high-potency medications are given intravenously, they must be delivered at a constant rate. It is not always possible to regulate roller clamps on the tubing to deliver an exact number

of drops per minute constantly. For this reason there are infusion pumps that can be used to deliver a uniform flow rate. The use of these pumps eliminates the need to count drops and adjust flow rates. The rate is set initially, and the pump delivers the medication at that rate. Some are set by milliliters per hour and others by drops per minute. There is a sensor in the machine that counts the drops. If the proper amount is not being infused, an alarm sounds (see Fig. 16-3).

Controllers are also used to deliver a uniform flow rate. These operate by gravity. A sensor is placed on the drip chamber of the intravenous tubing to detect the drop rate. If the actual rate is different than the set rate, the machine makes an adjustment. If this is unsuccessful, or if there is a blockage in the system, an alarm sounds. These machines have made the administration of intravenous medications easier for nurses.

NURSING IMPLICATIONS

With intravenous therapy there are general implications for nursing care, no matter what solution is administered: calculation and proper regulation of

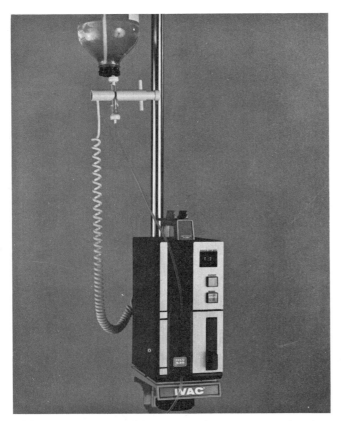

Figure 16-3. The infusion pump is a device that automatically delivers an infusion at a constant rate. (Wolff L, Weitzel MH, Zornow RA, Zsohar H: Fundamentals of Nursing, 7th ed. Philadelphia, JB Lippincott, 1983)

flow rate is very important; there should always be two clamps on the intravenous tubing as a safety precaution; the flow rate should be checked at least every hour; bottles should be time-taped for quick visual assessment; no intravenous solution should hang for more than 24 hours; and tubing should be changed every 48 hours. A label with the date of change should be affixed to the fresh tubing.

Observe the insertion site frequently for redness or swelling, which may indicate infiltration, and note whether the patient reports pain at the site. Other complications to watch for are extravasation (leakage into surrounding tissue), thrombosis (clotting), necrosis (tissue destruction), and infection. Be sure electrolyte solutions are diluted properly and administered slowly. Keep track of the patient's current electrolyte levels by checking on the laboratory work at regular intervals.

A time strip or other label that shows at a glance how the IV solution is running in relation to time should be affixed to the bottle of solution. In this way the nurse can tell at a glance if the proper rate is being maintained. If the rate falls behind what is ordered, *never* speed up the rate; rather, adjust the rate and retape the time label.

With hyperalimentation it is necessary to observe strict sterile technique in all stages of administration. The solutions used are extremely unstable and are excellent mediums for growth of microorganisms. These solutions should be used immediately after preparation and given slowly into large veins that will allow quick dilution.

When polystyrene sulfonate (Kayexalate) is given orally to treat hyperkalemia, it is essential that laxatives are ordered. Otherwise, constipation and fecal impaction may occur.

PRACTICE PROBLEMS—VITAMINS, MINERALS, FLUIDS, AND ELECTROLYTES

1. The order reads: 1000 ml $D_5 \frac{1}{2}$ NS to run for 8 hr. The set delivers 10 gtt/ml.

$$\frac{\text{total amount of solution} \times \text{drop factor}}{\text{hours} \times 60 \text{ min/hr}}$$
$$= \text{gtt/min}$$
$$\frac{1000 \text{ ml} \times 10 \text{ gtt/ml}}{8 \text{ hr} \times 60 \text{ min/hr}} = \text{gtt/min}$$

$$\frac{10,000 \text{ gtt}}{480 \text{ min}} = 20.83 = 21 \text{ gtt/min}$$

The IV drip will be adjusted to deliver 21 gtt/min.

2. The order reads: Ampicillin 500 mg intravenous piggyback (IVPB) in 100 ml D_5W to run for $1\frac{1}{2}$ hr. The drop factor is 60 gtt/ml.

$$\frac{\text{total amount of solution} \times \text{drop factor}}{\text{hours} \times 60 \text{ min/hour}}$$

$$= \text{gtt/min}$$

$$\frac{100 \text{ ml} \times 60 \text{ gtt/ml}}{1.5 \text{ hr} \times 60 \text{ min/hr}} = \text{gtt/min}$$

$$\frac{100 \text{ gtt}}{1.5 \text{ min}} = 66.7 = 67 \text{ gtt/min}$$

The IV drip will be adjusted to deliver 67 gtt/min.

3. The order reads 500 ml NS at 15 gtt/min. The drop factor is 10 gtt/ml. How long will the solution run?

$$\frac{\text{total amount of solution} \times \text{drop factor}}{\times \text{minutes}}$$

$$= 15 \text{ gtt/min}$$

$$\frac{500 \text{ ml} \times 10 \text{ gtt/ml}}{\times \text{min}} = 15 \text{ gtt/min}$$

$$15x = 5000$$

$$x = \frac{5000}{15 \text{ min}} = 333.3 \text{ minutes}$$

$$333.3 \text{ min} \div 60 \text{ min/hr} = 5.6 \text{ hr}$$

The IV drip will be adjusted so that the infusion runs for 5.6 hours, or 5 hours and 36 minutes.

Work the following problems:

1. The order reads: Ringer's lactate 1000 ml to run at 75 ml/hr. The drop factor is 10 gtt/ml. How many drops per minute should be delivered? At this rate how many hours will the solution run?

2. The order reads: 1000 ml D_5W q10h. The drop factor is 15 gtt/ml. How many drops per minute should be delivered?

3. The order reads: 1000 ml NS to run over 6 hours. The administration set delivers 10 gtt/ml. How many drops per minute will need to run?

4. Five hundred milliliters of D_5W with 20 mEq KCl is to run for 20 hours. The drop factor for the administration set is 60 gtt/ml. How many drops per minute should be delivered?

5. Cephalothin (Keflin) 500 mg is to run IVPB over 1 hour. It is mixed in 100 ml D_5W. The set delivers 15 gtt/ml. At how many drops per minute will you set the rate?

6. The order reads: Run 250 ml NS at 10 gtt/min. How long will the IV infusion run? (The drop factor is 15 gtt/ml.)

Answers are given on p. 283.

CHAPTER 17
Antacids, digestants, demulcents, and carminatives

Too much hydrochloric acid (HCl) in the stomach is called *hyperchlorhydria*. It can cause a feeling of fullness after meals, usually referred to as indigestion, with belching and gastric distention. To relieve these symptoms, the acid must be neutralized with antacids. These drugs are available without a prescription and are widely used and often abused.

The mucous membrane that lines the stomach and the entire digestive tract normally provides sufficient protection against gastric secretions. When this protection is lost because of disease, however, the mucosa may be destroyed by the acid juices. In these cases antacids are used to relieve heartburn, esophagitis, and gastritis caused by the irritation by HCl. If the condition remains untreated, peptic ulcer may develop.

Antacids act by buffering (chemically altering) the gastric secretions, so they are not irritating, and by absorbing the excess acid. Antacid therapy should decrease stomach acidity while preventing electrolyte imbalance, constipation, and diarrhea.

CLASSIFICATION OF ANTACIDS

Antacids are classified as *systemic* and *nonsystemic* (see Table 17-1). *Systemic* antacids are taken by mouth and dissolve easily in the gastric and intestinal secretions. They are rapidly absorbed into the bloodstream. They may cause electrolyte and acid–base imbalances, as well as *acid rebound* (higher levels of HCl). Although patients claim they have greater relief with the systemic antacids, physicians generally do not prescribe them because of their adverse effects.

The *nonsystemic* antacids are also taken by mouth, but once in the stomach they are not readily absorbed. Thus they have no direct effect on either electrolyte or acid–base balance, and there is no acid rebound. Nonsystemic antacids are further divided into groups according to their main ingredient.

Aluminum compounds are mixtures of aluminum and other substances. They are slow to act but have a lengthy buffering action on the gastric juices. They are available in both tablet and liquid form. Most patients prefer the tablets, although the liquid has a better antacid effect. Magnesium is the major ingredient in magnesium compounds. One of these compounds, magaldrate (Riopan), a combination of magnesium and aluminum hydroxide, has the additional advantage of being a nonsystemic antacid that is low in sodium.

The first antacid used was calcium carbonate, or chalk. It has a high capability of neutralizing stomach acid, and its action is rapid and prolonged. It does, however, cause acid rebound similar to the systemic antacids, but this is relatively slight and occurs only after long-term use. Pepto-Bismol and Tums are two widely used medications that contain chalk.

In addition to the neutralizing antacids discussed above, there are newer anti-ulcer agents

TABLE 17-1　ANTACIDS

DRUG	ROUTE AND DOSAGE RANGE	USE	ADVERSE EFFECTS	NURSING IMPLICATIONS
aluminum hydroxide (AlternaGel, Amphogel)	PO—1–2 tsp or 1–2 tablets 4–6 times/ day	To relieve hyperacidity associated with peptic ulcer, gastritis, esophagitis, gastric hyperacidity, and hiatal hernia	Constipation	Tablets must be chewed well and taken with water or milk. Give between meals and at bedtime, followed by a sip of water. Antacids must not be taken by anyone also taking antibiotics containing any form of tetracycline. Keep stool chart.
aluminum hydroxide + magnesium hydroxide (Maalox)	PO—2–4 tsp or 1–4 tablets qid	See aluminum hydroxide.	Mild and usually infrequent	See aluminum hydroxide.
aluminum hydroxide + magnesium hydroxide + simethicone (Digel, Gelusil, Maalox Plus, Mylanta)	PO—2 tsp or 2 tablets prn (to a maximum of 12 qd)	See aluminum hydroxide, plus: to relieve gas and postoperative gas pain; to aid in endoscopic examinations	Mild and usually infrequent	See aluminum hydroxide.
calcium carbonate (Dicarbosil, Titralac)	PO—1–4 tablets prn (to a maximum of 16 qd)	To treat peptic ulcer, gastritis, gastric hyperacidity, heartburn, sour stomach, hiatal hernia, peptic esophagitis, acid indigestion, and gas	Mild and usually infrequent	Tell patients that tablets should be chewed or dissolved slowly in the mouth.
cimetidine (Tagamet)	PO—300 mg qid or 400 mg bid (in severe conditions up to a maximum of 2400 mg qd) IM, IV—300 mg q6h	Use for short-term treatment of duodenal ulcer; to treat pathological hypersecretory diseases	Bitter taste, diarrhea, muscle pains, rash, dizziness, mild gynecomastia with long-term use, confusion, blood disorders, cardiac arrhythmias and cardiac arrest (following IV use)	Give with meals and at bedtime to decrease GI upset. Check skin for rash. Assist with activity if necessary. Evaluate mental status. Warn patient of possible breast enlargement. Keep stool chart. Blood tests should be done at regular intervals. Monitor apical pulse. No antacids should be given within 1 hr of administration.
magaldrate (Riopan)	PO—1–2 tsp or tablets qid	See aluminum hydroxide.	Mild and usually infrequent	
magnesium hydroxide mixture (Milk of magnesia)	PO—5 ml–30 ml prn	See aluminum hydroxide, plus: Use as a laxative and treatment for mild hypomagnesemia	Nausea, diarrhea, abdominal pain, possible hypermagnesemia	See aluminum hydroxide, plus: Offer the patient a small amount of water if given for antacid effect, and a large amount of water if taken for laxative effect.

(continued on page 145)

metoclopramide HCl

for Ernie

	USE	ADVERSE EFFECTS	NURSING IMPLICATIONS
...g q6–	In short-term treatment of active duodenal ulcer and to treat certain conditions of hypersecretion	Headache, malaise, dizziness, nausea, constipation, rash, abdominal pain, (rare) elevated liver function test results	Do not use Multistix to test urine. Assist patient with activities if necessary. Keep stool chart.
...O—1 g qid	For short-term treatment of duodenal ulcer	Constipation, rare: diarrhea, nausea, gastric upset, indigestion, dry mouth, rash, itching, back pain, dizziness, sleepiness, vertigo	Tetracycline, phenytoin or cimetidine should not be given within 2 hours of administration. Give when stomach is empty (1 hour before meals and at hs).

(technically *not* antacids) that decrease gastric acid secretions by inhibiting the cells that produce the secretions. They are called histamine antagonists, and examples are cimetidine (Tagamet) and ranitidine (Zantac). Anticholinergic drugs (see Chapter 18) are also helpful in decreasing gastric secretions.

NURSING IMPLICATIONS

The aluminum compounds tend to cause constipation, while the magnesium compounds tend to cause diarrhea. Therefore, you should check the frequency and consistency of the patient's stools. Keeping a stool chart will show, at a glance, whether a problem is developing. Sometimes the physician will order different antacids to be given throughout the day, for example, a magnesium compound at midnight, 8 AM, and 4 PM and an aluminum compound at 4 AM, noon, and 8 PM. Thus, the patient receives antacids every 4 hours but is less likely to suffer from diarrhea or constipation.

Instruct the patient to chew antacid tablets slowly and thoroughly, so that the particles are small before being swallowed. This helps ensure maximum antacid effect. Liquid antacids should be taken with a small amount of milk or water so that the antacid will reach and enter the stomach rather than merely coat the esophagus. If a large amount of water is taken, the antacid will be diluted and less effective.

Shake antacid suspensions well before you pour them. This will ensure that the drug particles are properly distributed throughout the suspension.

Patients should be cautioned against long-term self-medication with antacids because this practice may mask the underlying problem. Persistent indigestion or gastric pain requires medical investigation. If hospitalized patients need to be given antacids frequently, for example, every 1 or 2 hours, have them help. Teach them how to measure the medication and to observe the proper time intervals. Participation in his own care will often help the patient feel better.

Many antacids contain sodium and should not be given to patients on sodium-restricted diets. Patients with cardiac and renal disease, and those with high blood pressure, should also be sure their sodium intake is within prescribed limits.

DIGESTANTS

Digestants are drugs that aid digestion when the presence of a disease might affect this normal process (Table 17-2). Most often in such cases, one of the enzymes or other chemicals required for normal digestion is lacking.

If it is digestive enzymes that are lacking, pancreatic preparations may be given. These mixtures of pancreatic enzymes are usually prescribed when the pancreas has been surgically removed and to treat cystic fibrosis. Examples of these enzyme preparations are Viokase, Pancrease, and Cotazym. Bile salts, necessary for digestion of fats and absorption of fat-soluble vitamins, may be missing in the patient with biliary disease. In this case, ox bile extract and dehydrocholic acid (Decholin) may be needed. A deficiency of HCl is corrected by giv-

TABLE 17-2   DIGESTANTS

DRUG	ROUTE AND DOSAGE RANGE	USE	ADVERSE EFFECTS	NURSING IMPLICATIONS
pancreatic preparations (Cotazym, Pancrease, Viokase)	PO—¼–¾ tsp, 1–2 packets or 1–3 tablets or capsules prior to each meal or snack	To aid digestion in patients with cystic fibrosis and pancreatic enzyme deficiencies due to pancreatitis, pancreatectomy, or obstruction caused by malignant growth	Allergic reactions, indigestion	Patients must be taught to keep their diets in proper balance of fat, protein, and starch to avoid indigestion. Watch for any allergic reaction.

ing glutamic acid HCl (Acidulin), availabe in capsules, tablets, or dilute solutions. A mixture of barley, enzymes, and sugars, called malt extract, is occasionally given as a digestant to patients who are not able to digest carbohydrates well.

NURSING IMPLICATIONS

There are few problems related to giving digestants, as they are a form of replacement therapy for substances that are normally found in the body. Hydrochloric acid preparations have a very sour taste. Encourage your patient to eat or drink something palatable afterward. Also keep in mind that the acid can damage tooth enamel if not diluted sufficiently.

DEMULCENTS

Demulcents are drugs given for their soothing action. They relieve irritation of the mucous membrane in the digestive tract. Demulcents are found in preparations that soothe oral or intestinal mucosa.

Boiled starch and boiled milk are common household demulcents. Certain drugs act like demulcents by binding (attracting) and thus removing irritant materials. This process is called adsorbent action. Activated charcoal and kaolin are examples of absorbents. Other demulcent medications are acacia gum, glycerin, and kaolin-pectin mixture (Kaopectate).

CARMINATIVES

Carminatives are antiflatulent or flatus-expelling drugs that relieve discomfort due to gas. The active ingredients are usually substances that act as irritants to the gastrointestinal tract, thus increasing intestinal motility and promoting exit of gas from the stomach and the intestine.

Household substances used for their carminative effects are whiskey, brandy, and peppermint oil in hot water. Medications with antiflatulent effect usually contain simethicone (Table 17-3).

TABLE 17-3   CARMINATIVE

DRUG	ROUTE AND DOSAGE RANGE	USE	ADVERSE EFFECTS	NURSING IMPLICATIONS
simethicone (Mylicon, Si-lain)	PO—150 mg–400 mg qd in divided doses	To treat flatulence (gas), functional gastric bloating, and postoperative gas pains; used prior to diagnostic GI procedures to enhance visualization	None	None

CHAPTER 18
Antispasmodics

In order to understand how gastrointestinal and genitourinary functions are affected by drugs, it is necessary to review the function of a part of the nervous system, the autonomic nervous system (ANS). The ANS is one of the systems responsible for maintenance of homeostasis. It regulates digestion, heart rate, blood pressure, and other essential life processes. The ANS is divided into parasympathetic and sympathetic portions, which act in opposite ways.

In the gastrointestinal (GI) tract there are mostly parasympathetic fibers that stimulate both muscle and sensory secretory organs. ANS actions on GI function are as follows: metabolic rate is slowed; salivary gland and abdominal organ vessels are dilated, thereby increasing secretions; stomach and pyloric muscles contract; intestinal tone and motility are increased; and gastric, pancreatic, and islets cells are stimulated to produce further secretions.

In the genitourinary (GU) tract, parasympathetic fibers control contraction of the detrusor muscle, which allows emptying of the bladder. Examination of the individual parasympathetic nerve cell fibers would reveal a tiny space between one nerve cell fiber and the next, as well as between those fibers and the muscles they affect. In order for the impulse to cross this space, a special substance called a *transmitter* must be present. In the parasympathetic nervous system this transmitter substance is called *acetylcholine* (ACh).

Once the nerve impulse has been transmitted to the next nerve cell fiber or muscle fiber, a substance that inactivates ACh, cholinesterase, is produced. If the cholinesterase is not present to prevent re-excitation of the muscle, the muscle will be in a constant state of excitation.

Drugs that are either chemically related to ACh or evoke similar effects are called *cholinergic* drugs. Those medications that block the action of cholinergic drugs are called *anticholinergic* or *cholinergic-blocking* agents (see Table 18-1).

CHOLINERGIC DRUGS

Since cholinergics behave much like ACh and act at the same sites (mimics), they are often referred to as parasympathomimetic drugs. These drugs act in one of two ways: (1) direct action, which means they act like ACh, or (2) indirect action, which means they inhibit cholinesterase, the enzyme that inactivates ACh, and thus prolong the action of ACh. In either case, the end result is the same—action similar to that of acetylcholine.

In gastrointestinal disease the cholinergics are used to treat paralytic ileus, to stimulate both large and small intestine after surgery, and to promote salivation. They are helpful, too, in cases of postoperative and postpartum urinary retention. They have other uses, as well, including treatment of glaucoma, and circulatory, muscle, and neurologic diseases. These uses shall be discussed in other chapters.

(*Text continues on p. 150.*)

TABLE 18-1 ANTISPASMODICS

DRUG	ROUTE AND DOSAGE RANGE	USE	ADVERSE EFFECTS	NURSING IMPLICATIONS
isopropamide + prochlor- perazine (Combid)	PO—1–2 capsules q12h	Use with other therapy in treatment of pep- tic ulcer, the irrita- ble bowel syn- drome, and functional diarrhea	See prochlorperazine (Chapter 6), *plus:* *Cardiovascular:* tachy- cardia, palpitations *GI:* dry mouth, nausea, constipation, bloated feeling, difficulty swallowing *GU:* urinary hesitancy and retention *Eyes:* dilated pupils, blurred vision *Others:* fever, nasal congestion	See prochlorperazine, *plus:* Monitor apical pulse and note any complaints of palpita- tions. Keep stool chart. Note any complaints of GI discomfort or difficulty swallowing. Record I&O (note any de- crease in urinary output or difficulty with urination). Assess visual acuity. Monitor temperature. Note complaints of nasal congestion.
CHOLINERGICS				
bethanechol (Duvoid, Ure- choline)	PO—10 mg–30 mg tid to qid SC—2.5 mg–5 mg tid to qid	To treat acute postop- erative and postpar- tum urinary reten- tion; to treat urinary retention due to neurogenic bladder conditions	*GI:* abdominal discom- fort, nausea, diarrhea, gas *ANS:* flushed skin, in- creased salivation, sweating *Others:* headache, leth- argy, hypotension, asthmatic attacks	Give when stomach is empty to avoid nausea and vomit- ing. Watch for increased saliva- tion and perspiration. Note skin color. Monitor blood pressure. Evaluate respiratory function in case of asthma attack.
neostigmine (Prostigmin)	PO—15 mg–375 mg qd IM, SC—0.25 mg–1 mg qd IV—0.5 mg–2 mg	To control the symp- toms of myasthenia gravis; to prevent and treat postopera- tive distention and urinary retention	*GI:* nausea, vomiting, diarrhea, bowel cramps *ANS:* increased saliva- tion, sweating, bron- chial secretions, and peristalsis *Others:* fasciculations, muscle weakness (overdose can lead to death)	Be sure to give medications exactly on time as ordered. Check for increased secre- tions. Keep a stool chart. Note any abnormal muscle movements or complaints of muscle weakness.
pyridostigmine (Mestinon)	PO—60 mg–1.5 g qd IM, IV—(for myas- thenia) ⅟₃₀ the PO dose (to re- verse drug action) 10 mg–20 mg	To treat myasthenia gravis and to re- verse the action of nondepolarizing muscle relaxants	See neostigmine.	See neostigmine.
ANTICHOLINERGICS				
atropine	PO—0.3 mg–0.6 mg 30 minutes before meals (dose may be individualized) IM, IV, SC—0.4 mg– 0.6 mg	To control excess motor activity in GI diseases, such as pylorospasm, spas- tic constipation, ul- cerative colitis; to treat spasms of the urinary tract; use in the management of gastric, duodenal, or intestinal ulcers; use as a preoperative medication to re- duce salivation and bronchial secre- tions; to relieve symptoms of poi- soning by insecti- cides and nerve gas	*ANS:* dry nose and mouth, thirst, flushed and dry skin *Cardiovascular:* tachy- cardia or bradycardia, palpitations *Others:* pupil dilation, difficulty with speech and swallowing, headache, restless- ness, weakness, rash, fever	Offer fluids as necessary for comfort. Evaluate skin condition. Evaluate ability to talk and swallow. Monitor pulse, BP, and pupil size. Check temperature. Keep stool chart.

(continued on page 149)

TABLE 18-1 (continued)

DRUG	ROUTE AND DOSAGE RANGE	USE	ADVERSE EFFECTS	NURSING IMPLICATIONS
oxybutynin (Ditropan)	PO—5 mg q6–12h	To relieve symptoms associated with voiding in patients with neurogenic bladder	See atropine, *plus:* *CNS:* drowsiness, dizziness, insomnia *Endocrine:* impotence, suppressed lactation *GU:* urinary hesitancy and retention *GI:* nausea, vomiting, bloated feeling, constipation *Eyes:* blurred vision, increased ocular tension	See atropine, *plus:* Assist with activities as necessary. Assess sleep pattern. Warn patients about possible impotence and interference with lactation. Evaluate voiding pattern and keep record of daily I&O.
scopolamine (Hyoscine)	PO—0.4 mg–1 mg tid to qid IM, SC, IV—0.3 mg–0.6 mg tid to qid	To sedate and decrease salivation in parkinsonism, spastic states and cases of cerebral excitation, such as delirium tremens, hysteria, and mania; use as a preoperative medication with morphine or meperidine to inhibit secretions of the respiratory tract and salivary glands; to prevent motion sickness	Disorientation, delirium, increased pulse, dilated pupils, dry mouth and throat, decreased respirations	Evaluate mental status. Monitor pulse and respiratory rate. Note pupil size. Offer fluids if allowed.
propantheline (Pro-Banthine)	PO—15 mg 30 minutes berore meals and 30 mg at hs	Use with other drugs in treatment of peptic ulcer; to reduce GI and urinary tract motility	*GI:* nausea, vomiting, diarrhea or constipation *ANS:* drying of salivary secretions, blurred vision, decreased perspiration, urinary retention. *CNS:* headache, dizziness, drowsiness, insomnia, nervousness, confusion, loss of sense of taste *Cardiovascular:* tachycardia, palpitations *Endocrine:* impotence, suppressed lactation *Others:* weakness, allergic reactions	Caution the patient not to engage in dangerous activities. Keep stool chart. Assist with activities as necessary. Evaluate mental status. Note any change in sleep pattern. Evaluate visual acuity. Note changes in body secretions. Monitor pulse. Warn patients of possible change in sexual function and milk production. Watch for allergic reactions. Record I&O.
dicyclomine (Bentyl)	PO—10 mg–20 mg tid to qid IM—20 mg q4–6h	Use with other drugs in the treatment of peptic ulcer; to treat irritable colon, spastic colon, mucous colitis, acute enterocolitis, and infant colic	See propantheline.	See propantheline.
phenobarbital + hyoscyamine + atropine + scopolamine (Donnatal)	PO—1–2 tablets, capsules, or tsp q6–8h	Use to treat peptic ulcer, irritable and spastic colon, mucous colitis, and acute enterocolitis	*With high doses:* blurred vision, dysuria, flushed, dry skin, dry mouth	

The most commonly used cholinergic drug with direct action is bethanechol chloride (Urecholine). Bethanechol is given to relieve the postoperative distention due to lack of motility, which causes gas to accumulate in the intestine. It is also helpful in relieving urinary retention. It does this by increasing parasympathetic constriction of the bladder detrusor and opening the bladder sphincter.

Indirect cholinergic drugs, such as neostigmine (Prostigmin) and pyridostigmine (Mestinon), are used mainly to treat neurologic disease.

Adverse effects

Cholinergic drugs affect so many body structures that adverse effects are many and varied. Nausea, vomiting, diarrhea, abdominal cramps, sweating, and increased salivation are common. Flushing is due to dilation of surface blood vessels. Blood pressure and heart rate may drop. The patient may complain of difficulty in breathing. It is these adverse effects that limit the use of cholinergics.

NURSING IMPLICATIONS

Cholinergics are contraindicated if any obstruction is suspected or present in the gastrointestinal or genitourinary system. Urinary output should be measured carefully after each voiding to assess the effectiveness of cholinergics given to relieve urinary retention. Listen for bowel sounds, and keep a stool chart.

ANTICHOLINERGIC OR CHOLINERGIC-BLOCKING DRUGS

The anticholinergic drugs inhibit ACh. Because they negate parasympathetic action they are sometimes referred to as parasympatholytic drugs. These drugs prevent parasympathetic impulses from traveling from one neuron to another or to muscle fibers. The result is an action that mimics the function of the sympathetic nervous system.

Anticholinergics relax smooth muscle, inhibit secretion of glands, and dilate the pupils (see Table 18-1). Thus, they are widely used as antispasmodics in diseases and disorders of the gastrointestinal system. They decrease both the secretions and motility of the stomach and intestine and relieve smooth muscle spasms. In the genitourinary system these drugs relax the ureters and decrease the tone of the bladder fundus, as well as the detrusor muscle. Specific conditions that respond to this antispasmodic action are peptic ulcer, spastic colon, gastritis, ulcerative colitis, pylorospasm, enuresis (bed wetting), hypertonicity of the urinary bladder and ureters, and renal colic. They may also be used to reverse the action of cholinergic drugs in cases of overdose.

Anticholinergics are derived from natural plant sources or are synthesized. The natural anticholinergics are belladonna (tincture, extract, and fluid extract), atropine, and scopolamine. Because these natural drugs have such widespread effects in the body, their use as antispasmodics is limited. In an effort to decrease the adverse effects and at the same time produce stable drugs with specific action, chemists developed synthetic anticholinergics. Methantheline bromide (Banthine) and propantheline bromide (Pro-Banthine) are synthetic anticholinergics given to diminish gastric hypermotility and hypersecretion. They slow stomach action, secretions, and peristalsis, causing delayed emptying.

Adverse effects

The adverse effects experienced with the anticholinergic drugs may be annoying and uncomfortable but are not often serious. Drowsiness and dry mouth are common. There may be photophobia and blurred vision. Constipation can easily occur due to the decrease in gastrointestinal motility.

Although there is a wide margin of safety with drugs in the belladonna group, occasionally overdose or atropinism occurs. It may result from either incorrect measurement or, in children, overingestion. The signs and symptoms are dry, burning mouth with increased thirst; hot, dry, flushed skin with or without rash; elevated temperature; and a weak and rapid pulse. The patient is restless, weak, and confused. He may complain of urgency, frequency, or difficulty in voiding.

NURSING IMPLICATIONS

Anticholinergics should not be used when prostatic hypertrophy is present, since they can cause urinary retention that would aggravate the problem. It is important to measure these medications (especially those in liquid form) carefully, since overdosing can be serious.

To relieve dry mouth, offer ice chips, hard candies, and frequent mouth care. Be sure to check the patient's diet order before giving water or candy. Patients with photophobia should be encouraged to wear dark glasses. In the hospital, turn overhead lights off and draw the shades. Try to use indirect lighting whenever possible. Keep accurate output records of urine and stools. Watch for constipation or urinary retention.

Persons taking anticholinergics should be warned about driving or operating heavy machinery, since drowsiness may create a safety hazard. Blurred vision may also increase the possibility of an auto accident.

PRACTICE PROBLEMS—ANTISPASMODICS

1. The order reads: propantheline (Pro-Banthine) 15 mg PO $\frac{1}{2}$ h $\overline{ac}$ and hs.

    The label reads: propantheline 7.5 mg/tablet. How many tablets will you give?

    $$\frac{D}{H} = G$$

    $$\frac{2 \; \cancel{15 \; mg}}{1 \; \cancel{7.5 \; mg}} = 2 \text{ tablets}$$

    You would give 2 tablets of propantheline (Pro-Banthine).

2. Neostigmine (Prostigmin) 0.5 mg IM is ordered to be given daily. Neostigmine comes 0.25 mg/ml. How many milliliters will be given?

    $$\frac{D}{H} \times A = G$$

    $$\frac{0.5 \; \cancel{mg}}{0.25 \; \cancel{mg}} \times 1 \text{ ml} = G$$

    $$2 \times 1 \text{ ml} = 2 \text{ ml}$$

    You will give 2 ml of neostigmine (Prostigmin).

Work the following problems:

1. The order reads: dicyclomine (Bentyl) 15 mg PO tid.
    The label reads: dicyclomine 10 mg/tablet.
    How many tablets will you give?

2. The order reads: bethanechol (Urecholine) 2.5 mg SC qid.
    The label reads: bethanechol 5 mg/ml.
    How much would you give?

Answers are given on p. 283.

CHAPTER 19
Emetics and antiemetics

EMETICS

Emetics are substances that induce vomiting, thus their primary use is in cases of poisoning. Although gastric lavage has become the treatment of choice in such situations, emetics are still used in the home. The danger associated with emetics is that there are certain situations when vomiting should not be induced:

> If the poison swallowed is caustic (example—lye)
>
> If the patient is comatose or has difficulty in swallowing
>
> If the ingested substance has petroleum as an ingredient

Common household substances may often serve as emetics. For example, plain starch, salt, mustard, mild soapsuds in warm water, or simply large amounts of warm water will induce vomiting. In the hospital, apomorphine, an opium preparation, may be given by injection and is generally effective within 2 minutes (in children) to 15 minutes (adults). Ipecac syrup is an emetic available without a prescription (see Table 19-1).

NURSING IMPLICATIONS

When giving an emetic, be sure the patient is positioned correctly to avoid aspiration of any vomitus. If vomiting has not occurred within 30 minutes of administration, the patient should have gastric lavage.

ANTIEMETICS

Antiemetics are drugs given to relieve the symptoms of nausea and vomiting. Vomiting may be caused by many factors from strong emotion to gastrointestinal or ear diseases. In any case, either the stomach or the inner ear sends impulses to the brain's vomiting center, and the stomach empties. Antiemetics work to block the impulses from the stomach or inner ear.

Household remedies for vomiting include plain hot tea, room-temperature carbonated soft drinks, and cola syrup. Over-the-counter medications, such as Pepto-Bismol and Alka-Seltzer, may also help relieve the nausea that usually precedes vomiting.

Many groups of drugs have antiemetic properties in addition to their major pharmacologic action. Sedatives, hypnotics, and anticholinergics can all have an antiemetic effect, but due to their other adverse effects, they are not usually given. Antihistamines, like dimenhydrinate (Dramamine), diphenhydramine (Benadryl), and cyclizine (Marezine) are given for their antiemetic effect (see Chapter 26). One of the most frequently used antiemetic drugs is a phenothiazine, prochlorperazine (Compazine, see Chapter 6). It is not very helpful in motion sickness but is highly effective in most other cases of nausea and vomiting. Promethazine

(Text continues on p. 156.)

TABLE 19-1 EMETICS AND ANTIEMETICS

DRUG	ROUTE AND DOSAGE RANGE	USE	ADVERSE EFFECTS	NURSING IMPLICATIONS
EMETICS				
apomorphine	SC—2 mg–10 mg; do not repeat	To induce vomiting	CNS depression, euphoria, increased respirations, restlessness, tremors	Stay with the patient. Vomiting will usually result after 10–15 minutes. Monitor vital signs. Evaluate mental status. Note abnormal muscle movements.
ipecac	PO Adult—15 ml Child less than 1 yr—5 ml–10 ml; repeat in 20 min if necessary Follow dose with ½–1 glassful (child) and 1–2 glassfuls (adult) of water	To induce vomiting in emergencies (drug overdose and certain types of poisoning)	Fluid and electrolyte imbalance from prolonged or severe vomiting	Do not give in cases in which poisoning was caused by a petroleum product (kerosene, gasoline, coal oil, fuel oil, paint thinner, cleaning fluid), lye, strong acid, or strychnine. Check electrolyte levels. Stay with the patient.
ANTIEMETICS				
benzquinamide (Emete-con)	IM—50 mg; may repeat in 1 hr, then q3–4h IV—25 mg administered slowly; subsequent doses should be given IM.	To prevent and treat nausea and vomiting associated with anesthesia and surgery	*ANS:* dry mouth, shivering, sweating, hiccoughs, flushing, salivation, blurred vision *Cardiovascular:* hypertension, hypotension, cardiac arrhythmias *CNS:* drowsiness, insomnia, restlessness, headache, nervousness, excitement *GI:* anorexia, nausea *Others:* twitching, shaking, tremors, weakness, hives, rash, chills, increased temperature	Inject well within a large muscle (do not inject into lower or mid-third of upper arm). Monitor BP, apical pulse, and temperature. Do not give IV to patient with cardiovascular disease. Observe patient for excessive CNS stimulation or depression (a sign of overdose). Assist with activities as necessary. Evaluate mental status. Note any unusual muscle movements. Check skin for color change, rash, or hives.
dimenhydrinate (Dramamine)	PO, IM—50 mg–100 mg q4h IV—50 mg in 10 ml NS	To prevent and treat nausea, vomiting, or vertigo due to motion sickness	Drowsiness	Caution patients not to drive or engage in other dangerous activities.
diphenhydramine (Benadryl)	PO—50 mg tid to qid IM, IV—10 mg–100 mg tid to qid	To prevent and treat motion sickness; to treat allergic conditions; to treat parkinsonism, including that caused by drugs	*CNS:* headache, sedation, dizziness, incoordination, confusion, lethargy, restlessness, excitement, irritability, tremor, insomnia, euphoria, paresthesias, blurred or double vision, vertigo, tinnitus, hysteria, convulsions *Cardiovascular:* hypotension, palpitations, tachycardia, arrhythmias	Caution patients not to drive or engage in other dangerous activities. Evaluate mental status. Keep stool chart. Record I&O. Evaluate appetite. Note changes in sleeping pattern. Offer fluids if allowed. Check skin for change in color, rash, or hives. Evaluate visual acuity. Monitor vital signs. Assist with activities as necessary.

(continued on page 155)

TABLE 19-1 (continued)

DRUG	ROUTE AND DOSAGE RANGE	USE	ADVERSE EFFECTS	NURSING IMPLICATIONS
diphenhydramine (*continued*)			*Respiratory:* thick bronchial secretions, tight feeling in the chest, wheezing, nasal stuffiness *GI:* GI distress, nausea, vomiting, anorexia, diarrhea or constipation, dry mouth, nose and throat *GU:* problems with urination, early menses *Skin:* rash, hives, increased perspiration, photosensitivity *Others:* anaphylaxis, chills, blood disorders	Record all emesis. Note any abnormal muscle movements. Evaluate hearing. Watch for respiratory difficulties due to increased thick secretions. Avoid brightly lit areas and direct sun. Blood tests should be ordered at regular intervals. Adverse effects are much more likely to occur in the elderly patient.
meclizine (Antivert, Bonine)	PO—25 mg–100 mg qd in divided doses	See dimenhydrinate, *plus:* To manage vertigo associated with vestibular disease	Drowsiness, dry mouth, blurred vision	See dimenhydrinate.
promethazine (Phenergan)	IM, IV, PO, PR—12.5 mg–25 mg q4–6h (up to 50 mg may be given for sedation)	To treat allergic reactions, motion sickness, and nausea and vomiting associated with certain types of surgery and anesthesia; use as a sedative for operative procedures, obstetrics, and apprehension; use in combination with analgesics to control postoperative pain	*CNS:* dizziness, drowsiness, lethargy, parkinsonism, incoordination, tinnitus, blurred or double vision, excitation, euphoria, insomnia, nervousness, tremors, seizures, hysteria, syncope *Respiratory:* asthma, nasal congestion *GI:* nausea, vomiting, jaundice *Skin:* allergic reactions, photosensitivity *Others:* BP and pulse changes, blood disorders	See dimenhydrinate, *plus:* Note any abnormal muscle movements. Assist with activities as necessary. Evaluate hearing and vision. Evaluate mental status. Note changes in sleep pattern. Institute seizure precautions. Monitor vital signs. Check skin for rash, hives, or change in color.
thiethylperazine (Torecan)	PO—10 mg qd–tid IM—10 mg qd–tid PR—suppository (10 mg) qd–tid	To relieve nausea and vomiting	See promethazine, *plus:* *ANS:* dry mouth, nose, tinnitus, alterations in saliva flow and taste *Others:* peripheral edema of arms, hands, and face	See promethazine, *plus:* Be alert to complaints of over- and/or undersecretion in mouth. Assess for edema. Weigh daily.
trimethobenzamide (Tigan)	PO—250 mg tid or qid PR—200 mg (1 suppository) tid or qid IM—200 mg tid or qid	To control nausea and vomiting	*CNS:* headache, dizziness, drowsiness, disorientation, depression, parkinsonism, blurred vision, muscle cramps and spasms, convulsions, coma *GI:* diarrhea, jaundice *Skin:* allergic reactions, irritation at injection site	Caution patients not to drive or engage in other dangerous activities. Assist with activities as necessary. Note any abnormal muscle movements. Monitor BP. Evaluate visual acuity. Blood tests should be done at regular intervals.

(continued on page 156)

TABLE 19-1 (continued)

DRUG	ROUTE AND DOSAGE RANGE	USE	ADVERSE EFFECTS	NURSING IMPLICATIONS
trimethobenzamide (continued)			Others: hypotension, blood disorders	Evaluate mental status. Check skin for change in color or rash. Minimize irritation at injection site by using and Z-track method of injecting medication. Encourage fluid replacement. Monitor gluteal site electrolyte levels.

(Phenergan) is a phenothiazine derivative that is also frequently used as an antiemetic (see Table 19-1).

NURSING IMPLICATIONS

These drugs have a very low incidence of adverse effects. Common to all is the drowsiness they cause. Persons who take antiemetics should not perform potentially dangerous activities that require alert behavior.

Remember that psychological factors may play a large part in your patient's sensations of nausea. You may take advantage of the power of suggestion by explaining that the antiemetic drug you are giving will make him feel better. Finding ways to reduce noise, odor, vibrations, and discomfort as much as possible will help alleviate discomfort and soothe your patient. Remember that nausea and vomiting are usually symptoms of underlying disease. Although antiemetics may make your patient more comfortable, they may also mask serious disease.

PRACTICE PROBLEMS—EMETICS AND ANTIEMETICS

1. The order reads trimethobenzamide (Tigan) 200 mg IM q6h prn nausea. The patient is complaining of nausea. Trimethobenzamide comes 100 mg/ml. How much would you give?

$$\frac{D}{H} \times A = G$$

$$\frac{\overset{2}{\cancel{200}\text{ mg}}}{\underset{1}{\cancel{100}\text{ mg}}} \times 1 \text{ ml} = G$$

$$\frac{2}{1} \times 1 \text{ ml} = 2 \text{ ml}$$

Thus, 2 ml of trimethobenzamide (Tigan) is given.

Work the following problems:
1. The order reads: meclizine (Antivert) 25 mg PO tid.

The label reads: meclizine 12.5 mg/tablet. How much meclizine would you give?

2. The physician orders promethazine (Phenergan) 25 mg IM on call to the operating room. Promethazine comes 50 mg/ml. How much would you give?

3. The order reads: trimethobenzamide (Tigan) 250 mg PO q6h prn nausea.
The label reads: Each capsule contains 250 mg trimethobenzamide.
How much would you give if the patient complained of nausea?

Answers are given on p. 283.

CHAPTER 20
Diuretics

A diuretic is any substance that stimulates the flow of urine. Diuretics include liquids that are thoroughly familiar to us (tea, coffee, water), as well as medications prescribed to rid the body of excess fluid accumulated in the tissues (edema) (see Table 20-1).

Diuretics are prescribed to treat edema resulting from conditions other than kidney disease. The abnormal kidney rarely responds to them. The goal of diuretic therapy is to move the extra fluid out of the body by promoting the excretion of sodium and water, at the same time maintaining electrolyte balance. Conditions that cause edema and are effectively treated with diuretics include congestive heart failure (CHF), liver disease (ascites), hypertension, pregnancy, and edema due to other drugs (principally the corticosteroids).

When used in patients suffering from CHF, diuretics reduce the edema and thus relieve severe dyspnea. This decreases the patient's fear of suffocation. The reduced fluid load also decreases the effort required for body movements and reduces the demands on the heart for oxygen.

When used to treat hypertension, diuretics have a dual effect. First, by getting rid of excess body fluid, they decrease the amount of blood in circulation. This lowers the blood pressure. If diuretics are given over long periods of time, they

This chapter is based on an article by the author, which originally appeared in *The Journal of Practical Nursing*. Part I, Diuretics: Uses and effects, 27:12, 1977; Part II, Diuretics: Nursing care for the patient on diuretics, 28:1, 1978.

cause dilation of the arterioles, which even further lowers blood pressure.

Diuretics are also used to treat conditions in which edema is not present, such as glaucoma, epilepsy, poisoning, and oliguria. Occasionally, diuretics are used to aid in weight reduction, especially if the person has a tendency to retain fluids.

Because each diuretic has advantages and disadvantages, the selection of a specific diuretic is influenced by its potency, its onset, its peak and duration of action, and its adverse effects. Diuretics are often classified by their mechanism of action, their chemical composition, or the site in the kidney nephron where they exert their effects. The electrolyte movements involved are extremely important, since they influence whether the patient recovers or gets worse due to electrolyte imbalance.

ELECTROLYTE IMBALANCES

Hypochloremia—Low chloride (Cl)
Hyperkalemia—Increased potassium (K)
Hypokalemia—Low potassium
Hypomagnesemia—Low magnesium (Mg)
Hyponatremia—Low sodium (Na)

OTHER IMBALANCES

Hyperglycemia—Increased sugar
Hyperuricemia—Increased uric acid

(*Text continues on p. 161.*)

TABLE 20-1 DIURETICS

DRUG	ROUTE AND DOSAGE RANGE	USE	ADVERSE EFFECTS	NURSING IMPLICATIONS
OSMOTIC				
mannitol (Osmitrol)	IV—50 g–200 g qd (may be a single dose)	To treat cerebral edema associated with increased intracranial pressure; oliguria due to surgery, burns, and trauma; increased intraocular pressure due to glaucoma, sedative overdose; mercury poisoning; preoperative medicine for brain or eye surgery	*CNS:* headache, mental confusion *Cardiovascular:* hypotension, circulatory overload *GI:* nausea, vomiting *Other:* hyponatremia	Onset of action is 30 minutes to 1 hour. Peak action is in 2 to 3 hours. Duration of action may be up to 10 hours. Administer carefully; extravasation causes tissue irritation and necrosis. Monitor BP and pulse. Check electrolyte levels. Assess mental status. Keep accurate I&O. Check weight daily.
THIAZIDES				
chlorothiazide (Diuril)	PO, IV—0.5 g–1 g qd or bid	To treat hypertension, CHF, edema associated with hepatic and renal disease; to treat edema secondary to corticosteroid and estrogen therapy; to treat premenstrual fluid retention, fluid retention during obesity, nephrotic syndrome, acute glomerular nephritis, chronic renal failure, edema and toxemia of pregnancy	*CNS:* weakness, lethargy, depression, drowsiness, restlessness, muscle pains or cramps, dizziness, dull headache, paresthesias *Cardiovascular:* orthostatic hypotension, irregular pulse, tachycardia, cardiac arrhythmias *GI:* dry mouth, thirst, anorexia, nausea, vomiting, decreased GI motility *GU:* oliguria, glycosuria *Others:* increased blood levels of sugar, uric acid, and urea, electrolyte imbalances, photosensitivity	Onset of action is 1 to 2 hours. Duration of action is 6 to 12 hours. Check electrolyte levels and blood work. Assess mental status. Ambulate with assistance if necessary. Check BP, pulse, and respiration. Check urine for sugar and blood. Strain urine. Assess nutritional status. Keep stool chart. Keep accurate I&O. Check weight daily. Avoid brightly lit areas and direct sunlight.
hydrochlorothiazide (Hydrodiuril, Esidrix, Oretic)	PO—25 mg–200 mg qd (single dose or divided)	See chlorothiazide.	See chlorothiazide.	See chlorothiazide.
methyclothiazide (Enduron)	PO—2.5 mg–10 mg qd (single dose or divided)	See chlorothiazide.	See chlorothiazide.	See chlorothiazide, *plus:* Duration of action is 24 hours.
metolazone (Zaroxolyn, Diulo)	PO—2.5 mg–20 mg qd as a single dose	To treat hypertension (either alone or with other antihypertensives in more serious disease): to treat salt and water retention in edema accompanying CHF and renal disease	*CNS:* dizziness, drowsiness, vertigo, headache, fatigue, weakness, restlessness *Cardiovascular:* chest pain, palpitations, orthostatic hypotension, increased volume depletion, hemoconcentration, venous thrombosis, blood disorders, syncope	Ambulate with assistance and assist with other activities as necessary. Monitor apical pulse and blood pressure (both lying and standing). Blood tests should be done at regular intervals to check liver function and for metabolic disorders. Assess appetite. Keep a stool chart.

(continued on page 159)

TABLE 20-1 (continued)

DRUG	ROUTE AND DOSAGE RANGE	USE	ADVERSE EFFECTS	NURSING IMPLICATIONS
metolazone (*continued*)			*GI:* dry mouth, anorexia, nausea, vomiting, diarrhea or constipation, abdominal bloating, epigastric distress, jaundice, hepatitis *Skin:* rash, hives *Others:* electrolyte imbalances, chills, sugar in the blood and urine, gout attacks, muscle cramps or pain, liver dysfunction	Note skin color. Observe skin for any rash or hives. Test urine for sugar. Note any complaints of muscle discomfort, or pain in joints, especially in the large toe.
chlorthalidone (Hygroton)	PO—25 mg–100 mg/day as a single dose	See chlorothiazide.	See chlorothiazide.	See chlorothiazide.
POTASSIUM-SPARING				
amiloride (Midamor)	PO—5 mg–20 mg/day	Used in combination with other diuretics in treating CHF or hypertension to restore and maintain normal serum potassium levels	*CNS:* headache, weakness, lethargy, dizziness, mental changes *GI:* nausea, anorexia, diarrhea, vomiting, abdominal pains, gas pains, changes in appetite, constipation *Others:* muscle cramps cough, dyspnea, impotence	Onset of action is within 2 hours. Peak action in 6–10 hours. Duration of action is 24 hours. Carefully monitor potassium levels. Observe for any change in mental status. Keep stool chart. Evaluate appetite. Note character of respirations. Warn patient of possible impotence. Note any complaints of muscle cramps. Always give with food. Weigh patient daily.
amiloride + hydrochlorothiazide (Moduretic)	PO—1–2 tablets/day with meals	See amiloride and hydrochlorothiazide.	See amiloride and hydrochlorothiazide.	See amiloride and hydrochlorothiazide.
spironolactone (Aldactone)	PO—25 mg–400 mg qd in divided doses	To treat conditions where increased aldosterone is produced; to treat nephrotic syndrome; to treat hepatic cirrhosis with ascites; to treat hypokalemia, CHF, and essential hypertension	*CNS:* drowsiness, ataxia, headache, mental changes *Endocrine:* gynecomastia, irregular menses, hirsutism *Others:* electrolyte imbalances, rash	Assist with activities as necessary. Evaluate mental status. Warn patients about possible changes in breast size and other hormonal problems. Check electrolyte levels at regular intervals. Inspect skin for any signs of rash.
spironolactone + hydrochlorothiazide (Aldactazide)	PO—1–2 tablets qd to qid	To treat edema in patients with CHF, hepatic cirrhosis accompanied by edema or ascites, and the nephrotic syndrome; to treat essential hypertension	See spironolactone and hydrochlorothiazide.	Onset of action is within 1 hour. Peak action is in 1 to 2 hours. Duration of action is 5 to 10 hours, *plus:* See spironolactone and hydrochlorothiazide.

(continued on page 160)

TABLE 20-1   (continued)

DRUG	ROUTE AND DOSAGE RANGE	USE	ADVERSE EFFECTS	NURSING IMPLICATIONS
triamterene (Dyrenium)	PO—100 mg–150 mg bid after meals	To treat edema associated with CHF, cirrhosis of the liver, nephrotic syndrome, corticosteroid-induced edema, idiopathic edema and hypertension (in combination)	*CNS:* weakness, headache, malaise, muscle irritation, flaccid paralysis *Cardiovascular:* cold extremities, serious ECG changes *GI:* nausea, vomiting, diarrhea, dry mouth, intestinal cramping *GU:* oliguria, anuria *Other:* electrolyte imbalances, especially hyperkalemia	Assist with activities as necessary. Evaluate mental status. Note complaints of muscle discomfort or weakness. Check temperature of extremities. Monitor apical pulse. Keep stool chart. Record I&O, and note changes in urinary output. Electrolyte levels should be checked at regular intervals.
triamterene + hydrochlorothiazide (Dyazide, Maxzide)	PO—1–2 capsules or tablets qd–bid after meals	See triamterene.	See triamterene and hydrochlorothiazide.	Onset of action is within 1 hour. Peak action is in 2 to 3 hours. Duration of action is 7 to 9 hours.

CARBONIC ANHYDRASE INHIBITORS

DRUG	ROUTE AND DOSAGE RANGE	USE	ADVERSE EFFECTS	NURSING IMPLICATIONS
acetazolamide (Diamox)	PO, IV—250 mg–1.5 g qd (amounts greater than 250 mg should be given in divided doses)	To treat glaucoma, CHF, and epilepsy (petit mal and grand mal)	*CNS:* fatigue, drowsiness, confusion, face and extremity paresthesias *Others:* anorexia, hives, metabolic acidosis, thirst, glycosuria	Assess mental status. Assist with activity if necessary. Inspect skin. Check urine for sugar. Keep accurate I&O. Check weight daily.

POTENT OR LOOP

DRUG	ROUTE AND DOSAGE RANGE	USE	ADVERSE EFFECTS	NURSING IMPLICATIONS
bumetanide (Bumex)	PO—0.5 mg–2 mg as a single dose (repeated if necessary) IM, IV—0.5 mg–1 mg (repeated if necessary) Maximum daily dosage is 10 mg.	To treat edema associated with CHF, hepatic and renal disease, nephrotic syndrome	*CNS:* dizziness, vertigo, headache, muscle cramps, changes in mental status, impaired hearing, weakness, fatigue *Cardiovascular:* hypotension, chest pain, changes in ECG *GI:* nausea, vomiting, diarrhea, abdominal pain, upset stomach *Others:* rash, hives, itching, joint pain, sweating, hyperventilation, dry mouth, premature ejaculation, impotence, electrolyte imbalance (especially hypokalemia)	Onset of action: PO—30–60 minutes IV—5 minutes Peak action: PO—1–2 hours IV—15–45 minutes Duration of action: PO—4–6 hours IV—3–6 hours Check electrolyte levels. Inspect skin for any changes. Evaluate mental status. Assess hearing. Keep stool chart. Keep accurate I&O. Weigh daily. Monitor B/P, respiration. Warn male patients about possible problems with sexual function.
furosemide (Lasix)	PO—20 mg–80 mg; repeat in 6–8 hr prn (in severe cases to a maximum of 600 mg qd) IV, IM—20 mg–40 mg injected slowly; if necessary, after 1–2 hr, repeat dose of 20 mg–80 mg	To treat edema of CHF, acute pulmonary edema, hepatic cirrhosis with ascites, nephrotic syndrome, lymphedema, and hypertension	*CNS:* dizziness, tinnitus, deafness *GI:* nausea, vomiting, diarrhea *Others:* electrolyte imbalance (especially hypokalemia), rash, dehydration	Onset of action: PO—within 1 hour IV—within 5 minutes Peak action: PO—within 2 hours IV—within 30 minutes Duration of action: PO—4–8 hours IV—2 hours Pain may be present at injection site. Check electrolyte levels.

(continued on page 161)

TABLE 20-1 (continued)

DRUG	ROUTE AND DOSAGE RANGE	USE	ADVERSE EFFECTS	NURSING IMPLICATIONS
furosemide (*continued*)				Inspect skin. Assess hearing. Keep accurate I&O. Check weight daily.
ethacrynic acid (Edecrin)	PO—50 mg–200 mg qd to bid IV—0.5 mg–1 mg/kg qd (to a maximum of 100 mg in critical situation)	See furosemide.	See furosemide, *plus:* decreased urinary urate excretion causing hyperuricemia; severe anorexia, tetany, severe diarrhea	See furosemide, *plus:* Strain urine. Assess appetite. Keep stool chart. Evaluate muscle tone.

A basic principle of fluid and electrolyte balance is that the flow of water follows the flow of sodium in the body. Whenever sodium is absorbed, so is water. If sodium leaves the body, water follows. Other electrolytes behave in predictable ways when diuretics cause changes in fluid balance. Possible electrolyte imbalances caused by diuretics are listed in the chart in this section.

CLASSIFICATION OF DIURETICS

Osmotic diuretics cause excretion of large amounts of urine but are rarely used to treat generalized edema. They are used in certain serious conditions, such as cerebral edema associated with increased intracranial pressure; oliguria due to surgery, burns and trauma; and increased intraocular pressure due to acute congestive glaucoma. Osmotic diuretics are also helpful in promoting the excretion of toxic substances resulting from sedative overdose. They are occasionally given as preoperative medications to patients undergoing brain or eye surgery. Mercurials, although highly effective as diuretics, are now usually replaced by oral diuretics.

Thiazides are the most commonly used diuretics. They are available in oral form and are considered safe, effective, and convenient. There are many different thiazide compounds, each differing mainly in potency. The major action of this group of diuretics is to prevent sodium from reentering the circulation in the kidney. Renal excretion of sodium, chloride, and water is thereby increased. The thiazides also significantly increase potassium excretion.

Conditions effectively treated with thiazide diuretics include the edema of CHF, edema and toxemia of pregnancy, premenstrual edema, edema caused by steroids, and mild to moderate hypertension. These diuretics are generally considered short-acting diuretics.

The most common and most dangerous adverse effect of the thiazides is hypokalemia, or potassium deficiency. This is because the drugs are often given over long periods of time and the body has no adequate way to conserve potassium. Hypokalemia may cause depression, generalized muscle weakness and cramps, progressive loss of appetite (anorexia), nausea, and irregular pulse.

Potassium-sparing diuretics, as the term suggests, prevent the loss of potassium. Diuretics in this group are seldom used alone. They are usually given with the thiazides, so maximum diuresis and conservation of potassium are achieved.

The potassium-sparing diuretics are prescribed in combination with thiazides for edema associated with liver and kidney diseases, in the management of hypertension, and to treat the edema associated with CHF. The most serious adverse effect of these drugs is hyperkalemia. If left untreated, it can lead to renal shutdown and complete heart block.

Carbonic anhydrase inhibitors are diuretics that block the action of the enzyme carbonic anhydrase. This enzyme functions to produce hydrogen ions and bicarbonate in the kidney. It is also involved in the production of aqueous humor in the eye. The drug used most often as a carbonic anhydrase inhibitor is acetazolamide. Conditions that are helped by this drug are glaucoma, epilepsy, and CHF.

Xanthine diuretics, such as theophylline, are seldom used since newer, more potent diuretics have proven as effective against pulmonary edema.

The *potent*, or *loop*, diuretics work in the kidney to promote the excretion of sodium, water, and large amounts of potassium. They are so potent that diuresis occurs within 1 hour of oral administration and within minutes of intravenous administration.

Potent diuretics are used to treat the edema of CHF, in hypertension (along with antihypertensive agents), and in renal disease. Severe imbalances of potassium, sodium, chlorine, calcium, and magnesium can occur during the course of therapy with these drugs. Tinnitus and deafness can occur following intravenous administration, although the oral route has also resulted in ototoxicity. If diuresis is too rapid, the patient may develop a rash and complain of lethargy, weakness, dizziness, anorexia, vomiting, diarrhea, leg cramps, abdominal discomfort, or mental confusion. These features can lead to circulatory collapse if left untreated.

Acidotic diuretics are salts that produce acidosis. When this happens, alkaline substances in the body move to fight the acidosis. This activity causes fluid to move out of the tissues and into the blood, resulting in diuresis. Acidotic diuretics are given by mouth.

NURSING IMPLICATIONS

Nurses play two fundamental roles in diuretic therapy. While the patient is in the hospital, medications must be administered and the patient carefully observed for his response to treatment. In the role of patient educator, the nurse must ensure that the patient understands why he has been placed on a diuretic regimen and is aware of the possible consequences of not following the doctor's orders. For example, a patient with "silent" hypertension may not perceive any reason to take his medication on the many days he feels well. The nurse must emphasize the importance of these drugs as part of the overall treatment. Although they cannot cure the disease, diuretics can prevent electrolyte imbalance, renal failure, and life-threatening arrhythmias.

Since the delicate balance of chemicals and fluids in the body is significantly affected by diuretics, their use must be carefully monitored. Regular doses are important. By helping the patient to understand the purpose of diuretics and the potential dangers they pose, the nurse increases the likelihood that they will be used most effectively.

The patient should be warned at the outset of therapy that the frequency and large quantities of urine are natural responses to the drug. Without this assurance he might become anixous or alarmed.

The nurse should also warn the patient that he may have to void several times during the night, although this nocturia usually ceases as the body stabilizes, after a few days of therapy. A bedpan or urinal should always be close by, even if the patient is ambulatory, since accurate measurement of all output is necessary. A calibrated device should be used to measure output. Strict and up-to-date recordings of intake and output should be kept near the patient's bedside.

The patient should be observed for signs of overhydration or dehydration. The nurse should carefully record these, as well as any changes in edema, such as the absence of pitting, decreased size of the abdomen, or decreased ascites. Frequent tests of specific gravity will show the relative concentration of urine as diuresis continues.

Vital signs, especially blood pressure, should be assessed regularly and a record made of any changes. If the patient has postural hypotension, he should be advised to get out of bed slowly or to wait for assistance. The patient should be weighed every day, preferably at the same time (before breakfast and after emptying the bladder), on the same scale, wearing the same clothes. It is not unusual for a patient to lose 10 to 20 pounds in one day of vigorous diuretic action.

Good nursing care of the patient receiving diuretics requires that special attention be paid to the skin covering edematous tissue, since it is poorly nourished and likely to break down. This can be avoided by frequent turning, range of motion exercises, and gentle massage with cream to bony prominences and weight-bearing areas of the body.

Because anorexia and fluid balance often go together, patients receiving diuretics need instruction regarding their special nutritional needs. The patient may need information about sodium-restricted diets. It is important that patients understand just what "salt restriction" means. Patients usually know they must avoid potato chips and extra salt from the shaker, but they often need instruction as to which other foods to avoid, such as ham, bacon, and sausage.

Another dietary concern is how to supplement potassium. Unfortunately, foods high in potassium are also high in calories, so it isn't possible to make up all potassium losses by increasing dietary potassium. One way to decrease salt intake and increase potassium intake at the same time is to have the patient use salt substitutes, which contain potassium, instead of table salt and cooking salt.

Patients on diuretics may suffer salt depletion

during the hot summer months, since sodium and potassium are lost in perspiration. In some cases the physician may discontinue diuretics during that time of the year.

Electrolyte levels should be closely watched, since even slight changes may have serious implications for the patient. Especially important are any changes in potassium, sodium chloride, and bicarbonate (HCO_3^-) levels. Blood urea nitrogen (BUN), creatinine, and uric acid levels should also be checked because they reflect renal function.

Potassium deficiency is often encountered during diuretic therapy, especially if the patient's diet is inadequate. The nurse should encourage patients to use salt substitutes, which contain potassium instead of sodium. A potassium drug supplement may be ordered (see Chapter 16).

Both nurse and patient should be familiar with the symptoms of hypokalemia, since it may lead to serious cardiac arrhythmias. Persons on diuretics who also take a digitalis preparation are at risk for digitalis toxicity, which may also cause cardiac arrhythmias. Since corticosteroids (see Chapter 34) also cause potassium loss, hypokalemia can easily occur if patients take both corticosteroids and diuretics. The physician should be notified at the first sign of dry mouth, thirst, weakness, drowsiness, restlessness, oliguria, muscle pain, or cramps.

Patients taking the potassium-sparing diuretics must avoid high potassium intake, since it may result in hyperkalemia. Commercial salt substitutes containing potassium should not be used by these patients. Symptoms of hyperkalemia include generalized weakness, nausea, cold extremities, diarrhea, intestinal cramping, flaccid paralysis, muscle irritation, and oliguria. These may lead to renal shutdown and complete heart block. The physician should be called immediately if any symptoms of hyperkalemia appear.

Patients with stomas should be watched carefully when receiving diuretics. Because these patients are already losing body fluid, their electrolyte balance is unstable. The administration of diuretics may make the fluid loss more forceful and cause serious illness. Blood tests to determine sugar content may be indicated if the patient has a family history of diabetes. His urine should be checked for sugar and acetone. Some diuretics are ototoxic. Special care must be taken when patients are receiving other ototoxic drugs, such as kanamycin and gentamicin.

PRACTICE PROBLEMS—DIURETICS

1. The order reads: hydrochlorothiazide (Esidrix) 25 mg PO daily.
   The label reads: 50 mg hydrochlorothiazide per tablet.
   How many tablets will you give?

   $$\frac{D}{H} = G$$

   $$\frac{1 \; \cancel{25} \; \cancel{mg}}{2 \; \cancel{50} \; \cancel{mg}} = \frac{1}{2} \; tablet$$

   You will give $\frac{1}{2}$ tablet of hydrochlorothiazide (Esidrix).

Work the following problems:

1. The order reads: furosemide (Lasix) 20 mg IM one time only.
   The label reads: furosemide 40 mg/4 ml.
   How many milliliters will be given?

2. The order reads: chlorthalidone (Hygroton) 50 mg PO daily.
   The label reads: chlorthalidone 50 mg/tablet.
   How many tablets will you give?

3. The order reads: furosemide (Lasix) 20 mg PO in AM.
   The label reads: furosemide 40 mg/tablet.
   How much will you give?

Answers are given on p. 283.

CHAPTER 21
Cathartics and stool softeners, enemas, and antidiarrheals

CATHARTICS AND STOOL SOFTENERS

Cathartics are medications given to induce bowel movements (see Table 21-1). Historically, they have been misused due to an early medical notion that the remedy for systemic disease was rapid and complete emptying of the bowel. Modern medicine discourages laxative use, since it is now understood that these drugs often cause problems rather than cure them.

Intermittent use of cathartics is indicated in a number of conditions, one common one being constipation. This condition exists when stools are abnormally hard in consistency and low in frequency. It can be the result of gastrointestinal disease, inadequate diet, lack of activity, emotional tension, the effect of drugs, or simply inattention to routine elimination. Cathartics may be given for the purpose of obtaining a stool specimen or to eliminate parasites responsible for intestinal infections. They may also be indicated when the bowel must be emptied and cleansed prior to diagnostic studies or operative procedures. Mild cathartics are given to patients who have undergone rectal or lower gastrointestinal surgery, to patients with cardiac disease or aneurysms, and to immobile patients to prevent impaction and straining that may aggravate their conditions.

Classification of cathartics

Cathartics are generally classified by degree of action and specifically classified by how they act. According to degree, or severity of action, cathartics are called *laxatives* (causing a few formed bowel movements with little or no cramping) or *purgatives* (causing many soft or liquid stools usually accompanied by cramping). There are five categories of cathartics classified according to how they act.

Irritant or *stimulant* cathartics cause increased peristalsis by irritating the sensory nerve endings in the bowel mucosa. One group of irritating cathartics are the anthraquinones, which act in the large intestine. They usually cause cramping and evacuation of the bowel in 6 to 24 hours. Examples of anthraquinones are cascara sagrada, senna, and danthron. These medications are available in powder, liquid, granule, tablet, and suppository form.

Another irritant substance is phenolphthalein. It is the major ingredient in popular over-the-counter cathartic preparations, such as Ex-Lax. It is a relatively mild, pleasant-tasting irritant. There is usually no cramping, with evacuation in 6 to 8 hours.

Castor oil is a fairly bland substance when taken by mouth, although the consistency is unpleasant. It has little cathartic action until it reaches the small intestine, where it breaks down to form irritating substances that continue down into the lower bowel. Great quantities of semiliquid stool are produced in 2 to 6 hours, with moderate cramping in most cases.

Bisacodyl (Dulcolax) is an irritant cathartic frequently used for thorough cleansing of the bowel prior to diagnostic tests or surgery. Bisacodyl sup-

TABLE 21-1 CATHARTICS AND STOOL SOFTENERS

DRUG	ROUTE AND DOSAGE RANGE	USE	ADVERSE EFFECTS	NURSING IMPLICATIONS
CATHARTICS				
biscodyl (Dulcolax)	PO—5 mg–30 mg qd PR—1 suppository (10 mg)	To treat acute and chronic constipation; to prepare the bowel for surgery, delivery, or diagnostic tests; use in bowel retraining programs and colostomy regulation	See cascara sagrada.	See cascara sagrada, *plus:* Do not give within 1 hour of antacids or milk.
cascara sagrada	PO—Powder—300 mg–1 g qd Extract—200 mg–400 mg qd Aromatic fluid extract 5 ml–15 ml qd	To promote bowel evacuation in post-surgical, postpartum, acute, and functional geriatric constipation, constipation due to drug effects, and constipation due to neurologic disease; to prepare the bowel for sigmoidoscopy	Occasional abdominal cramps, nausea, griping, loose stools; may discolor urine (pink, red, brown, or black)	Teach patients that frequent use of cathartics can result in dependence and loss of normal bowel function. Encourage fluid intake and dietary intake of bulk foods to promote good bowel habits. Keep stool chart. Warn patient of possible change in urine color.
castor oil (Neoloid)	PO—15 ml–60 ml qd	To treat isolated cases of constipation	See cascara sagrada.	See cascara sagrada.
glycerin	PR—1 suppository (3 g) qd	See mineral oil.	Rectal burning or itching, abdominal cramps, spasms of the rectal sphincter, increased mucus and possible bleeding from the rectum, dehydration	Encourage fluid intake. Keep stool chart. Test stool sample for presence of blood.
lactulose (Chronulac)	PO—15 ml–60 ml qd	To treat constipation, especially chronic cases	Gas pains, abdominal cramping, nausea, diarrhea	Reassure patient that abdominal discomfort is temporary. Keep a stool chart.
magnesium citrate	PO—100 ml–200 ml qd	To hasten the removal of poisons, parasites, and toxic anthelmintics from the GI tract; to prepare the bowel for surgery and diagnostic procedures	Possible electrolyte imbalance with prolonged use	Monitor electrolytes. Liquid should be kept chilled and served over ice.
mineral oil	PO—15 ml–45 ml qd	To relieve constipation in cases where straining at stool is contraindicated	May inhibit absorption of fat-soluble vitamins if taken within 2 hours of a meal	Offer at bedtime, on an empty stomach. Keep stool chart.
psyllium (Metamucil)	PO—2.5 g–30 g qd	To manage chronic constipation, irritable bowel syndrome, duodenal ulcer, diverticulitis, hemorrhoids, and constipation occurring during pregnancy, convalescence, and senility; use to increase the bulk of stools in patients with chronic watery diarrhea	Esophageal and bowel obstruction (if medication is given with insufficient amount of liquid)	Mix the powder by stirring it into a full glass of cool liquid and have the patient drink it immediately. (Follow with more liquid so at least 250 ml total is taken with each dose.) When given to treat chronic diarrhea, decrease the amount of liquid taken by ⅔. Keep stool chart.

(continued on page 167)

TABLE 21-1 (continued)

DRUG	ROUTE AND DOSAGE RANGE	USE	ADVERSE EFFECTS	NURSING IMPLICATIONS
psyllium + senna (PerDiem)	PO—1–2 rounded tsp taken with at least 8 oz of beverage qd–bid (at hs or before breakfast)	To treat constipation	None	Granules should be placed in the mouth and swallowed with a beverage. Do not chew granules. Keep a stool chart.
senna (Senokot)	PO—500 mg–2 g qd PR—1 suppository; repeat in 2 hr prn	See cascara sagrada	See cascara sagrada, *plus:* suppository may cause rectal burning or itching	See cascara sagrada.
sodium phosphate + sodium biphosphate (Fleet Phospho-Soda)	PO—20 ml–40 ml qd	See cascara sagrada	See cascara sagrada, *plus:* possible electrolyte imbalance	See cascara sagrada, *plus:* Monitor electrolytes. Liquid must be diluted with 3 to 4 ounces cold water and followed by 6 to 8 ounces cold water.
STOOL SOFTENERS				
docusate sodium (Colace)	PO—50 mg–200 mg qd	To soften hard stools in constipation, painful anorectal conditions, cardiac conditions, and when peristaltic stimulants are contraindicated	(Occasionally) bitter taste, throat irritation, nausea, rash	Liquid should be mixed in 3 to 4 ounces of milk or fruit juice to mask the taste. Check skin for rash. Keep stool chart.
docusate calcium (Surfak)	PO—50 mg–240 mg qd	See docusate sodium.	Mild abdominal cramps	Keep stool chart.
docusate sodium + casanthranol (Peri-Colace)	PO—1–4 capsule or tablet qd	To manage chronic or temporary constipation when peristaltic stimulation is needed	See docusate sodium, *plus:* abdominal cramps	Keep stool chart.

positories work in 15 to 60 minutes, while the tablets take from 6 to 12 hours to cause evacuation of bowel contents.

Saline cathartics work by osmotic action in the intestines. Hypertonic solutions draw water into the fecal material, while isotonic solutions inhibit water absorption from the fecal material. In either case, the increased bulk stimulates peristalsis and several loose stools result in 1 to 4 hours. These saline cathartics are used most often when powerful, quick action is desired to treat parasitic infection and poisoning and to obtain stool specimens.

Magnesium products mix in the stomach to form a cathartic substance, magnesium chloride. Sodium phosphate and sodium biphosphate are available in a solution, which is a relatively pleasant-tasting saline cathartic.

The *bulk* cathartics work in the most natural and least irritating way of all cathartics. They cause bowel distention by increasing the bulk of the fecal contents, which causes a reflex emptying of the bowel. They are slower acting (12 to 24 hours), but their action is prolonged (up to 3 days).

Household substances, such as bran, dried prunes, and figs, are bulk-forming cathartics. Methylcellulose, agar, carboxymethylcellulose, and psyllium seed are medicinal substances given orally that swell when in contact with fluid in the upper part of the intestine. They form a thick gel that increases the bulk and softness of stool. Psyllium seeds are sharp and cause irritation of the bowel mucosa, as well. These medications are available as powders, flakes, tablets, or syrups.

Lubricant or *emollient* cathartics soften the feces and reduce friction between them and the intestinal wall. The stool, therefore, slides more easily through the gastrointestinal tract. The lubricant cathartics are especially helpful in long-term therapy when the patient's condition necessitates passage of only soft stools. Rectal surgery, heart disease, and increased intracranial pressure are the types of situations that demand the passage of soft stools only. Mineral oil and olive oil are common examples of lubricant cathartics. Glycerin is another, available in both liquid and suppository form.

Stool softeners are sometimes refered to as "surface active agents" because they decrease the surface tension of the fecal mass, allowing water and fats to penetrate and soften it. The result is soft, formed stools. These cathartics take a few days to be effective, so they are not ordered when quick evacuation of the bowel is necessary.

NURSING IMPLICATIONS

Cathartics should not be given in a number of instances:

1. If the patient has had recent rectal surgery
2. In the presence of undiagnosed abdominal pain
3. If inflammation or obstruction of the bowel is suspected or present
4. In pregnancy
5. In the presence of gastrointestinal bleeding or anemia
6. If chronic or spastic constipation has been diagnosed

The misuse of cathartics can lead to the "laxative habit." When a laxative is taken and the bowel empties completely, there will be no bowel movement for 2 to 3 days. Persons overly concerned with bowel function will be alarmed at this and take more laxatives. With this continued laxative use, a normal stimulus for defecation does not occur and dependence on drug action rather than natural defecation reflex results. Patient teaching is, therefore, an important responsibility for the nurse who administers cathartics.

Patients need to be told that it is not necessary to have a bowel movement every day. There is no normal number of bowel movements per day or per week. What is important is that they receive adequate natural fiber (found in fruits, whole grains, and vegetables, such as carrots, beets, and cabbage),

water, and daily exercise and adhere to some sort of daily toilet routine.

The taste or consistency of some cathartic preparations is extremely unpleasant. There are several ways to make the medications more palatable. Agar, for instance, may be mixed with cereals, custards, or other foods. Citrus fruits or juices can mask the oily taste of mineral oil or castor oil. Magnesium solutions that are chilled and served over crushed ice are more pleasant to drink.

Bulk cathartics must be swallowed immediately. Tablets should not be chewed, and fluids must be drunk immediately after they are stirred to prevent obstruction in the upper gastrointestinal tract. Bulk cathartics should be administered with large amounts of water to ensure they pass quickly through the esophagus.

Timing is a factor to consider in giving cathartics. Do not give irritant cathartics that work quickly (*e.g.,* castor oil) at bedtime. Saline cathartics have the most rapid action when given in the morning after breakfast. They can cause gas and vomiting, however, and should be given with plenty of fluids.

If a cathartic produces complete bowel evacuation, there may be electrolyte imbalance due to loss of ions in the fecal contents. Hypokalemia, dehydration, alkalosis, or acidosis can be extremely dangerous, especially in the very young, elderly, or debilitated patient. Watch the electrolyte levels carefully in these patients.

Some irritant cathartics can cause the urine to turn red. Patients should be warned about this before it occurs.

The candy forms of laxatives available as over-the-counter medications may cause death if ingested in large amounts by children.

ENEMAS

An enema is any fluid introduced into the rectum for the purpose of aiding bowel movement. Enemas can be effective in evacuating the bowel without causing cramping or being absorbed systemically. Cleansing enemas are large amounts of fluid, usually plain water or soapsuds in water, which cause evacuation by irritant and bulk action.

Saline cathartics, such as sodium phosphate, are available in enema form as Fleets Enemas. Retention enemas contain small amounts of mineral, cottonseed, or olive oil. They soften the stool so it can readily pass out of the rectum. Docusate sodium

(Colace) is also available in an enema preparation to promote soft stools.

ANTIDIARRHEALS

Diarrhea is the rapid movement of feces through the intestine, resulting in abnormally frequent, watery stools. Absorption of water, nutritive elements, and electrolytes is decreased, and the patient usually complains of abdominal cramps and generalized weakness. The major causes of diarrhea are local irritation by infectious or chemical substances, and emotional disorders that increase peristalsis. Diarrhea is, therefore, a symptom of underlying disease.

Because the results of diarrhea can be serious

(dehydration, exhaustion, electrolyte imbalance, and malnutrition), medications are given to decrease the frequency of bowel movements. Diarrhea owing to intestinal parasites is usually self-limiting because the frequent stools carry the offending virus, bacteria, or other organism away. In these cases no medication is necessary. In other cases either systemic or locally acting antidiarrheals are ordered.

Systemic antidiarrheals belong to the narcotic analgesic, sedative, and antispasmodic groups of drugs discussed in previous chapters. Specifically used as antidiarrheals are the opium preparations and the anticholinergic drugs (Table 21-2). These substances act on intestinal smooth muscle to slow down peristalsis and relax the spasm caused by parasympathetic nerve stimulation.

TABLE 21-2 ANTIDIARRHEALS

DRUG	ROUTE AND DOSAGE RANGE	USE	ADVERSE EFFECTS	NURSING IMPLICATIONS
diphenoxylate + atropine (Lomotil)	PO—5 mg qd–qid	To treat diarrhea	*CNS:* numb extremities, drowsiness, restlessness, headache, dizziness, depression, malaise, euphoria, coma, possible dependency *GI:* anorexia, swollen gums, GI discomfort, paralytic ileus *Skin:* dry skin and mucous membranes, flushing, rash, itching, hives *Others:* increased temperature and decreased respiratory rate, tachycardia, urinary retention	Offer fluids as allowed. Monitor vital signs. Record and evaluate I&O. Check skin and inside of mouth for reactions. Evaluate mental status. Assist with activities as necessary. Keep stool chart. Check for dependency.
kaolin + pectin (Kaopectate)	PO—60 ml–120 ml tid or prn	To treat diarrhea	None	Keep stool chart.
loperamide (Imodium)	PO—initial dose—4 mg; then 2 mg after each unformed stool (to a maximum 16 mg qd) Maintenance—4 mg–8 mg qd as a single dose or in divided doses	To relieve acute nonspecific diarrhea and chronic diarrhea associated with inflammatory bowel disease; use to reduce the volume of ileostomy discharge	*CNS:* dizziness, drowsiness, fatigue *GI:* abdominal discomfort, nausea, vomiting, constipation, dry mouth *Other:* rash	Assist with activities as necessary. Keep a stool chart. Watch for signs of dependency.
paregoric (Camphorated opium tincture)	PO—5 ml–40 ml qd	To relieve diarrhea; to treat mild physical narcotic dependence in infants born to addicted mothers	Nausea, GI disturbances, physical dependence after prolonged use	Dilute in water. Keep stool chart (do not continue to give if stools become formed).

Many types of antidiarrheal drugs have a *local* effect. *Demulcent* preparations are given to soothe irritated mucosa. *Adsorbent* antidiarrheals attract the offending substances and carry them out of the body. If an irritant is suspected of causing the diarrhea, a cathartic is sometimes given to empty the entire bowel. In this way the causative substance shall be eliminated. *Astringents* work in a manner similar to that of the demulcents. They soothe but do not treat the cause of the diarrhea. These medications shrink the swollen mucosa and cover it with a protective coating. *Anti-infectives* are used to treat bacillary dysentery, "travelers' diarrhea," or other conditions where infectious organisms are the cause of the diarrhea.

Diarrhea can be caused by reduction in normal flora following long-term or vigorous anti-infective therapy. In these cases, drugs such as lactobacillus (Lactinex) that aid the regrowth of intestinal flora are given. Buttermilk will also promote regrowth of bacteria.

NURSING IMPLICATIONS

Since antidiarrheal drugs deal with a symptom of underlying disease, there is always the danger that serious problems will be masked. Any persistent diarrhea or prolonged use of antidiarrheal drugs should be evaluated by a physician.

In general, antidiarrheal drugs have few adverse effects when taken as ordered. Overzealous use, however, can cause constipation. An accurate recording of the number and character of stools should be kept, so that the effect of medications can be evaluated.

Some household products, such as buttermilk, yogurt, and raw apples, are helpful against diarrhea because they contain pectin.

PART 5
Drugs used to help meet patients' needs for the intake, transportation, and utilization of oxygen

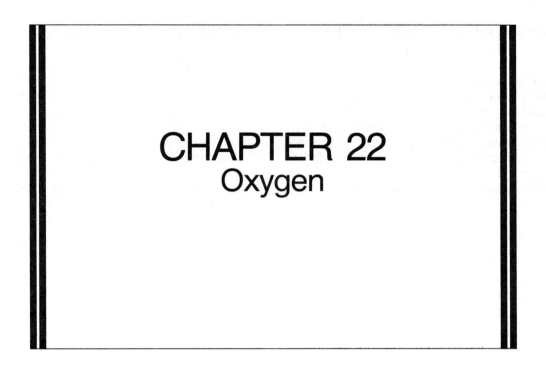

CHAPTER 22
Oxygen

Respiration is the process by which oxygen from the air breathed is taken into the body and used in the production of energy. It is almost always an involuntary function controlled by the respiratory center in the brain, although the rate and rhythm of respiration may be under voluntary control at times. Respiratory rate and rhythm are also affected by physical factors (blood levels of oxygen and carbon dioxide) and emotional states (fear, pain, stress).

A continuous supply of oxygen is necessary to maintain life. When oxygen intake is insufficient, all body systems may be affected. Especially vulnerable are the kidneys and brain, which need a constant supply of oxygen to carry out their essential functions.

Oxygen is given as a therapeutic substance when intake is low (hypoxia) or when there is an insufficient amount of oxygen in the blood (hypoxemia). It may also be given to increase the oxygen content of gases inhaled during general anesthesia and to treat some forms of headache.

The most frequent indication for oxygen administration is hypoxia. Hypoxia can be caused by a decreased respiratory rate (hypoventilation), blockage to air flow in the respiratory tract, disease involving the respiratory center in the brain, pneumothorax, heart and lung diseases, or lack of sufficient oxygen in the air being inhaled.

There are many methods of administering oxygen. The amount of oxygen delivered will depend on the efficiency of both administration and res-piration. Oxygen is ordered in liters per minute and is adjusted by means of a flowmeter attached to either a wall unit or a portable canister of oxygen.

Nasal prongs or a nasal cannula administer oxygen directly into the nostrils. Masks are more effective, often capable of delivering 90% to 100% oxygen. Oxygen tents or hoods have an advantage in that they regulate temperature and humidity of inspired air, as well as oxygen flow. Face tents are the most comfortable and convenient method of giving high concentrations of oxygen.

In addition to these methods, there is also the hyperbaric form, in which oxygen at high pressure is administered. This method has been found effective for treatment of infections such as gas gangrene and tetanus, to reverse carbon dioxide poisoning, and as an aid to radiation therapy of cancer.*

NURSING IMPLICATIONS

Smoking, using open flames, and using faulty electrical equipment that may spark are not allowed in rooms where oxygen is being administered. Make sure *no smoking* signs are posted outside and inside the patient's room.

When giving oxygen, be sure it is humidified so

* Cells with a high oxygen content are more susceptible to radiation.

the mucous membranes will not dry out. Most oxygen setups have nebulizers attached that bubble the gas through sterile warm water for this reason. Be sure the oxygen mask fits correctly so there is a tight seal over the nose and mouth. Use a disposable mask, if possible, and change it frequently to decrease the possibility of infection.

Oxygen is available in portable steel cylinders (green cylinders are used in the United States, white in Canada). The gas is under pressure, so care must be taken not to drop the cylinders or bump them together—either of which may cause an explosion.

Oxygen must be given with care to patients with chronic lung disease because their respiratory regulatory mechanism is disturbed. Giving too much oxygen to these patients may depress respirations.

CHAPTER 23
Respiratory stimulants

Respiratory stimulants were first mentioned in Chapter 12 as a type of CNS stimulant, or analeptic drug. They are called analeptic because in large doses they cause seizures.

Respiratory stimulants act on the respiratory center in the brain. Although they effectively stimulate rate and depth of respirations, respiratory depression is usually treated with artificial ventilation rather than drugs. The main use of respiratory stimulants is to treat respiratory depression due to anesthesia or chronic disease that causes respiratory insufficiency. The danger is that when given in doses large enough to produce the desired effect, these drugs also may cause convulsions, vomiting, and cardiovascular or respiratory problems.

A respiratory stimulant given by inhalation is ammonia (aromatic spirits of ammonia). A whiff of this drug stimulates the respiratory center. It is often referred to as "smelling salts" and is offered to the person who feels faint. Respiratory stimulants given by the parenteral route are usually administered in the operating room by an anesthetist.

CHAPTER 24
Bronchodilators

Bronchodilators are drugs that relieve bronchial constriction, thus promoting a freer flow of air into and out of the lungs. These drugs relax smooth muscle and decrease mucous membrane swelling and respiratory tract congestion by their vasoconstrictive action.

The three most common lung conditions that cause respiratory tract obstruction are chronic bronchitis, bronchial asthma, and emphysema. Together, these diseases are referred to as chronic obstructive lung disease (COLD) or chronic obstructive pulmonary disease (COPD).

Bronchodilators can be administered by mouth or parenterally, but perhaps the most effective method is by nebulization. To nebulize a medication, place the ordered amount of liquid medication in a machine (simple nebulizer, intermittent positive-pressure breathing device [IPPB], or ultrasonic nebulizer) that mixes the medication with air to form a fine mist. The patient inhales this mist, which applies the medication directly to the respiratory tract. The smaller the nebulized drops of medication (controlled by the machine), the farther they will travel into the lungs. The smallest drops will reach as far as the alveolar ducts and sacs.*

---

* Other drugs (antibiotics, mucolytics, and corticosteroids) can also be administered by nebulization.

CLASSIFICATION OF BRONCHODILATORS

There are two major groups of medications used to relax smooth muscle in the respiratory tract. Thus, we have two groups of bronchodilators: adrenergic drugs and xanthine substances (Table 24-1). *Adrenergic* drugs are discussed in Chapter 31. They act to inhibit smooth muscle, which leads to relaxation of the bronchial tree. This allows free flow of air and decreases dyspnea, shortness of breath, and wheezing. Epinephrine (Adrenalin) is the drug most commonly used to treat asthma. It is an adrenergic drug administered by nebulizer or parenterally but not orally, since it is destroyed by gastric secretions. Various preparations of epinephrine and epinephrine plus other medications are available in measured-dose aerosol inhalers for self-administration. Examples of these medications are Medihaler-Epi, AsthmaNefrin, Micronefrin, and Primatene Mist.

Isoetharine (Bronkosol) is an adrenergic drug administered by nebulizer to relieve bronchospasm. It is especially effective for relief of acute bronchial asthma attacks, chronic bronchitis, or emphysema. Albuterol (Proventil, Ventolin), isoproterenol (Isuprel), metaproterenol (Metaprel, Alupent), and terbutaline (Bricanyl, Brethine) are other adrenergic drugs that are available in many forms for use as bronchodilators.

(*Text continues on p. 180.*)

TABLE 24-1 BRONCHODILATORS

DRUG	ROUTE AND DOSAGE RANGE	USE	ADVERSE EFFECTS	NURSING IMPLICATIONS
albuterol (Proventil, Ventolin)	PO—2 mg–8 mg tid–qid Inhaler—2–4 inhalations q4–6h	To relieve bronchospasm in patients with reversible obstructive airway disease	*CNS:* nervousness, tremor, headache, insomnia, weakness, dizziness, drowsiness, flushing, restlessness, irritability, vertigo, stimulation *Cardiovascular:* tachycardia, palpitations, hypertension, angina *Others:* muscle cramps, nausea, vomiting, difficult urination, unusual taste, dry mouth/ throat	Assist with activities as necessary. Note any behavioral changes. Evaluate sleep pattern. Monitor BP and pulse. Note any complaints of chest discomfort or muscle cramps. Evaluate ease of urination.
aminophylline	PO—600 mg–1600 mg qd in divided doses Rectal—500 mg qd or bid IM—500 mg prn IV—Initial dose— 250 mg–500 mg (5 mg–6 mg/kg) over 20 min, then 0.1 mg–1 mg/kg/hr in continuous infusion	To treat acute bronchial asthma and reversible bronchospasm associated with chronic bronchitis and emphysema	*CNS:* dizziness, headache, lightheadedness, nervousness, insomnia, agitation *Cardiovascular:* palpitations, tachycardia, arrhythmias *GI:* anorexia, nausea, vomiting, bitter aftertaste, GI distress *Skin:* flushing, hives *Other:* increased respiratory rate	Evaluate appetite. Caution patients to avoid dangerous activities. Assist with activities as necessary. Assess sleep pattern. Monitor vital signs. Check skin for color and hives.
cromolyn (Intal)	Inhaler—Contents of one capsule tid to qid at regular intervals Solution—20 mg via nebulizer qid	To treat patients with severe asthma who need regular, long-term medication with symptomatic drugs	*CNS:* dizziness, headache *Respiratory:* bronchospasm, cough, laryngeal edema, nasal congestion, throat irritation, wheezing *GI:* nausea, swollen parotid glands *GU:* difficult or frequent urination *Musculoskeletal:* joint swelling or joint pain *Skin:* rash, hives *Other:* increased tearing of eyes	Administer with the inhaler designed for this particular drug. Ambulate with assistance if necessary. Watch for any respiratory difficulty. Monitor rate and rhythm of respirations. Note any swelling or discomfort in parotid area. Record I&O, and note any problems with urination. Note complaints of muscular aches, pain, swelling. Observe skin for any reactions. Note increased tearing of eyes.
epinephrine (Adrenalin, Medihaler-Epi)	Inhaler—1–2 inhalations 2 min apart SC, IM, IV, IC—0.1 mg–1.5 mg prn (to a maximum of 5 mg in 24 hr)	To relieve acute or chronic paroxysms of bronchial asthma, to treat drug sensitivity reactions and severe acute allergic reactions; added to local anesthetic solutions to decrease absorption of the anesthetic; used topically to control superficial bleeding; used with other therapy to treat cardiac arrest	*CNS:* fear, nervousness, tremor, dizziness, headache, anxiety, excitability, insomnia, weakness, mental changes *Cardiovascular:* tachycardia, palpitations, arrhythmias *GI:* nausea, vomiting *Skin:* sweating, pallor, tissue necrosis with repeated injections *Other:* respiratory distress	Evaluate mental status and level of anxiety. Monitor vital signs. Assess skin color and moisture. Evaluate sleep pattern. Watch for skin irritation at injection sites.

(continued on page 179)

TABLE 24-1 (continued)

DRUG	ROUTE AND DOSAGE RANGE	USE	ADVERSE EFFECTS	NURSING IMPLICATIONS
isoetharine (Bronkosol)	Inhaler—3–7 inhalations q4h In IPPB or Oxygen—0.25 ml–1 ml q4h (dilute 1:3 with saline)	To relieve acute bronchial asthma and other conditions, such as chronic bronchitis or emphysema, in which bronchospasm is a complicating factor	*If used too frequently:* *CNS:* headache, anxiety, tension, restlessness, insomnia, weakness, dizziness, excitement *Cardiovascular:* tachycardia, palpitations, changes in BP *GI:* nausea, vomiting	Excessive use can lead to decreased effect and may even cause a paradoxical airway obstruction. Warn patient about prolonged use and its dangers. Monitor vital signs. Evaluate mental status. Assess sleep patterns. For use in IPPB, dilute 1:3 with NS or other diluent.
isoproterenol (Isuprel, Medihaler-Iso)	SC, IM, IV—highly individualized doses Inhaler—Initial dose—1–2 inhalations Maintenance—1–2 inhalations q4–6h	To aid in treatment of shock; to treat cardiac arrest; to treat ventricular arrhythmias and bronchospasm associated with acute and chronic bronchial asthma, pulmonary emphysema, bronchitis, and bronchiectasis	*CNS:* nervousness, tremors, headache, dizziness, weakness *Cardiovascular:* palpitations, tachycardia, anginal pain *Others:* nausea, sweating, flushing	Monitor vital signs at frequent intervals. Reassure patients who are upset by the "pounding in the chest." Note any abnormal muscle movements. Assist with activities as necessary.
metaproterenol (Alupent, Metaprel)	PO—20 mg tid to qid Inhaler—2–3 inhalations prn (to a maximum of 12 qd)	See isoetharine.	*CNS:* nervousness, tremor *Cardiovascular:* tachycardia, hypertension, palpitations *GI:* nausea, vomiting, bad taste in mouth	Excessive use can lead to decreased effect and possible paradoxic airway obstruction. Warn patients not to use long-term. Monitor vital signs. Note abnormal muscle movements.
oxtriphylline (Choledyl)	PO—200 mg qid	See aminophylline.	*CNS:* headache, irritability, restlessness, insomnia, agitation, muscle twitching, convulsions *Cardiovascular:* palpitations, tachycardia, arrhythmias, hypotension, circulatory failure *GI:* nausea, vomiting, diarrhea, epigastric pain *Others:* flushing, fever, rapid respirations, increased excretion of albumin, diuresis, dehydration	Best drug effect is if taken on an empty stomach, but encourage patient to take the medication with meals or immediately afterward, if GI upset is a problem. Keep stool chart. Evaluate mental status. Note abnormal muscle movements. Monitor vital signs. Record I&O, and note any fluid imbalances. Check urine for albumin.
terbutaline (Brethaire, Brethine, Bricanyl)	PO—2.5 mg–5 mg tid SC—0.25 mg; repeat in 15–30 min if necessary Inhaler—2 inhalations q4–6h	See isoetharine.	See epinephrine.	See epinephrine, *plus:* Give injections in lateral deltoid.

(continued on page 180)

TABLE 24-1 (continued)

DRUG	ROUTE AND DOSAGE RANGE	USE	ADVERSE EFFECTS	NURSING IMPLICATIONS
theophylline (Elixophyllin, Slo-bid, Theolair, Theo-Dur)	PO—Highly individualized Loading dose—6 mg/kg Maintenance—1 mg–4 mg/kg q6–12h Maximum daily dose is 900 mg	See aminophylline.	See oxtriphylline.	See oxtriphylline.
theophylline + guaifenesin (Quibron)	PO—150 mg–300 mg q6–8h	For symptomatic relief in conditions such as bronchial asthma, chronic bronchitis and pulmonary emphysema, where bronchospasms are a problem	See oxtriphylline, *plus:* blood in vomitus, hyperglycemia	See oxtriphylline, *plus:* Test any emesis for blood. Tests for blood sugar should be done at regular intervals.
theophylline + ephedrine + phenobarbital (Tedral)	PO—1–2 tablet q4h	See isoetharine, *plus:* to prevent or minimize asthmatic attacks	See oxtriphylline, *plus:* drowsiness, dependence	See oxtriphylline, *plus:* Encourage patients to avoid potentially dangerous activities, such as driving an automobile. Observe for possible dependence.

The *xanthine* group includes caffeine, theophylline, and theobromine. Their diuretic action was discussed in Chapter 20. In addition to this effect, xanthine drugs relax bronchial smooth muscle. Theophylline and drugs derived from theophylline are the xanthines most commonly used as bronchodilators. Tedral, a combination of theophylline, ephedrine, and phenobarbital, combines the actions of xanthine, adrenergic, and sedative drugs. Over-the-counter medications with combined bronchodilating and expectorant action are also available.

Cromolyn (Aarane or Intal) is not a bronchodilator, but it is used to prevent asthma attacks. It is usually prescribed as part of long-term therapy for the asthmatic and is taken in regular daily doses.

NURSING IMPLICATIONS

With nebulized medications, the rate and depth of respirations have an important effect on drug action. Quick, shallow breaths will result in fewer droplets of medication reaching the alveoli and more medication escaping on expiration. Slow, deep breathing will be most effective. The breath should be held after deep inspiration to provide the most effective drug action deep in the lungs.

If a measured-dose oral inhaler is used, the patient should be taught to fully exhale, tilt the head backward and hold the inhaler above the head. He should then inhale the mist deeply and hold his breath for a few seconds before removing the inhaler from his lips. Exhalation should be done through pursed lips. The ordered number of inhalations should not be exceeded because tolerance may develop, and this may lead to decreased effectiveness. Patients should be reminded to inhale the smallest amount possible that relieves their symptoms. If the prescribed dose is no longer effective, notify the physician. Do not increase the dosage.

If medication is administered by the IV route, a steady flow rate must be maintained. If an infusion pump is not used, rate of flow must be checked carefully and *very* frequently.

There is a great potential for abuse of the over-the-counter bronchodilators. These drugs can have serious adverse effects and should be taken only as directed. If misused they can cause eventual heart failure.

Mouthpieces on nebulizers and inhalers must be kept clean. If microorganisms are not removed, they may be sprayed into the bronchi, leading to respiratory infections.

One of the most common reactions to bronchodilators is tachycardia. The patient may complain of palpitations as he feels his heart beat rapidly. The apical pulse should be taken before, during, and after medication with a bronchodilating drug. Any pulse rate greater than 120 beats per minute should be reported immediately.

The most frequent cause of chronic bronchitis is smoking. Any person with lung disease must be strongly warned against smoking, since it can only aggravate the condition.

PRACTICE PROBLEMS—BRONCHODILATORS

1. The order reads: theophylline (Elixophyllin) elixir 200 mg PO q6h.
   The label reads: theophylline 80 mg/15 ml.
   How much elixir will be given?

   $$\frac{D}{H} \times A = G$$

   $$\frac{5 \ \cancel{200} \text{ mg}}{2 \ \cancel{80} \text{ mg}} \times 15 \text{ ml} = G$$

   $$\frac{5}{2} \times 15 \text{ ml} = \frac{75}{2} = 37.5 \text{ ml}$$

   Thus, 37.5 ml of theophylline elixir will be given.

Work the following problems:

1. The order reads isoproterenol (Isuprel) 5 mg SL q4h. Isoproterenol comes in 10-mg tablets. How many tablets will you give?

2. The order reads: oxtriphylline (Choledyl) 200 mg PO qid.
   The label reads: oxtriphylline 100 mg/tablet.
   How many tablets will you give?

3. The order reads: theophylline (Elixophyllin) elixir 150 mg PO qid.
   The label reads: theophylline 20 mg/5 ml.
   How many milliliters of theophylline will be given?

Answers are given on p. 283.

CHAPTER 25
Mucolytics, expectorants, and antitussives

MUCOLYTICS AND EXPECTORANTS

The lining of the normal respiratory tract is coated with a layer of mucus that helps to entrap foreign particles and dust. The accumulated debris then travels upward, aided by ciliary action, smooth muscle movements, and coughing. Eventually, the mucus is either expectorated (spit out) or swallowed. If increased amounts of mucus are produced, or the mucus is unusually thick and sticky, patients may have difficulty removing their secretions.

The safest and simplest way to get secretions loose and thinned so they can be removed from the respiratory tract is to give plain water. The local (by drinking) or systemic (intravenous fluids) route may be used. If it is not possible to use either method, drug therapy is indicated.

Classification of drugs

Two groups of drugs are useful in removing secretions from the respiratory tract—the mucolytic and expectorant drugs (see Table 25-1). *Mucolytic* agents dissolve mucus, thinning its sticky consistency so it is easier to remove. These agents are usually administered by nebulizer to promote more effective respiration in patients with bronchial disease, cystic fibrosis, emphysema, and pneumonia. They are also frequently included as part of tracheostomy care. With the mucolytic drug, most patients will be able to cough up secretions; however, if the patient is too weak or too ill, or is paralyzed,

it may be necessary to remove secretions by suctioning. Postural drainage can also help to remove secretions from the lungs.

Expectorant drugs cause production of a lubricating fluid deep in the lungs. As it is pushed upward by muscle and ciliary action, this fluid helps to thin out secretions along the route, so they are easier to expel. Potassium iodide, a popular expectorant, is usually given as a saturated solution of potassium iodide (SSKI).

Guaifenesin (Robitussin) is an expectorant mixed with many other drugs in preparations given to relieve congestion and coughs. It is often given to make an unproductive cough productive, in hopes of diminishing the cough.

NURSING IMPLICATIONS

Encourage patients to drink large amounts of water every day to aid systemic hydration. Iodide substances must be given cautiously because they can cause sensitivity reactions. The resulting toxic symptoms can be fatal. Watch for any unusual rash or reaction.

ANTITUSSIVES

Coughing is a reflex mechanism by which the body cleanses the respiratory tract. A productive cough

TABLE 25-1 MUCOLYTICS AND EXPECTORANTS

DRUG	ROUTE AND DOSAGE RANGE	USE	ADVERSE EFFECTS	NURSING IMPLICATIONS
acetylcysteine (Mucomyst)	Given by nebulizer q2–6h 10% solution—2 ml–20 ml undiluted 20% solution—1 ml–10 ml diluted with NS or sterile water	Used with other therapy to treat diseases characterized by abnormal, thick or dry secretions; to treat atelectasis caused by mucous obstruction; used as an aid in diagnostic bronchial studies; used during tracheostomy care and anesthesia	Stomatitis, nausea, runny nose, possible bronchospasm (usually in sensitive asthmatics)	Be sure patient has a clean airway so the increased secretions can be removed, either by cough or suctioning. Inspect mouth for reaction.
codeine + triprolidine + pseudoephedrine (Actifed with codeine)	PO—10 ml (at intervals individualized according to needs and response of the patient)	For symptomatic relief of cough in conditions such as the common cold, acute bronchitis, allergic asthma, bronchiolitis, croup, emphysema, tracheobronchitis	*CNS/ANS:* sedation, sleepiness, dizziness, incoordination, fatigue, confusion, restlessness, excitation, nervousness, tremor, irritability, insomnia, euphoria, paresthesias, blurred vision, diplopia, vertigo, tinnitus, acute labyrinthitis, hysteria, neuritis, convulsions, hallucinations, physical dependence *Cardiovascular:* hypotension, headache, palpitations, tachycardia, extrasystoles *Respiratory:* thick secretions, tightness of chest and wheezing, nasal stuffiness *GI:* nausea, vomiting, anorexia, diarrhea or constipation, epigastric distress *GU:* urinary frequency, difficult urination, urinary retention, early menses *Others:* blood abnormalities, rash, itching, anaphylactic shock, photosensitivity, excessive perspiration, chills, dryness of mouth, nose, or throat	Evaluate mental status. Assist with activities if necessary. Caution patient not to engage in potentially dangerous activities. Note behavioral changes. Evaluate sleep pattern. Note any complaints of altered sensation. Assess visual acuity. Monitor BP and pulse. Note character of secretions. Keep a stool chart. Assess appetite. Observe skin for any reaction. Keep record of I&O. Note any difficulty with urination. Note any unusual perspiration. Blood tests should be done at regular intervals.
guaifenesin (Robitussin)	PO—100 mg–200 mg (1–2 tsp) q3–4h to a maximum 12 tsp qd	To treat cases of dry, unproductive cough	GI upset, nausea, drowsiness	This is a common ingredient in many cough medicines. Caution patients not to engage in dangerous activities. Do not take on an empty stomach if GI upset is a problem.

(continued on page 185)

TABLE 25-1 (continued)

DRUG	ROUTE AND DOSAGE RANGE	USE	ADVERSE EFFECTS	NURSING IMPLICATIONS
potassium iodide oral solution (SSKI)	PO—0.3 ml–0.6 ml (diluted in glassful of water) q6–8h	As an expectorant to treat chronic lung disease (including bronchial asthma, bronchitis and pulmonary emphysema) complicated by tenacious mucus	*GI:* stomach upset, nausea, vomiting, epigastric pain, metallic taste *Other:* rash	Question patient about any previous sensitivity to iodine products. Note any rash. Note any complaints of GI discomfort.
terpin hydrate	PO—5 ml–10 ml q3–4h	To facilitate expectoration; use as a vehicle for codeine	Possible GI distress if taken on an empty stomach	Take with food if GI upset occurs.

results in material being removed from the respiratory tract. Nonproductive coughing is dry and irritating. It can exhaust the patient and affect the general circulation as well as lung function.

Antitussives are drugs that relieve coughing, and they are commonly called cough medicines. The objective of treatment with antitussives is to decrease coughing that is extremely nonproduc-

tive, yet allow some coughing for the elimination of secretions. Suppression of cough will often lead to rest and comfort for the exhausted patient.

Classification of antitussives

Drugs that relieve coughing can work in two ways. One group of drugs depresses the cough center in

TABLE 25-2 ANTITUSSIVES

DRUG	ROUTE AND DOSAGE RANGE	USE	ADVERSE EFFECTS	NURSING IMPLICATIONS
caramiphen + phenylpropanolamine (Tuss-Ornade)	PO—1 capsule q12h	To relieve cough and nasal congestion associated with common colds	*CNS:* dizziness, drowsiness, nervousness, insomnia, weakness, irritability, headache, tremor, incoordination *Cardiovascular:* chest tightness/pain, palpitations, hypo- or hypertension *GI:* nausea, diarrhea, constipation, gastric upset, anorexia *Others:* visual disturbances, difficult or painful urination	Caution patient not to engage in potentially dangerous activities. Assess sleep patterns. Note any complaints of chest discomfort. Monitor BP, pulse, and respiration. Keep stool chart. Evaluate appetite. Assess visual acuity. Note any complaints of urinary symptoms. Note any unusual muscle movements.
benzonatate (Tessalon)	PO—100 mg–200 mg tid	For symptomatic relief of cough	*CNS:* sedation, headache, mild dizziness *GI:* nausea, GI upset, constipation *Skin:* rash, itching, hypersensitivity reactions, burning eyes, temporary local anesthesia in the mouth if not swallowed immediately *Others:* nasal congestion, "chilly" sensation, feeling of numbness in chest	Tell patient to swallow medication at once without chewing or sucking. Avoid dangerous activities. Assist with ambulation and other activities as needed. Observe skin for any reactions. Keep a stool chart. Note any complaints of chest discomfort.

(continued on page 186)

TABLE 25-2   (continued)

DRUG	ROUTE AND DOSAGE RANGE	USE	ADVERSE EFFECTS	NURSING IMPLICATIONS
dextromethor-phan (Romilar)	PO—10 mg–20 mg q4h or 30 mg q6–8h	To relieve cough	Rare—nausea, dizziness	
diphenhydra-mine + alcohol (Benylin)	PO—2 tsp q4h (to a maximum of 8 tsp q24h)	To control cough due to colds or allergy	See diphenhydramine.	See diphenhydramine.
hydrocodone + phenyltolox-amine (Tussionex)	PO—1 capsule, tsp, or tablet q8–12h	To relieve cough	Mild and infrequent—constipation, nausea, rash on face, drowsiness; may be habit forming	Watch for respiratory depression, especially in child. Action lasts for 12 hours. Caution patient not to engage in potentially dangerous activities.

the brain. These drugs have central action. Antitussives with peripheral action act in one of three basic ways: respiratory demulcents soothe the irritated throat; expectorants help to make a cough productive and decrease its frequency; drugs in the third group temporarily abolish the cough reflex (see Table 25-2).

Centrally acting antitussives. The narcotic analgesics morphine and codeine are both effective antitussives. The main disadvantage of narcotics is that they may cause respiratory depression and can lead to drug dependence. Popular antitussives that contain narcotics are Tussionex and Robitussin AC.

A non-narcotic medication somewhat less effective than morphine as an antitussive is dextromethorphan (Romilar). Its advantages are that it does not depress respirations or cause dependence, and it has no analgesic effect. Dextromethorphan is found in many mixtures and in many over-the-counter cough drugs.

Peripherally acting antitussives. *Demulcents* were introduced in Chapter 17 in relation to the gastrointestinal system. There are also specific respiratory demulcents that have a soothing effect on the lining of the respiratory tract. They are usually thick, sticky substances, similar to the over-the-counter cough syrups. Household respiratory demulcents are honey and hard candy. Steam can also be used for its soothing effect on irritated respiratory mucosa.

The lubricating fluid produced by *expectorants* not only soothes the mucosa but also helps to pro-

mote productive coughing. Guaifenesin, an expectorant, is often mixed with dextromethorphan and codeine to combine the effects of central and peripheral antitussive medications.

Benzonatate (Tessalon) has both peripheral and central actions. It depresses the cough center in the brain and numbs the stretch receptors in the lungs that are responsible for the cough reflex.

NURSING IMPLICATIONS

When used as directed, antitussives have a low incidence of adverse effects. Many preparations contain combinations of drugs, so the nursing implications depend on the constituents.

Over-the-counter antitussives should be used only as directed. They should not be used when a cough persists, since it may be a symptom of serious disease, such as lung cancer.

Patients who smoke will further irritate their respiratory tract. They need to stop smoking. The humidity of the inspired air should be increased, and patients should be encouraged to increase their fluid intake to aid in liquefying secretions.

Help the patient to change his position frequently. Deep breathing exercises and postural drainage will also help to raise secretions. Observe and record the amount and quality of sputum produced.

Liquid antitussives should not be diluted. Water should not be taken for at least 30 minutes after administration, so full demulcent effect can take place.

CHAPTER 26
Antihistamines

In order to understand how antihistamines work, we must first look at what histamine is and how it affects the body. Histamine is a substance occurring naturally in the body. Allergic reactions to food or environmental insults (bee stings, dust, pollen, snake bites); skin injury; and some medications and enzymes cause histamine to be released into the bloodstream. When this happens, three reactions occur: (1) blood vessels dilate; (2) smooth muscle in the bronchial tree, intestines, and uterus contracts; and (3) secretions from glands in the stomach and respiratory tract increase. The resulting conditions may be mildly discomforting, such as a rash or itching, or potentially fatal, as in angioneurotic edema and anaphylactic shock.

Dilation of the blood vessels causes skin flushing, increased temperature of the skin, itching or burning sensations, and a fall in blood pressure. The engorged blood vessels in the mucous membranes of the nose cause nasal and sinus congestion. If the skin has been injured, histamine release causes a raised red area of local edema called a *wheal*. Histamine is used as a diagnostic agent to test for achlorhydria (lack of hydrochloric acid).

Antihistamines are given to prevent histamine from acting and thus prevent the "histamine response." Their main use is in the treatment of allergies (seasonal, household, or drug) and colds (Table 26-1). Since antihistamines block the circulatory and pulmonary effects of histamine, they relieve congestion resulting from allergies or colds and are commonly known as decongestants.

Adrenergic drugs oppose the action of histamine by producing opposite effects, such as constriction of arteries and bronchodilation. Examples of these drugs are oxymetazoline (Afrin), ephedrine plus phenylephrine (Neo-Synephrine), pseudoephedrine (Sudafed), and triprolidine plus pseudoephedrine (Actifed). Cimetidine (Tagamet) inhibits gastric secretions, and for this reason, it is classified as an antihistamine.

There are antihistamines whose side-effects such as sedation are the main reason for their use. They relieve motion sickness, nausea, and vomiting. Diphenhydramine (Benadryl), for example, is an antihistamine with mild antispasmodic, sedative, antiemetic, and antiparkinsonian actions. A variation of diphenhydramine is dimenhydrinate (Dramamine), which is used to treat motion sickness.

NURSING IMPLICATIONS

If histamine is being given as a diagnostic agent, be sure to take the patient's pulse and blood pressure immediately after administration and at frequent intervals thereafter since severe reactions can occur. Epinephrine should be available to treat possible anaphylaxis.

The major adverse effect of antihistamines is drowsiness. Persons taking these medications should be warned not to perform dangerous activities, such as driving an automobile or operating heavy machinery.

TABLE 26-1   ANTIHISTAMINES

DRUG	ROUTE AND DOSAGE RANGE	USE	ADVERSE EFFECTS	NURSING IMPLICATIONS
brompheniramine maleate (Dimetane)	PO—4 mg–8 mg tid to qid or 8 mg–12 mg sustained action q8–12h IM, SC, IV—5 mg–20 mg bid	To treat allergic conditions and vasomotor rhinitis	*CNS:* headache, sedation, dizziness, incoordination, fatigue, confusion, restlessness, excitation, nervousness, tremor, irritability, insomnia, euphoria, paresthesias, visual changes, vertigo, tinnitus, hysteria, convulsions *Cardiovascular:* hypotension, palpitations, tachycardia, arrhythmias *Respiratory:* thick bronchial secretions, tight chest, wheezing, nasal stuffiness *GI:* anorexia, nausea, vomiting, diarrhea or constipation, dry mouth, nose, and throat *Skin:* rash, hives, increased perspiration, photosensitivity *Others:* anaphylaxis, chills, blood disorders, problems with urination, early menses	Warn patients not to engage in dangerous activities. Check skin for rash or hives. Warn patient to stay out of direct sunlight and to avoid brightly lit areas. Monitor vital signs. Offer fluids if allowed. Blood tests should be done at regular intervals. Assist with activity as necessary. Evaluate mental status and mood. Note any abnormal muscle movements. Question the patient about unusual sensations in the extremities. Assess visual acuity. If GI upset occurs, give when stomach is full. Keep stool chart. Record I&O and check for problems with output. Warn female patient that she may experience early menses. Assess respiratory quality and note unusual mucus production.
brompheniramine maleate + phenylephrine + phenylpropanolamine (Dimetapp)	PO—elixir—1–2 tsp tid to qid Extentabs—1 q8–12h	See brompheniramine, *plus:* to treat acute sinusitis, nasal congestion, and otitis	See brompheniramine.	See brompheniramine.
chlorpheniramine maleate (Chlor-Trimeton, Teldrin)	PO—4 mg q4–6h (to a maximum of 24 mg qd); sustained action 8 mg–12 mg q8–12h IM, SC, IV—5 mg–20 mg (to a maximum 40 mg qd)	To treat allergic reactions and anaphylaxis	See brompheniramine.	See brompheniramine.
chlorpheniramine maleate + phenylpropanolamine (Ornade)	PO—1 spansule q12h	For prolonged relief of upper respiratory tract congestion and hypersecretion associated with vasomotor and allergic rhinitis	See brompheniramine.	See brompheniramine.
cyproheptadine (Periactin)	PO—4 mg–32 mg qd in divided doses	To treat allergic conditions, vasomotor rhinitis, cold urticaria, dermatographism; to treat anaphylaxis (along with other measures)	See brompheniramine.	See brompheniramine.

(continued on page 189)

TABLE 26-1 (continued)

DRUG	ROUTE AND DOSAGE RANGE	USE	ADVERSE EFFECTS	NURSING IMPLICATIONS
tripelennamine (Pyribenzamine, PBZ, PBZ-SR)	PO—25 mg–50 mg q4–6h (to a maximum of 600 mg qd in divided doses); long acting—100 mg q8–12h Topical—2% cream or ointment	To relieve symptoms of allergic conditions and anaphylaxis; use topically to relieve itching	See brompheniramine.	See brompheniramine.
triprolidine + pseudo-ephedrine (Actifed)	PO—1 tablet or 2 tsp tid–qid	See brompheniramine, *plus:* may be effective in treating symptoms associated with the common cold	See brompheniramine.	See brompheniramine.

CHAPTER 27
Blood products

Blood transfusions are given to restore blood volume in conditions such as acute hemorrhage, burns, blood vessel injury, shock, anemia, and leukemia. The entire blood supply may be exchanged when diseases such as erythroblastosis fetalis or acute fulminating hepatitis occur. In most cases, only the specific parts or fractions of blood required are given rather than whole blood. This is more economical, since only the needed product is used and the remainder can be used for another purpose. Blood products used for transfusion include whole blood, packed or frozen red blood cells, platelets, granulocytes, plasma, and albumin.

Plasma expanders are not blood products but serve to expand the blood volume. They do this by osmotic action, drawing fluid into the blood vessels. Plasma expanders are cheaper and more easily available than blood. Furthermore, they do not pose the threats of incompatibility reactions and infection.

NURSING IMPLICATIONS

The two major complications of blood administration are blood group incompatibility reactions and transmission of viral hepatitis. Circulatory overload is also possible if blood is given too quickly or in large amounts.

Viral hepatitis is transmitted when donor blood contains antibodies for the disease. Careful testing of donated blood has decreased this occurrence. Symptoms of blood group incompatibility reaction can range from mild (rash, itching, chills and fever) to severe (shock, renal failure, and death). During transfusion of whole blood or cells (plasma contains no cells and, therefore, cannot cause incompatibility reactions) the temperature, pulse, and blood pressure should be closely monitored. Any rash or difficulty in breathing should be reported at once, since these could be the first signs of a fatal anaphylactic reaction.

Acquired immune deficiency syndrome (AIDS) is considered by some to be another complication of blood transfusions. The incidence of this is less than 1% of all persons receiving blood transfusions. All donated blood is tested for the virus that causes AIDS. If the virus is present, the blood is discarded.

CHAPTER 28
Antianemics

Anemia is a decrease in the number of red blood cells, a decrease in the amount of hemoglobin in the red blood cells, or both. Three types of anemias are treated with antianemic drug therapy: iron-deficiency anemia, pernicious anemia, and megaloblastic anemia.

In *iron-deficiency anemia* the red blood cells are smaller than normal and lighter in color because they contain less hemoglobin. Iron is necessary for the body's manufacture of hemoglobin, and inadequate iron intake is the major cause of iron-deficiency anemia. Even a normal intake of iron may be insufficient during certain periods in the life cycle when there is greatly increased demand for iron. Examples of such periods are infancy, adolescence, and pregnancy. Another cause of iron-deficiency anemia is internal bleeding due to disease, trauma, or unusually heavy menstrual flow. The person with this type of anemia complains of fatigue, headache, and anorexia and appears pale and weak.

The iron compounds are classified as antianemic agents because this is their major use (see Table 28-1). They are usually given orally. Parenteral administration of iron is dangerous because of the possibility of overdose* and anaphylaxis. This route is used only when oral administration is impossible, when rapid replacement is necessary, or when absorption is diminished due to intestinal disease.

* The body has no way to eliminate excess iron.

Pernicious anemia is no longer "pernicious" (deadly), as it was when first named in the early 1900s. It results from the lack of a substance in the body called "intrinsic factor," which is necessary for the formation of red blood cells and absorption of vitamin B_{12} (cyanocobalamin). This deficiency may be linked to illness and hereditary factors but is often idiopathic (without apparent cause). The treatment is life-long administration of cyanocobalamin by intramuscular injection.

Megaloblastic anemia is a condition in which large, immature red blood cells are present in the bone marrow. It may be due to deficiency of vitamin B_{12} or deficiency of folic acid, another B-complex vitamin. The treatment is usually oral administration of folic acid.

NURSING IMPLICATIONS

Oral iron preparations should be given with or after meals to decrease gastrointestinal upset. Absorption is increased if orange juice or ascorbic acid is given at the same time. Liquid iron preparations can stain the teeth and should be taken through a straw.

Warn the patient receiving iron that it causes stools to appear very dark (tarry). Pain and skin discoloration at the injection site are common when iron must be given parenterally, and a method of intramuscular administration called the "Z-track" method has been introduced to prevent leakage of iron into

193

the subcutaneous layer. In this technique the skin is pulled sideways, then the needle with medication is introduced. After the medication has been injected, the needle is withdrawn and the skin is released. This effectively seals the medication in the intramuscular layer (see Fig. 28-1).

No serious adverse effects occur with vitamin B$_{12}$ or folic acid therapy, but allergic reactions may occur. Watch for nausea, vomiting, headache, fever, muscle aches, and urticaria.

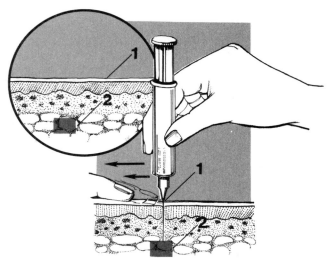

Figure 28-1. The Z-track method of giving an intramuscular injection. The skin is pulled laterally (arrows) before the needle is inserted—the insertion site (1), the site where the medication will be placed (2). (Inset) The relationship of the insertion site (1) to the medication site (2) after injection. (Wolff L, Weitzel MH, Zornow RA, Zsohar H: Fundamentals of Nursing, 7th ed. Philadelphia, JB Lippincott, 1983)

TABLE 28-1   ANTIANEMICS

DRUG	ROUTE AND DOSAGE RANGE	USE	ADVERSE EFFECTS	NURSING IMPLICATIONS
cyanocobalamin (vitamin B$_{12}$)	PO—1 mcg–1 mg qd SC, IM—30 mcg qd for 5–10 days; then 100 mcg–200 mcg every month	To treat pernicious anemia and other vitamin B$_{12}$ deficiency states	Usually none; rare diarrhea, itch, hives, anaphylaxis	Note any loose stools. Watch for allergic skin reactions. Monitor temperature.
folic acid (Folvite)	PO—0.1 mg–1 mg qd	To treat megaloblastic and macrocytic anemias due to folic acid deficiency; to treat anemias of malnutrition, pregnancy, infancy, or childhood; to treat anemia of sprue	Rare allergic reactions	Watch for allergic skin reactions. Monitor temperature.
ferrous sulfate (Feosol)	PO—1 tablet q6–8h (p̄c and hs)	To treat simple iron deficiency and iron-deficiency anemia	GI discomfort, nausea, diarrhea or constipation, staining of teeth	Offer at mealtime to avoid GI upset. Avoid staining of teeth by diluting the liquid and having patient drink it through a straw.

(continued on page 195)

TABLE 28-1   (continued)

DRUG	ROUTE AND DOSAGE RANGE	USE	ADVERSE EFFECTS	NURSING IMPLICATIONS
ferrous gluco- nate (Fergon)	PO—1–2 tablet or tsp qd	To treat hypochromic anemia of childhood and pregnancy, idi- opathic hypochro- mic anemia, and anemia associated with chronic blood loss	Rare	
ferrous fumarate (Feostat, Ircon)	PO—100 mg–400 mg qd	To treat iron-defi- ciency anemia	Rare	
iron dextran (Imferon)	IM, IV—test dose on first day—0.5 ml; then 5 ml IM qd until required amount is given; or 2 ml IV qd until total dose given	To treat iron-defi- ciency anemia that cannot be treated by oral iron therapy	*CNS:* headache, pares- thesias, shivering *Musculoskeletal:* muscle and joint aches, flare- up of rheumatoid ar- thritis *Others:* severe febrile reactions, fatal ana- phylaxis, hypotension, rash, itching, irritation at injection site, nau- sea	Check skin for allergic reac- tions. Monitor temperature and BP. Question patient about mus- cle and joint movement. Inject only into upper outer quadrant of the buttocks. (Inject deeply, using Z- track method to avoid tis- sue irritation.)

CHAPTER 29
Drugs that affect blood clotting

The process by which blood clots is complex. More than 12 "clotting factors" are involved in the various stages of clot formation. There are also anti-clotting substances circulating in the bloodstream that keep blood from clotting inside the blood vessels and dissolve any small clots that happen to form. When the balance of clotting and anti-clotting factors is upset either uncontrolled bleeding or thromboembolic* disorders can result. Thromboembolic disorders are the most common cause of death in the United States. They are treated by administration of anticoagulant drugs.

Anticoagulants are drugs used to prevent the formation of blood clots (see Table 29-1). They do not dissolve clots that have already formed, so their use is primarily as preventive therapy. The major uses of anticoagulants are (1) to treat occlusive vascular disease, such as venous thrombosis, coronary artery disease (CAD), congestive heart failure (CHF), cerebrovascular diseases (stroke, transient ischemic attacks), pulmonary thrombosis, and myocardial infarction (MI); (2) as prophylactic therapy during major surgery (especially pelvic), for patients on prolonged bed rest, and those with rheumatic heart diseases (RHD); and (3) to prevent clots in blood sent to the laboratory for study, used in transfusions (including hemodialysis and heart-lung machine), or experiments.

* A thrombus is a blood clot formed in a blood vessel or the heart. An embolus is all or part of a thrombus that travels from one blood vessel to a smaller one where it lodges and obstructs blood flow.

CLASSIFICATION OF ANTICOAGULANT DRUGS

Heparin and the coumarin preparations are the two main anticoagulant drugs used today. They both keep new clots from forming but differ significantly in other ways.

Heparin acts in the bloodstream and is used when rapid anticoagulation is necessary. It is quickly absorbed; the response to it is almost immediate; and it is rapidly excreted. There are few toxic reactions. The disadvantages of heparin are its short (3 to 4 hours) duration of action, its expense, and the fact that it must be injected, which often causes local reactions.

Coumarin drugs act in the liver. This indirect action is slower than that of heparin. They are used for long-term anticoagulation, such as in treatment of MI, recurrent phlebitis, and chronic occlusive disease. In addition to their effectiveness when given orally, coumarin drugs are less expensive than heparin. Another advantage is that once the dose is adjusted, coumarin preparations can be given just once a day.

Thrombolytic drugs, such as streptokinase (Streptase), break down existing clots. *Antiplatelet* drugs keep platelets from clumping together, which is an essential part of the clotting process. These drugs are used to prevent clots. Examples are aspirin, dipyridamole (Persantine), and sulfinpyrazone (Anturane). *Hemostatic* agents stop active bleeding. They are also called *coagulants*. Ex-

TABLE 29-1 DRUGS THAT AFFECT BLOOD CLOTTING

DRUG	ROUTE AND DOSAGE RANGE	USE	ADVERSE EFFECTS	NURSING IMPLICATIONS
aminocaproic acid (Amicar)	PO, IV—Initial dose—5 g; then 1.0 g–1.25 g qh (to a maximum 30 g in 24 hr)	To treat excessive bleeding resulting from systemic hyperfibrinolysis and urinary fibrinolysis	*CNS:* dizziness, tinnitus, malaise, headache *GI:* nausea, abdominal cramps, diarrhea *Others:* orbital swelling, nasal stuffiness, rash	Assist with activities as necessary. Keep stool chart. Check eyes and skin for reactions.
dicumarol	PO—25 mg–300 mg (according to prothrombin time)	To prevent and treat pulmonary embolism, venous thrombosis, atrial fibrillation with embolization, and coronary occlusion	*GI:* anorexia, nausea, vomiting, diarrhea, abdominal cramps *GU:* hematuria, kidney damage, orange-red urine *Skin:* petechiae, skin inflammations, itching, hair loss, mouth ulcers *Others:* fever, blood disorders	Watch for any signs of bleeding, such as under the skin, through dressings, in urine, stools or vomitus, and in mucosa. Test all stool, vomitus, and urine samples for the presence of blood. Warn patients to be careful when shaving or brushing teeth so they do not injure skin and mucous membranes, causing bleeding. Evaluate appetite. Monitor temperature and blood pressure. Keep stool chart. Warn patient that his urine may change in color. Blood tests should be done at regular intervals to check for disorders and kidney damage.
heparin	SC, IV—5,000 U–40,000 U in 24 hr (according to test results)	See dicumarol, *plus:* for diagnosis and treatment of acute and chronic coagulation disorders, to prevent clot formation during arterial and cardiac surgery; to prevent cerebral thrombosis in evolving stroke; to treat coronary occlusion-caused MI; used as an anticoagulant during blood transfusions, extracorporeal circulation, dialysis, and in blood samples for laboratory purposes	Hemorrhage, local irritation, pain, hematuria, occasional histamine-like reactions following injection (chills, fever, hives, anaphylaxis, asthma, tearing, rhinitis)	Watch for any signs of bleeding (under dressings, in skin and mucous membranes, urine, vomitus and stools). Test all stool, vomitus, and urine samples for the presence of blood. Warn patients to shave and brush their teeth carefully. Evaluate injection site for irritation. Monitor temperature and BP. Check skin for rash. Evaluate respiratory rate and rhythm.
warfarin (Coumadin)	PO—individualized according to prothrombin time IM, IV—Initial dose—20 mg–60 mg Maintenance—2 mg–10 mg qd	See dicumarol, *plus:* with other drugs in the treatment of transient cerebral ischemic attacks	*GI:* nausea, diarrhea, abdominal cramps *Skin:* hair loss, hives, dermatitis, purple toes, skin necrosis *Others:* hemorrhage, fever, hypersensitivity reactions, hemorrhagic infarction	See heparin, *plus:* Warn patients about possible change in skin color of toes.

amples are vitamin K preparations and amino-caproic acid (Amicar).

NURSING IMPLICATIONS

The most serious adverse effect of anticoagulant drug therapy is bleeding tendencies, with symptoms of hematuria, epistaxis (nosebleed), easy bruising, bleeding gums, or blood in the stool. Hospitalized patients should have their urine and stools checked regularly for the presence of blood.

All patients receiving anticoagulants need to be warned to avoid situations that could cause injury and bleeding. Male patients should shave carefully, using an electric razor whenever possible. Teeth should be brushed gently. Knives should be used with caution. If dental care is necessary, the dentist must be aware of the medication being taken.

Patients on long-term anticoagulant therapy should carry an identification card or wear a Medic-Alert tag stating their name, the name and telephone number of their physician, and the name and dose of the drug they take.

Occasionally, too much of an anticoagulant is given and bleeding becomes a problem. To reverse the action of heparin, protamine sulfate is given. It acts within minutes to stop anticoagulant effect. Menadione (vitamin K) and phytonadione are two preparations that can reverse the action of coumarin drugs. Unlike the immediate action of protamine, however, reversal with these drugs takes hours.

Periodic checks on clotting time must be done if anticoagulants are taken on a long-term basis. Patients must be taught the importance of having these tests done so they will go to the laboratory at the appointed times.

Diet teaching may be indicated. High ingestion of fat is thought to be associated with the tendency to form thrombi.

Anticoagulants should not be given to patients with blood, liver, or kidney disease; peptic ulcer; colitis; or those who are already bleeding. Patients who have had spinal cord or brain surgery should not receive anticoagulants, since even minor bleeding in these areas can be extremely dangerous.

PRACTICE PROBLEMS—DRUGS THAT AFFECT BLOOD CLOTTING

1. The order reads: heparin 15,000 U SC q12h.
    The label reads: heparin 20,000 U/ml.
    How much heparin will be given?

    $$\frac{D}{H} \times A = G$$

    $$\frac{3 \; \cancel{15,000} \; \cancel{U}}{4 \; \cancel{20,000} \; \cancel{U}} \times 1 \; ml = G$$

    $$\frac{15}{20} \times 1 \; ml = G$$

    $$\frac{3}{4} \times 1 \; ml = \frac{3}{4} \; ml$$

    Thus, $\frac{3}{4}$ ml (0.75 ml) of heparin will be given.

Work the following problems:
1. The order reads: heparin 4000 U SC q6h.
    The label reads: heparin 5000 U/ml.
    How many milliliters will be given?

2. The order reads: warfarin (Coumadin) 5 mg PO daily.
    The label reads: warfarin 2.5 mg/tablet.
    How many tablets will you give?

3. The order reads: heparin 2500 U SC q6h.
    The label reads: 10,000 U heparin/ml.
    How much would you give?

Answers are given on pp. 283–284.

CHAPTER 30
Antilipemics

Atherosclerosis is a condition characterized by the formation of fat deposits (plaques) on the inside walls of arteries. It is sometimes referred to as "hardening of the arteries." Atherosclerosis is known to cause occlusion of arteries throughout the body, which can lead to many serious diseases, such as cerebrovascular accident (CVA), myocardial infarction (MI), and renal insufficiency. Although no absolute relationship has been demonstrated between high lipid levels and increased incidence of atherosclerosis, many researchers are of the opinion that if lipid levels are lowered, there will be less likelihood of atherosclerosis.

Antilipemic drugs are used to treat a group of metabolic disorders called hyperlipidemias, in which blood levels of lipids (triglycerides and cholesterol) are elevated. They cannot remove existing atherosclerotic plaque; what they do is to prevent the formation of additional plaque (see Table 30-1).

NURSING IMPLICATIONS

While antilipemic drugs will decrease levels of blood lipids, other causes of hyperlipidemia may need attention as well. A diet high in saturated fats will defeat the purpose of drug therapy. Inherited predisposition to atherosclerosis is also thought to be a factor.

Before drug therapy is begun, changes in the patient's diet need to be made. The intake of saturated fats (found mainly in animal meats, milk, and milk products) should be decreased. Alcohol, concentrated sweets, and cholesterol should also be limited. The use of polyunsaturated fats (found in plant and fish oils) should be encouraged.

Cholestyramine has an extremely unpleasant (fishy) taste, yet must be taken in large amounts. Patients become very ingenious in their attempts to mask the taste. The powdered medication can be mixed in fruit juices or soft foods such as custard or applesauce. The dry powder should never be swallowed alone since it could block the esophagus.

Cholestyramine cannot be given with other drugs, especially drugs that contain acids, because it causes them to be inactivated. Other medications may be given either 1 hour before or 4 hours afterward. Fat-soluble vitamins will not be absorbed if they are given with cholestyramine and may need to be administered by the intramuscular route.

TABLE 30-1 ANTILIPEMICS

DRUG	ROUTE AND DOSAGE RANGE	USE	ADVERSE EFFECTS	NURSING IMPLICATIONS
clofibrate (Atromid S)	PO—500 mg qid	To treat hyperlipidemia and disorders in patients at high risk of coronary artery disease when treatment with weight reduction, exercise, control of diabetes mellitus, and other drug therapy has been unsuccessful	*CNS:* headache, dizziness, fatigue, weakness *Endocrine:* impotence, decreased sex drive *GI:* nausea, vomiting, diarrhea, weight loss, indigestion, gas, stomatitis, increased appetite, liver damage, gallstones *Skin:* rash, itching, hives, dry brittle hair (in females), hair loss *Others:* muscle aches, cramps, blood disorders, renal dysfunction, cardiac arrhythmias, dyspnea, interference with blood clotting mechanisms	Diet teaching may be necessary to help patients avoid high cholesterol intake. Blood tests to determine lipid levels should be done and reviewed frequently. Keep stool chart. Evaluate appetite. Record weight daily. Check skin for reactions. Assess condition and amount of hair. Note bleeding time. Check mouth for inflammation. Take apical pulse, and note any arrhythmias. Warn patients of possible impotence and change in sexual drive. Monitor I&O.
cholestyramine (Questran)	PO—1 packet or 1 scoop tid or qid	To help decrease elevated cholesterol levels; to relieve itching associated with partial biliary obstruction	*GI:* interference with absorption of fat-soluble vitamins, as well as other medications, constipation, impaction, nausea, vomiting, diarrhea, gas, heartburn, anorexia, steatorrhea, gallstones *Skin:* rash, itching (especially tongue or perianal itch) *Others:* osteoporosis, acidosis, increased bleeding tendency	Give other drugs at least 1 hour before or 4 to 6 hours after cholestyramine. The powder must always be mixed in water, soup, or other fluid (2 oz to 6 oz), or with a pulpy fruit. Note any unusually prolonged bleeding. Keep stool chart, and note presence of fat in stools. Evaluate appetite. Check skin for reactions. Watch for itching.
colestipol (Colestid)	PO—15 g–30 g in 2–4 divided doses qd	See cholestyramine, *plus:* to treat digitoxin overdose	See cholestyramine.	See cholestyramine.

CHAPTER 31
Cardiac stimulants and cardiac depressants

CARDIAC STIMULANTS

The heart may be weakened by age, disease, or a combination of the two. The failing heart is unable to work efficiently; cardiac output falls; and the vital organs (kidneys, brain, gut, lungs) do not receive adequate nourishment. Compensatory mechanisms such as increased heart rate may result in further problems.

Drugs that stimulate the heart are called *cardiotonics*. These drugs enable the heart to pump more efficiently, thus increasing cardiac output to the other organs.

Classification of cardiac stimulants

The drugs that stimulate heart action may be divided into two major groups (see Table 31-1). First, there are the *digitalis* preparations obtained from the foxglove plant. They have been used for centuries to treat hearts weakened by age or disease. The other group of drugs that stimulate heart action is the *adrenergic* drugs.

Digitalis preparations. The active ingredients of the digitalis plant are called *glycosides* and have been used in medicine since the time of the Egyptians and Romans. Digitalis glycosides work directly on the heart muscle (myocardium). They improve the strength of heart contraction, thus increasing cardiac output. By slowing conduction through the atrioventricular (A-V) node, they slow heart rate. The net result of medication with digitalis glycosides is a slower, stronger heart action.

The primary use of digitalis preparations is to treat congestive heart failure. Another use is in the treatment of specific cardiac arrhythmias. Although cardiac depressants are the drugs of choice in most of these cases, arrhythmias that respond to digitalis are atrial fibrillation, atrial flutter, and paroxysmal atrial tachycardia (PAT).

The preferred route of administration for digitalis preparations is by mouth. Digitalis is safe, inexpensive, and, if given at appropriate times, causes little gastrointestinal upset. Subcutaneous injection is irritating and its adverse effects are unpredictable. Digitalis preparations may be given intravenously but only in emergency situations or when other routes cannot be used. All digitalis glycoside preparations have similar functions but differ in onset and duration of action.

Adrenergic drugs. The function of the autonomic nervous system is reviewed in Chapter 18. It is divided into sympathetic and parasympathetic systems, which have different (usually opposite) functions. Transmission of nerve impulses from one fiber to the next was discussed. It was explained that certain substances called transmitters are necessary for this transmission to occur. In the parasympathetic nervous system the transmitter substance is *acetylcholine* (ACh). Fibers that liberate acetylcholine are called *cholinergic* fibers. Drugs that produce a similar action are called *cholinergic*

TABLE 31-1 CARDIAC STIMULANTS

DRUG	ROUTE AND DOSAGE RANGE	USE	ADVERSE EFFECTS	NURSING IMPLICATIONS
DIGITALIS PREPARATIONS				
digitoxin (Crystodigin)	PO, IM, IV—Digitalization—1.2 mg–1.6 mg qd (First dose 0.6 mg, then 0.4 mg in 4–6 hours, then 0.2 mg q4–6h until therapeutic effect) Maintenance—0.05–0.3 mg qd	To treat congestive heart failure, atrial fibrillation, atrial flutter, paroxysmal atrial tachycardia and supraventricular tachycardia	*CNS:* headache, weakness, apathy, mental changes, visual disturbances (blurred or yellow or green vision) *Cardiovascular:* arrhythmias, heart block, bradycardia *GI:* anorexia, nausea, vomiting, abdominal pain, diarrhea *Others:* blood disorders, skin reactions, gynecomastia, local discomfort with IM injection	Evaluate appetite. Keep stool chart. Evaluate vision and color discrimination. Evaluate mental status. Take apical pulse before administering—note rate and rhythm. (If rate is less than 60 *do not give* medicine but report to nurse in charge or to physician.) Warn males of possible breast enlargement. Give IM only when both PO and IV routes are impossible. Inject deep into muscle and follow by firm massage. No more than 0.5 mg should be injected at one time.
digoxin (Lanoxin)	PO—Digitalization—1 mg–1.5 mg qd in divided doses q6–8h Maintenance—0.125 mg–0.5 mg qd IM, IV—Digitalization—0.5 mg–1 mg qd in divided doses q4–6h Maintenance—0.125 mg–0.5 mg qd	See digitoxin, *plus:* to treat cardiogenic shock	See digitoxin.	See digitoxin.
ADRENERGIC DRUG				
levarterenol or norepinephrine (Levophed)	IV—4 ml mixed in 1000 ml D$_5$W (flow rate is adjusted to establish and maintain a low normal blood pressure)	To restore blood pressure in acute hypotension; used with other therapy in the treatment of cardiac arrest and profound hypotension	Possible bradycardia Adverse effects only when overdosage occurs—severe hypertension, reflex bradycardia, headache, increased peripheral resistance, decreased cardiac output, extravasation may lead to tissue necrosis and sloughing	Monitor apical pulse and blood pressure frequently throughout administration. Inspect infusion site for any sign of extravasation.

drugs. Drugs that block cholinergic action are called *anticholinergic* or *cholinergic-blocking* agents.

In the sympathetic division of the autonomic nervous system the transmitter substance that is liberated at most nerve endings is called *norepinephrine,* which is a close relative of epinephrine. Fibers that liberate norepinephrine are called *adrenergic* fibers. Drugs that are chemically related to norepinephrine or produce a similar action are called *adrenergic drugs.* Drugs that block adrenergic action are called *adrenergic blockers.*

Looking at the circulatory system, we see the opposite effects of parasympathetic and sympathetic innervation. The parasympathetic actions (which would also be caused by administration of *cholinergic* drugs) are a decrease in heart rate and blood pressure, relaxation of cardiac muscle, and (usually) dilation of coronary blood vessels. Sympathetic nerve stimulation (or administration of *adrenergic* drugs) causes increased heart rate and blood pressure, contraction of heart muscle, and (usually) dilation of coronary blood vessels.

Since adrenergic drugs have basically the same stimulating effect as the functioning sympathetic nervous system they are sometimes called sympathomimetic drugs (they "mimic" the sympathetic). Individual adrenergic drugs differ, however, in their ability to produce action similar to that of the sympathetic nervous system. Some, for instance, stimulate the heart and dilate blood vessels while others constrict blood vessels and have no stimulating effect on the heart. This chapter discusses adrenergic drugs that affect the heart. Those used for their effects on other areas of the body are dealt with in Chapter 32 (vasoconstrictors), Chapter 12 (central nervous system stimulants), Chapter 18 (smooth muscle relaxants), and Chapter 24 (bronchodilators).

The models for adrenergic drugs are the natural *catecholamines*—epinephrine, norepinephrine, and dopamine. Epinephrine (Adrenalin) and norepinephrine (Levophed) are adrenergic drugs that are sometimes injected directly into the heart when it has stopped beating. They act immediately to increase the strength and rate of heart action.

Isoproterenol (Isuprel) is a synthetic catecholamine useful in treating heart block, cardiac arrest, pulmonary hypertension, and pulmonary embolism. It produces greater increase in heart action and rate than epinephrine. It is also a potent vasodilator, thus increasing cardiac output and coronary blood flow.

NURSING IMPLICATIONS

When digitalis preparations are first prescribed a period of digitalization takes place, consisting of high doses of the drug given until toxic symptoms appear. A smaller maintenance dose is then ordered.

The most frequent cause of complications in digitalis therapy is overdose (digitalis toxicity). Careful observation for adverse effects, especially during digitalization, is important. Certain conditions, such as hypokalemia, metabolic disorders, and old age, can predispose the patient to digitalis toxicity.

The apical pulse must be taken for one full minute before any digitalis preparation is given, and if the rate is less than 60 beats per minute, the drug should not be given. Both the head nurse and the doctor must be notified of the situation. Patients who will be taking digitalis preparations at home should be taught to check their own pulses regularly. They should also be encouraged to establish a routine to ensure that their pill is taken every day without fail.

Nurses in the hospital need to be very careful about dosage when digitalis preparations are ordered. The placement of decimal points can cause confusion, and dosage errors may be very dangerous. Check carefully to differentiate, for example, between 0.25-mg and 0.025-mg doses.

CARDIAC DEPRESSANTS

The stimulus for each heart beat travels from the sinoatrial node in the right atrium through the muscles of the atria, to the atrioventricular node, and from there through the muscles of the ventricles. This activity results in a heart beat with regular rhythm. Any change in this normal heart rhythm is called an *arrhythmia*. Arrhythmias can be due to malfunction in the atria (atrial arrhythmias) or in the ventricles (ventricular arrhythmias).

Drugs used to treat cardiac arrhythmias are called *cardiac depressants* (see Table 31-2). Their purpose is to depress the stimuli that give rise to abnormal beats and to depress activity of an irritated heart muscle. They are also called *antiarrhythmic* drugs.

Classification of cardiac depressants

The drugs used to treat cardiac arrhythmias may be divided into two groups according to their use. In the first group are drugs for *emergency* situations, when potentially fatal arrhythmias have occurred. Other cardiac depressants are available for treatment of arrhythmias that are not immediately life threatening.

Emergency cardiac depressants. Lidocaine (Xylocaine), discussed in Chapter 11 as a topical anesthetic, may be given intravenously to correct ventricular arrhythmias, such as premature ventricular contractions (PVCs) and ventricular tachycardia. Lidocaine is usually the first drug used to

(*Text continues on p. 208.*)

TABLE 31-2 CARDIAC DEPRESSANTS

DRUG	ROUTE AND DOSAGE RANGE	USE	ADVERSE EFFECTS	NURSING IMPLICATIONS
disopyramide (Norpace, Norpace CR)	PO—400 mg–800 mg qd in divided doses (individualized, based on response and tolerance)	To suppress and prevent the recurrence of ventricular arrhythmias	*CNS/ANS:* Insomnia, blurred vision, depression, dizziness, nervousness, numbness/tingling, dry mouth, eyes, nose, and throat *Cardiovascular:* hypotension, CHF, conduction disturbances, edema, weight gain, shortness of breath, chest pain *GI:* nausea, vomiting, diarrhea, anorexia, epigastric pain, bloating, gas pains, constipation *GU:* urinary retention or hesitancy, impotence *Others:* generalized weakness, malaise, headache, aches/pains, rash, itching, changes in liver function, low potassium, hemoglobin and hematocrit, increased cholesterol and triglyceride levels, hypoglycemia	Assess visual acuity. Note any behavioral changes. Monitor BP and apical pulse. Note any complaints of unusual sensations or pains. Record weight daily. Keep stool chart. Evaluate appetite and sleep pattern. Note any difficulty with urination. Warn patient about possible impotence. Assess skin for rash. Liver function tests and other blood tests should be done at regular intervals to assess for changes.
lidocaine (Xylocaine)	IM—4.3 mg/kg IV—50 mg–100 mg; repeat after 5 min if necessary at ⅓ to ½ of initial dose	To treat cardiac arrhythmias, especially those originating in the ventricles, such as in acute myocardial infarction	*CNS:* dizziness, drowsiness, anxiety, euphoria, tinnitus, blurred or double vision, twitching, tremors, convulsions, unconsciousness, sensations of heat, cold, or numbness *Cardiovascular:* bradycardia, hypotension, possible cardiac arrest *Respiratory:* respiratory depression, respiratory arrest *Others:* vomiting, soreness at injection site	ECGs should be done frequently during administration. Evaluate mental status. Assess vision and hearing. Note any complaints of abnormal sensations. Note any unusual muscle movements. Evaluate level of consciousness. Monitor vital signs closely.
procainamide (Pronestyl)	PO—Initial dose—1 g–1.25 g Maintenance—50 mg/kg qd in divided doses at 3-hr intervals or 0.5 g–1 g q4–6h IM—0.5 g—1 g q4–8h IV—100 mg q5 min (to maximum of 1 g), then IV infusion of 2 mg–6 mg/min	To treat premature ventricular contractions, ventricular tachycardia, atrial fibrillation, paroxysmal atrial tachycardia, cardiac arrhythmias associated with anesthesia and surgery	*CNS:* weakness, mental depression, giddiness, psychosis with hallucinations *Cardiovascular:* cardiac arrhythmias, hypotension *GI:* anorexia, nausea, bitter taste, diarrhea *Others:* hives, itching skin, fever, chills, blood disorders, lupus-like syndrome	Check apical pulse frequently and report irregularities. Evaluate appetite. Check skin for reactions. Monitor temperature. Keep stool chart. Monitor BP. Evaluate mental status. Blood tests should be done at regular intervals.

(continued on page 207)

TABLE 31-2 (continued)

DRUG	ROUTE AND DOSAGE RANGE	USE	ADVERSE EFFECTS	NURSING IMPLICATIONS
propranolol (Inderal)	PO—30 mg–640 mg qd in divided doses IV—1 mg–3 mg; repeat after 2 min if necessary	To treat angina pectoris caused by coronary atherosclerosis; to treat cardiac arrhythmias (supraventricular, ventricular, and tachycardic), and hypertrophic subaortic stenosis; to treat migraine headache; used along with other drugs to treat hypertension	*CNS:* lightheadedness, mental depression, insomnia, lethargy, visual disturbances, hallucinations, memory loss, disorientation, mood swings, paresthesias in hands *Cardiovascular:* bradycardia, CHF, hypotension *Respiratory:* respiratory distress, bronchospasm *GI:* nausea, vomiting, diarrhea or constipation, abdominal cramping, sore and aching throat *Others:* blood disorders, fever, rash	Check apical pulse frequently and report irregularities. Monitor blood pressure. Evaluate mental status. Assess sleep pattern. Evaluate visual acuity. Blood tests should be done at regular intervals. Check orientation. Keep stool chart. Assist with activities if necessary. Monitor temperature. Note respiratory rate and quality.
quinidine gluconate (Quinaglute, Duraquin)	PO—324 mg–660 mg q8–12h IM—Test dose—200 mg; then 400 mg–600 mg q2h prn IV—330 mg–750 mg	To treat premature atrial and ventricular contractions, paroxysmal atrial tachycardia, paroxysmal AV junctional rhythm, atrial fibrillation and flutter, paroxysmal ventricular tachycardia; use for maintenance therapy after electrical conversion of atrial fibrillation or flutter	*CNS:* vertigo, blurred or double vision, disturbed color vision, night blindness *Cardiovascular:* arrhythmias, hypotension *GI:* nausea, vomiting, abdominal pain, diarrhea *Skin:* rashes with intense itching, photosensitivity *Others:* blood disorders, respiratory distress, cinchonism (headache, nausea, disturbed vision, tinnitus)	Evaluate hearing and vision. Caution patients to avoid direct sunlight and brightly lit rooms. Monitor all vital signs closely. Keep stool chart. Check for rashes, and note any itching. Blood tests should be done at regular intervals. Give with food to decrease GI upset.
quinidine sulfate (Quinora)	PO—0.2 g–0.6 g q2–8h	See quinidine gluconate.	See quinidine gluconate, *plus:* bitter taste	See quinidine gluconate.
tocainide (Tonocard)	PO—1200 mg–2400 mg/day in 3 divided doses	To suppress and prevent the recurrence of ventricular arrhythmias	*CNS:* stuttering, slurred speech, coma, seizures, depression, diplopia, dysarthria, insomnia, nightmares, psychosis, weakness *Cardiovascular:* ventricular fibrillation, AV block, hypertension, cardiomegaly, syncope, sinus arrest *Respiratory:* respiratory arrest, pulmonary edema and embolism, dyspnea, pneumonia *GI:* abdominal pain, constipation, dysphagia, upset stomach, thirst, dry mouth *Others:* blood disorders, fever, rash, muscle spasms	Note any speech abnormality. Assess visual acuity. Note any behavioral changes and evaluate mental status. Evaluate sleep pattern. Note any complaints of muscle weakness or pain. Monitor apical pulse, temperature, and BP closely. Note character and rate of respirations. Keep stool chart. Monitor I&O. Check skin for rash. Blood tests should be done at regular intervals.

treat arrhythmias, since its ability to act immediately makes it an ideal emergency drug. Phenytoin (Dilantin) is also useful in serious ventricular arrhythmias, as well as in arrhythmias caused by digitalis toxicity. Atropine sulfate may be given in a cardiac emergency to correct sinus bradycardia or heart block. The intravenous route is used with all of these drugs because it ensures rapid absorption.

Cardiac depressants for less critical situations. Quinidine, often considered to be a model antiarrhythmic drug, is widely used to treat atrial fibrillation, atrial flutter, and ventricular arrhythmias. It may be given by mouth or parenterally.

Procainamide (Pronestyl) is less effective than quinidine in treating atrial fibrillation and flutter, but it is quite effective in treating arrhythmias due to ectopic beats (heartbeats originating in areas other than the sinoatrial node).

Propranolol (Inderal) is an adrenergic blocker that decreases heart rate and cardiac muscle contraction. It is a cardiac depressant useful in the treatment of both ventricular and atrial arrhythmias.

NURSING IMPLICATIONS

Emergency cardiac depressants are usually given in an emergency setting. Patients receiving these drugs intravenously should be placed on a cardiac monitor so the situation can be continuously assessed. Emergency equipment such as an airway, oxygen, and defibrillator should be kept nearby.

Cardiac depressants are given to treat arrhythmias, but they may have the reverse effect of causing arrhythmias and tachycardia. For these reasons, the apical pulse must be checked periodically so that heart rate and rhythm can be measured. Patients can be taught to take their own pulses.

In addition to its antiarrhythmic action, quinidine is also a vasodilator and therefore may cause a drop in blood pressure. For this reason, the blood pressure, as well as the pulse, must be measured in patients receiving quinidine preparations.

A frequent toxic effect of quinidine is cinchonism, with symptoms of nausea, vomiting, diarrhea, vertigo, visual disturbances, and ringing in the ears (tinnitus).

Procainamide has a bitter taste that can be masked by a strongly flavored juice. Mouthwash or hard candy can also help to disguise the aftertaste.

As with other heart medications, the patient taking an antiarrhythmic drug should be instructed never to skip a dose. The prescribed amount and schedule should never be changed without specific instructions from the physician.

PRACTICE PROBLEMS—CARDIAC STIMULANTS AND CARDIAC DEPRESSANTS

1. The order reads: digoxin (Lanoxin) elixir 0.25 mg via NG tube.
   The label reads: digoxin 0.05 mg/ml.
   How many milliliters will you give?

$$\frac{D}{H} \times A = G$$

$$\overset{5}{\cancel{\frac{0.25 \text{ mg}}{0.05 \text{ mg}}}} \times 1 \text{ ml} = G$$

$$5 \times 1 \text{ ml} = 5 \text{ ml}$$

Thus, 5 ml of digoxin (Lanoxin) elixir is given.

2. The order reads: propranolol (Inderal) 80 mg PO tid.
   The label reads: propranolol 40 mg/tablet.
   How many tablets will you give?

$$\frac{D}{H} = G$$

$$\overset{2}{\cancel{\frac{80 \text{ mg}}{40 \text{ mg}}}} = 2$$

You will give 2 tablets of propranolol (Inderal).

Work the following problems:

1. The order reads: quinidine gluconate 200 mg IM one time.
   The label reads: quinidine gluconate 80 mg/ml.
   How many milliliters will you give?

2. The order reads: digitoxin 0.05 mg daily.
   The label reads: digitoxin 0.1 mg/tablet.
   How many tablets will you give?

3. The physician orders quinidine sulfate 0.4 g. The drug comes from the pharmacy labeled 200 mg quinidine sulfate per tablet. How many tablets would you give?

Answers are given on p. 284.

CHAPTER 32
Vasodilators and vasoconstrictors

VASODILATORS

Drugs that produce dilation of blood vessels are called *vasodilators*. They are valuable in the treatment of hypertension and also in increasing blood flow to the heart or the extremities. Vasodilators may have their effect in the central nervous system or locally, and some of them combine both actions. The use of centrally acting vasodilators in hypertension is discussed in Chapter 33. Those having local action are discussed here (see Table 32-1).

Coronary vasodilators

As their name suggests, the coronary vasodilators are used in the treatment of heart disease (angina pectoris, coronary artery insufficiency, and ischemia). They produce dilation of coronary arteries that are in spasm and thus relax the arterial smooth muscle. The *nitrates* or *nitrites* are the most commonly used coronary vasodilators. Short-acting nitrates, such as amyl nitrite, sublingual nitroglycerin (TNG), and isosorbide (Isordil), act within minutes to relieve chest pain. These drugs may also be taken prophylactically before exercise that is known to cause chest pain. Long-acting nitrates are used mainly in prevention of pain.

Dipyridamole (Persantine) is a short-acting coronary vasodilator that is not a nitrate. Its vasodilating action occurs within approximately 20 minutes of oral administration.

Propranolol (see Chapter 31 for its use as a cardiac depressant) and nadolol (Corgard) are adrenergic blocking agents used to treat angina pectoris. They do so by blocking sympathetic nervous stimulation, thereby causing the coronary blood vessels to dilate. This relieves myocardial pain by increasing the supply of oxygen. Ethyl alcohol (see Chapter 10) and the xanthines (see Chapter 20) are other effective coronary vasodilators.

The calcium channel blockers are a new group of vasodilators that work by altering the flow of calcium into certain "channels" in cardiac and vascular smooth muscle. The result is relaxation (dilation) of cardiac arteries and arterioles. Examples of these drugs are diltiazem (Cardizem), nifedipine (Procardia), and verapamil (Calan, Isoptin).

Peripheral vasodilators

Some of the drugs that produce peripheral vasodilation are classified as adrenergic-blocking agents. By blocking the activities of the sympathetic nervous system, they cause vasodilation. These drugs are occasionally helpful in the treatment of chronic arterial occlusion and peripheral vascular disease (PVD).

NURSING IMPLICATIONS

Since the effects of the vasodilators are widespread, hypotension, flushed face (the patient may say his

(*Text continues on p. 214.*)

TABLE 32-1 VASODILATORS

DRUG	ROUTE AND DOSAGE RANGE	USE	ADVERSE EFFECTS	NURSING IMPLICATIONS
amyl nitrite	Inhalation—0.18 ml– 0.3 ml prn	To relieve angina pectoris	*CNS:* increased intra-ocular and intracranial pressure, headache, dizziness, weakness, restlessness, fainting *Cardiovascular:* tachycardia, hypotension *GI:* nausea, vomiting *Skin:* flushed face, pallor, cold sweat *Others:* incontinence of urine and feces	Monitor vital signs. Assist with activity as necessary. Observe skin for color and hydration. Watch for incontinence, and record all I&O.
cyclandelate (Cyclospasmol)	PO—400 mg–1600 mg qd in divided doses	Along with other therapy to treat intermittent claudication, arteriosclerosis obliterans, thrombophlebitis, nocturnal leg cramps, Raynaud's phenomenon, and certain cases of ischemic cerebral vascular disease	GI distress, belching, mild flushing, headache, weakness, tachycardia	Take medication with meals or antacids to decrease GI distress. Monitor pulse rate.
diltiazem (Cardizem)	PO—120 mg–240 mg/day in divided doses tid–qid	To treat angina pectoris due to coronary artery spasm and chronic stable angina	*CNS:* headache, drowsiness, dizziness, lightheadedness, nervousness, depression, weakness, insomnia, confusion, hallucinations, fatigue, paresthesias *Cardiovascular:* flushing, CHF, arrhythmias, bradycardia, syncope, hypotension, pounding heart, swelling or edema *GI:* nausea, vomiting, diarrhea or constipation, indigestion *Skin:* rash, itching, petechiae *Others:* photosensitivity, nocturia, thirst, polyuria, joint pain	Assist patient with activities if necessary. Evaluate mental status. Assess sleep patterns. Note any complaint of unusual sensations. Monitor vital signs. Note any flushing or swelling/edema. Weigh daily. Keep stool chart. Check skin for rash or itching. Note complaints of unusual thirst and/or frequent urination.
dipyridamole (Persantine)	PO—50 mg tid	Long-term therapy for chronic angina pectoris	Headache, dizziness, nausea, flushing, weakness, fainting, mild GI distress, rash	Medication should be taken at least 1 hour before meal. Check skin for change in color or rash. Assist with activities as necessary.
isosorbide (Isordil, IsoBid, Sorbitrate)	SL—2.5 mg–10 mg q2–3h PO—5 mg–30 mg qid Sustained release—40 mg q6–12h	To prevent and treat acute anginal attacks; to relieve the pain of coronary artery disease	*CNS:* headache (may be persistent and severe), dizziness, weakness, restlessness, collapse *GI:* nausea, vomiting *Skin:* rashes, flushed skin, increased sweating *Others:* postural hypotension	Observe skin for color and any rash. Note complaints of headache. Assist with activity as necessary. Monitor BP—warn patient to change position (getting out of bed especially) carefully and slowly. Note any behavioral change. PO tablets should be taken on an empty stomach. Be sure to give proper form of the medication (do not confuse SL with PO).

(continued on page 213)

TABLE 32-1 (continued)

DRUG	ROUTE AND DOSAGE RANGE	USE	ADVERSE EFFECTS	NURSING IMPLICATIONS
isoxsuprine (Vasodilan)	PO—10 mg–20 mg q6–8h IM—5 mg–10 mg q8–12h	To relieve symptoms associated with cerebral vascular insufficiency; to treat peripheral vascular diseases, such as arteriosclerosis obliterans, Buerger's disease, and Raynaud's disease; use in threatened abortion	Hypotension, dizziness, tachycardia, nausea, vomiting, abdominal distress, severe rash	Monitor BP and pulse. Assist with activity as necessary. Check skin for rash.
nadolol (Corgard)	PO—40 mg–320 mg once daily	For long-term management of angina pectoris, alone or in combination with other drugs to treat hypertension	See propranolol, *plus:* *CNS/ANS:* dizziness, fatigue, sedation, memory loss, dry mouth, eyes, or skin *Cardiovascular:* peripheral vascular insufficiency, rhythm/conduction disturbances *GI:* anorexia, indigestion, bloating, gas, colitis *GU:* impotence, or decreased libido *Others:* headache, facial swelling, weight gain, slurred speech, cough, nasal stuffiness, sweating, tinnitus, blurred vision, alopecia	See propranolol, *plus:* Warn patient of possible change in sexual drive and/or function.
nifedipine (Procardia)	PO—10 mg–30 mg tid–qid	To manage both vasospastic and chronic stable angina	*CNS/ANS:* dizziness, lightheadedness, giddiness, headache, weakness, tremor, nervousness, mood changes, sleep disturbances, imbalance, flushing, hot sensations, sweating, chills *Cardiovascular:* peripheral edema, palpitations, hypotension, syncope *Respiratory:* dyspnea, cough, wheezing, nasal and chest congestion *GI:* nausea, heartburn, diarrhea or constipation, cramps, gas pains *GU:* sexual difficulties *Musculoskeletal:* muscle cramps, inflammation, joint stiffness *Others:* rash, itching, fever	BP must be carefully monitored, especially during initial treatment phase. Assist with ambulation if necessary. Note any behavioral changes. Assess sleep pattern. Note any complaints of altered sensation. Monitor temperature, apical pulse, and respiratory rate and character. Keep stool chart. Warn patient about possible difficulties with sexual function. Note any complaints of muscle/joint discomfort. Assess skin for rash.

(continued on page 214)

TABLE 32-1 (continued)

DRUG	ROUTE AND DOSAGE RANGE	USE	ADVERSE EFFECTS	NURSING IMPLICATIONS
nitroglycerin (Nitro-Bid, Nitrodisc, Nitro-Dur, Nitrol, Nitrostat, TNG, Transderm-Nitro, Tridil)	PO—2.5 mg–9 mg q8–12h SL—0.15 mg–0.6 mg prn Topical ointment— 1–5 inches q3–4h Transdermal system—one system q24h IV—8 mg per 250 ml diluent (5 mcg–50 mcg/min)	To manage, prevent, or treat angina pectoris	*CNS:* headache, dizziness, vertigo, weakness, fainting *Cardiovascular:* tachycardia, palpitations, postural hypotension *Others:* flushed skin, nausea, vomiting, dermatitis	Follow orders carefully as to the route of administration. Topical route is effective wherever it is applied on the body. Chest, abdomen, and anterior thigh are common areas. Avoid distal extremities. Ointment should be applied and spread thinly but not rubbed in. Avoid getting paste on fingers when applying. Monitor BP and pulse. Assist with activities as necessary. Observe for flushing. Transdermal system should be removed 1 hour before next one is applied. Apply subsequent systems to a different area.
pentaerythritol (Peritrate)	PO—40 mg–160 mg qd	To reduce the incidence and severity of anginal attacks	See isosorbide.	See isosorbide, *plus:* Give ½ hour before or 1 hour after meals.
verapamil (Calan, Isoptin)	PO—240 mg–480 mg/day in divided doses IV—1st dose: 0.075 mg–0.15 mg/kg *over 2 minutes* Repeat doses—0.15 mg/kg 30 min after initial dose	IV—to treat supraventricular tachyarrhythmias PO—to treat angina at rest and chronic stable angina	*CNS:* dizziness, fatigue, headache *Cardiovascular:* hypotension, bradycardia, severe tachycardia, peripheral edema, AV block, CHF, or pulmonary edema *GI:* nausea, abdominal discomfort, constipation *Rare:* bronchospasm, laryngospasm, rash, and itching	When administered IV, continuous ECG monitoring is necessary. Monitor BP and pulse. Keep stool chart. Watch for signs of edema. Check skin for rash.

head feels "full"), and vertigo are common. Be sure to measure the patient's blood pressure before any vasodilator is administered; if the systolic pressure is below 100 mm Hg, the medication should be withheld and the physician notified.

If the drug is being administered to relieve chest pain, be sure to assess the location and degree of pain before you give the medication—without this baseline it is difficult to evaluate the effectiveness of the drug.

If the drug is prescribed for PVD, you need to observe the patient and note any sensation of increased warmth, as well as change in color and in the character of the pain in the extremities. Relief may be of a temporary nature, therefore assess for return of symptoms.

Nitroglycerin tablets are often kept at the patient's bedside so he may take one immediately when he has chest pain. The tablets should be stored in tightly stoppered dark glass containers to ensure potency, and they should be replaced every 3 months.

You may need to demonstrate to the patient just what is meant by the term *sublingual.* Instruct the patient not to drink water after placing the tablet under his tongue. Remind him that if he does not get relief, he may take a second and a third tablet at 5-minute intervals. If these measures fail to provide relief, measure the blood pressure, and notify the nurse in charge.

Nitropaste is prescribed in inches. The appropriate amount is squeezed from the tube onto specially marked measuring paper, which is then applied anywhere on the body. Most patients apply it to the chest area because of its proximity to the heart. The paste should not be rubbed in. Remind the patient to wear gloves to avoid getting it on his fingers.

The transdermal system of administering nitroglycerin requires placement of a "patch" every 24 hours. The different-sized "patches" (measured in centimeters) release different dosages of drug per 24-hour period in a controlled manner. Be sure the area is clean, dry, and free of hair so the adhesive will adhere. Do not apply subsequent systems to the same area. The "patch" may be applied to any body area except the hands or feet, although most patients prefer to apply it to the chest.

VASOCONSTRICTORS

Vasoconstrictors, also called *vasopressors* or simply *pressors*, are drugs that constrict the blood vessels. Their action may be either systemic or local (see Table 32-2).

Systemic vasoconstrictors

Drugs in this category are used to control acute hypotension caused by circulatory shock or anaphylactic reaction. They are adrenergic drugs, both catecholamines (epinephrine, dopamine, and lev-

TABLE 32-2 VASOCONSTRICTORS

DRUG	ROUTE AND DOSAGE RANGE	USE	ADVERSE EFFECTS	NURSING IMPLICATIONS
SYSTEMIC				
dopamine HCl (Intropin)	IV—200 mg–400 mg in 250 ml–500 ml IV solution (administer 2 mcg–50 mcg/kg/min)	To restore BP in shock syndromes due to myocardial infarctions, trauma, endotoxic septicemia, open heart surgery, renal failure, and CHF	*Cardiovascular:* arrhythmias, tachycardia, anginal pain, palpitations, hypotension *GI:* nausea, vomiting *Others:* headache, dyspnea	Monitor BP and pulse closely. Note difficulties with respiration. Note complaints of chest pain and headache.
metaraminol (Aramine)	IM, SC—2 mg–10 mg IV—15 mg–500 mg in 500 ml IV solution	To prevent and treat acute hypotensive states occurring with spinal anesthesia; used with other drugs to treat hypotension due to hemorrhage, cardiogenic shock, drug reactions, septicemia, surgical complications; to treat shock with brain damage due to trauma or tumor	Arrhythmias, possible cardiac arrest, abscess and tissue necrosis at injection sites, pulmonary edema, relapse in patients with malaria	Monitor BP frequently during administration. Note injection site (appearance and color). Take apical pulse, and note any irregularities.
norepinephrine or levarterenol (Levophed)	IV—4 mg–68 mg/1000 ml IV solution	To restore BP in acute hypotensive states (poliomyelitis, spinal anesthesia, myocardial infarction, septicemia, blood transfusion and drug reactions, removal of pheochromocytoma, and after sympathectomy); used with other medication to treat cardiac arrest	Bradycardia, headache, increased peripheral resistance, decreased cardiac output, depleted plasma volume	Monitor BP and pulse. Avoid extravasation. Check infusion site frequently for free flow.

(continued on page 216)

TABLE 32-2 (continued)

DRUG	ROUTE AND DOSAGE RANGE	USE	ADVERSE EFFECTS	NURSING IMPLICATIONS
ergotamine tartrate (Ergostat, Ergomar)	SL—1–3 tablets prn (Not to exceed 5 tablets/week or 3/24 hr)	To treat cluster, migraine, or other vascular headaches	*CNS:* numbness or tingling in fingers and toes, pain in muscles of extremities and heart *Cardiovascular:* brady- or tachycardia *GI:* nausea, vomiting *Others:* itching, localized edema	Medication must be protected from light and heat. Note any complaints of muscle pain. Monitor pulse rate. Note itching or local edema. Initiate therapy at first sign of headache.
LOCAL				
dexbrompheniramine maleate + pseudoephedrine sulfate (Drixoral)	PO—1 tablet bid in AM and at hs (In severe cases to a maximum of 3 tablets qd)	To relieve symptoms of upper respiratory mucosal congestion in nasal allergies, acute rhinitis, rhinosinusitis, and blocked eustachian tubes	*CNS:* headache, drowsiness, confusion, vertigo, restlessness, anxiety, insomnia, tension, weakness *Cardiovascular:* tachycardia, palpitations, angina, hypertension, circulatory collapse *GI:* anorexia, GI distress, abdominal cramps, nausea, vomiting *Others:* difficult urination, pupillary dilation, rash, increased perspiration	Evaluate mental status. Assist with activities as necessary. Assess sleeping pattern. Monitor apical pulse and blood pressure. Note any complaints of chest pain or discomfort. Assess appetite. Record I&O, and note complaints of urinary problems. Observe skin for rash or increased perspiration.
methysergide maleate (Sansert)	PO—4 mg–8 mg qd c̄ meals	To reduce the frequency of severe vascular headaches	*CNS:* insomnia, drowsiness, mild euphoria, ataxia, dizziness, hallucinations, weakness *GI:* nausea, vomiting, diarrhea or constipation, heartburn, abdominal pain, weight gain *Skin:* facial flushing, rash, hair loss *Others:* fibrotic changes in tissues, edema, blood disorders, muscle and joint pain	Give with meals to avoid GI upset and pain. Assess sleeping pattern. Evaluate mental status. Keep stool chart. Assist with ambulation and other activities as needed. Check skin for flushing and rash. Note any hair loss. Check weight daily. Keep record of I&O. Note complaints of joint and muscle pain. There should be a drug-free interval of 3 to 4 weeks after each 6 month course of therapy.
oxymetazoline (Afrin)	Nasal drops or spray—(0.05% solution)—2–3 sprays or drops into each nostril bid	To relieve nasal congestion in upper respiratory disorders; used to treat and prevent middle ear infections	*CNS:* headache, light-headedness, insomnia *Respiratory:* dryness of nasal mucosa, possible rebound congestion with overuse *Others:* palpitations, burning and stinging of nasal mucosa	Warn patients not to use more than the ordered amount. Monitor pulse. Assess sleeping pattern.

(continued on page 217)

TABLE 32-2 (continued)

DRUG	ROUTE AND DOSAGE RANGE	USE	ADVERSE EFFECTS	NURSING IMPLICATIONS
phenylpro-panolamine + phenyleph-rine + phen-yltoloxamine citrate + chlorphenira-mine maleate (Naldecon)	PO—1 tsp or 1 tab-let tid to qid	To relieve nasal congestion associ-ated with pollen al-lergy and minor in-fections of the upper respiratory tract	See brompheniramine.	See brompheniramine.
pseudo-ephedrine (Sudafed)	PO—60 mg tid to qid	To treat acute head colds, ear infec-tions, croup, sinus infections, tracheo-bronchitis, and asthma	Possible mild CNS stim-ulation (nervousness, dizziness, insomnia, nausea, headache)	Evaluate behavior and sleep pattern. Assist with activities if dizzi-ness is a problem.
tetrahydrozoline (Tyzine, Vis-ine)	Nasal solution—(0.1%) 2 gtt–4 gtt q3h prn Drops—(0.05%) 1 gtt–2 gtt OU q8–12h	To relieve congestion of the nasal and na-sopharyngeal mu-cosa; to relieve eye irritation due to al-lergies, strain, swimming, glare, or minor irritants	See oxymetazoline, *plus:* burning and stinging of the eyes	See oxymetazoline.

arterenol) and noncatecholamines (ephedrine, phenylephrine, and metaraminol). Their general-ized vasoconstrictive action leads to a rise in ar-terial blood pressure and increased blood flow to the heart and brain. These drugs are usually given in emergency situations by intravenous routes, al-though they can be injected directly into the heart (intracardiac route).

The ergot alkaloids are vasoconstrictors whose chief use in the past was as oxytocic drugs (see Chapter 39). They are now used primarily in the treatment of vascular (migraine) headache. The most commonly used ergot preparation is ergota-mine plus caffeine (Cafergot). Methysergide (San-sert) is related chemically to the ergot alkaloids and is used in the prophylactic treatment of vas-cular headache.

Local vasoconstrictors

Drugs that cause local vasoconstriction control su-perficial bleeding and shrink swollen nasal mem-branes. These drugs are sometimes combined with antihistamines and used as nasal decongestants (see Chapter 26). Tetrahydrozoline (Visine, Tyzine) is a local vasoconstrictor that relieves eye irrita-tion.

NURSING IMPLICATIONS

Blood pressure must be taken every 2 to 5 minutes when vasoconstrictors are being given intrave-nously, since overdose can cause severe hyperten-sion. Headache, photophobia, chest pain, and vom-iting may also occur. If these medications infiltrate the subcutaneous tissue, serious cell damage with sloughing will occur; therefore, needle placement must be checked frequently.

In addition to the medications discussed as vasoconstrictors, there are other substances that are also vasoconstrictive, such as nicotine in tobacco and also tyramine, a chemical found in many foods (see Chapter 6). Patients who smoke or ingest ty-ramine while receiving vasoconstrictors must be watched for possible additive hypertensive effects.

A patient taking ergotamine tartrate to relieve vascular headache should go to bed in a darkened room for the next several hours.

PRACTICE PROBLEMS—VASODILATORS AND VASOCONSTRICTORS

1. The order reads: dipyridamole (Persantine) 50 mg PO tid.
   The label reads: dipyridamole 25 mg/tablet.
   How many tablets will be given?

   $$\frac{D}{H} = G$$

   $$\frac{2 \, \cancel{50} \, \cancel{mg}}{1 \, \cancel{25} \, \cancel{mg}} = 2$$

   Thus, 2 tablets of dipyridamole (Persantine) will be given.

2. Metaraminol (Aramine) 6 mg IM one time is ordered for a patient with low blood pressure. Metaraminol comes in a vial containing 10 mg/ml. How much will be given?

   $$\frac{D}{H} \times A = G$$

   $$\frac{3 \, \cancel{6} \, \cancel{mg}}{5 \, \cancel{10} \, \cancel{mg}} \times 1 \, ml = G$$

   $$\frac{3}{5} \times 1 \, ml = \frac{3}{5} \, ml \text{ or } 0.6 \, ml$$

Thus, $\frac{3}{5}$ ml (0.6 ml) of metaraminol (Aramine) will be given.

Work the following problems:

1. The order reads: methysergide (Sansert) 2 mg PO tid with meals.
   The label reads: methysergide 2 mg/tablet.
   How many tablets will be given?

2. The order reads: isosorbide (Isordil) 10 mg PO qid.
   The label reads: isosorbide 5 mg/tablet.
   How many tablets will be given?

3. The order reads: isoxsuprine (Vasodilan) 8 mg IM q8h.
   The label reads: isoxsuprine 10 mg/ml.
   How much will be given?

Answers are given on p. 284.

CHAPTER 33
Antihypertensives

With any condition causing an increase in peripheral vascular resistance, the heart has to work harder to pump blood and the diastolic blood pressure rises above normal. This condition is called *arterial hypertension*, and it is associated with disorders of the cardiovascular, renal, and cerebrovascular systems.

In most cases of hypertension no cause can be found. This type of hypertension, called *essential* or *primary* hypertension, can be controlled by medication. In the remaining cases, the hypertension is traceable to a specific cause and the disease is termed *secondary* hypertension.

Malignant hypertension is an uncommon but extremely serious type of hypertension. It can be fatal unless it is treated as soon as symptoms develop, because the blood vessels are so quickly damaged that repair is not possible. With proper medications, malignant hypertension can be kept under control.

CLASSIFICATION OF ANTIHYPERTENSIVE DRUGS

The aim of antihypertensive drugs is to keep the blood pressure within normal limits, regardless of whether the patient is in a standing, sitting, or reclining position. Furthermore, blood flow to any part of the body must not be compromised. The drugs act by either decreasing peripheral resistance or decreasing the volume of circulating blood. Some drugs have a combined action, but the net result is the same—the heart does not work as hard, and the blood pressure falls.

Many drugs have antihypertensive action (see Table 33-1). *Vasodilators* increase the diameter of blood vessels, which causes a drop in the pressure of circulating blood. Thus, they may be used as a specific treatment for hypertension. *Adrenergic blockers* act in a way that is not yet completely understood, but they do lower blood pressure. As with vasodilators, the general action of all adrenergic blockers is to lower blood pressure, thus members of the group are used specifically to treat hypertension. Examples of such drugs are guanethidine (Ismelin), prazosin (Minipress), and phentolamine (Regitine). All *diuretics* cause excretion of water and sodium, thereby reducing blood volume. This, in turn, lowers the blood pressure. The thiazide diuretics are especially effective as antihypertensives. Captopril (Capoten) is one of a new class of antihypertensives that inhibits an enzyme system involved in fluid retention, thereby lowering blood pressure.

Sedatives, tranquilizers, and antidepressants are *psychotropic* drugs used to treat hypertension. Although most of them do not relieve the hypertension itself, they do allay the anxiety and apprehension that often cause blood pressure to rise. These medications are used with other drugs in combination therapy for hypertension. Some psychotropics have specific antihypertensive action, such as the *Rauwolfia alkaloids*. Newer psycho-

(*Text continues on p. 224.*)

TABLE 33-1   ANTIHYPERTENSIVES

DRUG	ROUTE AND DOSAGE RANGE	USE	ADVERSE EFFECTS	NURSING IMPLICATIONS
atenolol (Tenormin)	PO—50 mg–100 mg qd	To manage hypertension either alone or along with other agents	*CNS:* vertigo, dizziness, fatigue, depression, headache, nightmares, insomnia *Cardiovascular:* bradycardia, shortness of breath, cold extremities, Raynaud's disease, palpitations, CHF, hypotension *Respiratory:* dyspnea, bronchospasm, wheezing *GI:* gastric pain, nausea, diarrhea or constipation, gas, heartburn *Skin:* itching	Evaluate mental status. Assist with activities as necessary. Assess sleep pattern. Monitor apical pulse, BP, and respiratory rate and rhythm. Note any cold extremities or abnormal circulation in extremities. Keep a stool chart. Observe for any itching.
captopril (Capoten)	PO—25 mg–150 mg tid	Used along with other drugs to treat hypertension and heart failure in patients who have not responded well to other drug regimens	*CNS:* dizziness, headache, malaise, fatigue, insomnia, fever, paresthesias *ANS:* flushing, pallor, dry mouth *Cardiovascular:* hypotension, edema (face, extremities, mucous membranes), tachycardia, chest pain, palpitations, myocardial infarction, CHF, Raynaud's disease *GI:* nausea, vomiting, diarrhea, constipation, anorexia, abdominal pain, ulcers, gastric irritation, loss of sense of taste *GU:* polyuria, oliguria, proteinuria, impotence *Skin:* rash, itching *Others:* dyspnea, photosensitivity, blood disorders	Give 1 hour before meals. Assist patient with activities if necessary. Note complaints of fatigue and/or any unusual sensations. Note skin color. Assess sleep patterns. Monitor BP, pulse, and respirations frequently. Note any swelling. Keep stool chart. Evaluate appetite. Keep strict I&O records. Note any changes in urinary output/frequency. Check for protein in urine at regular intervals. Blood tests should be done at regular intervals. Warn patients to report any signs of infection and to avoid excessive perspiration that could lead to dehydration. Warn male patient about possible change in sexual function.
clonidine (Catapres)	PO—Initial dose— 0.1 mg bid Maintenance—0.2 mg–0.8 mg qd in divided doses	To treat mild to moderate hypertension	*CNS:* drowsiness, dizziness, sedation, headache, fatigue, vivid dreams or insomnia, behavioral changes, nervousness, restlessness, anxiety, depression *Cardiovascular:* CHF, arrhythmias *Endocrine:* weight gain, gynecomastia, impotence	BP should be monitored frequently during administration. Warn patient to avoid dangerous activities. Warn patient not to stop taking the drug abruptly. Assist with ambulation as necessary. Keep stool chart. Evaluate mental status and any behavioral changes. Assess appetite.

(continued on page 221)

TABLE 33-1 (continued)

DRUG	ROUTE AND DOSAGE RANGE	USE	ADVERSE EFFECTS	NURSING IMPLICATIONS
clonidine (*continued*)			*GI:* anorexia, nausea, vomiting, parotid pain, constipation, liver damage *Skin:* rash, itching, hives, thinning hair *Others:* dry mouth and nose, urinary retention, increased sensitivity to alcohol, itchy and burning eyes	Check weight daily. Keep accurate I&O record. Warn males of possible breast enlargement and impotence. Evaluate sleeping patterns. Check skin for rash, itch, or hives. Note thinning hair. Encourage patients to avoid alcohol. Patients should be encouraged to have periodic eye examinations.
guanethidine (Ismelin)	PO—10 mg–50 mg daily as a single dose	To treat moderate and severe hypertension and renal hypertension	*CNS:* dizziness, weakness, lethargy, fainting, blurred vision, droopy eyelids, muscle tremor and aches, mental depression *Cardiovascular:* postural and exertional hypotension, bradycardia, CHF, angina *Respiratory:* dyspnea, asthma, nasal congestion *Endocrine:* weight gain, impotence *GI:* diarrhea, vomiting, nausea, dry mouth, parotid pain *Skin:* rash, hair loss *Others:* fluid retention, incontinence	Monitor BP frequently in standing and lying positions and after exercise. Instruct patients to sit or lie down as soon as they feel dizzy or weak. Monitor pulse and respirations, noting any difficulty with breathing. Keep stool chart. Record I&O. Check weight daily. Warn males of possible impotence. Note any hair loss. Check skin for rash. Evaluate visual acuity. Note any complaints of muscular aches and pains or pain near parotid glands.
hydralazine (Apresoline)	PO—40 mg–400 mg qd in 4 divided doses IM, IV—20 mg–40 mg prn	To treat essential hypertension	*CNS:* headache, paresthesias in extremities, muscle cramps or tremors, mental changes *Cardiovascular:* palpitations, tachycardia, angina, hypotension *Respiratory:* nasal congestion, dyspnea *GI:* anorexia, nausea, vomiting, diarrhea, constipation *Skin:* flushing, hypersensitivity reactions, conjunctivitis *Others:* increased tearing, edema, problems with urination, blood disorders, lupuslike syndrome	Monitor BP, pulse, and respirations carefully. Assess appetite. Keep stool chart. Note complaints of chest pain. Check eyes for inflammation and increased tears. Note any abnormal muscle movements. Keep accurate I&O record. Check weight daily. Evaluate mental status. Check skin for reactions. Blood tests should be done at regular intervals.
labetalol (Normodyne, Trandate)	PO—400 mg–2400 mg/day in 2–3 divided doses IV—50 mg–300 mg	Used alone or in combination with other medications to manage hypertension	See atenolol.	See atenolol.

(continued on page 222)

TABLE 33-1 (continued)

DRUG	ROUTE AND DOSAGE RANGE	USE	ADVERSE EFFECTS	NURSING IMPLICATIONS
methyldopa (Aldomet)	PO—500 mg–3 g qd in 2–4 divided doses IV—250 mg–1 g q6h	To treat hypertension	*CNS:* headache, sedation, weakness, dizziness, lightheadedness, Parkinsonism, mental disorders *Endocrine:* gynecomastia, lactation, impotence, decreased libido *Cardiovascular:* bradycardia, angina, orthostatic hypotension *GI:* nausea, vomiting, diarrhea or constipation, abdominal distention, gas, dry mouth, weight gain, "black" tongue, inflammed salivary glands and pancreas, liver dysfunction *Others:* edema, lupus-like syndrome, anemias, nasal stuffiness, rash	See hydralazine, *plus:* Assist with activities as necessary. Observe tongue for change in color and texture. Warn patients of possible breast changes, impotence, and change in sexual drive.
methyldopa + hydrochlorothiazide (Aldoril)	PO—Initially—1 tablet bid–tid for 2 days; then individualized to a maximum of 3 g methyldopa and 100 mg–200 mg hydrochlorothiazide	To treat hypertension	See methyldopa and Table 20-1.	See methyldopa and Table 20-1.
metolazone (Diulo, Zaroxolyn)	PO—2.5 mg–20 mg qd as a single dose	To treat hypertension (either alone or with other antihypertensives in more serious disease); to treat salt and water retention in edema accompanying CHF and renal disease	*CNS:* dizziness, drowsiness, vertigo, headache, fatigue, weakness, restlessness *Cardiovascular:* chest pain, palpitations, orthostatic hypotension, increased volume depletion, hemoconcentration, venous thrombosis, blood disorders, syncope *GI:* dry mouth, anorexia, nausea, vomiting, diarrhea or constipation, abdominal bloating, epigastric distress, jaundice, hepatitis *Skin:* rash, hives *Others:* electrolyte imbalances, chills, sugar in the blood and urine, gout attacks, muscle cramps or pain, liver dysfunction	Ambulate with assistance and assist with other activities as necessary. Monitor apical pulse and blood pressure (both lying and standing). Blood tests should be done at regular intervals to check liver function and for metabolic disorders. Assess appetite. Keep a stool chart. Note skin color. Observe skin for any rash or hives. Test urine for sugar. Note any complaints of muscle discomfort, or pain in joints, especially the large toe.

(continued on page 223)

TABLE 33-1 (continued)

DRUG	ROUTE AND DOSAGE RANGE	USE	ADVERSE EFFECTS	NURSING IMPLICATIONS
metoprolol tartrate (Lopressor)	PO—50 mg–450 mg qd in 2–3 divided doses	Use alone or in combination with other drugs to manage hypertension	See atenolol.	See atenolol.
minoxidil (Loniten)	PO—10 mg–40 mg qd in 1–2 divided doses (to a maximum of 100 mg qd)	To treat severe hypertension that has not been responsive to other drug/diuretic therapy	*Cardiovascular:* tachycardia, angina, pericardial effusion, possible cardiac tamponade, arrhythmias *Others:* salt and water retention, increased hair growth, breast sensitivity	Monitor apical pulse carefully and frequently. Record I&O. Check weight daily. Warn patient about new hair growth. Give reassurance that it will stop when the drug is discontinued. Warn patient about breast tenderness.
prazosin (Minipress)	PO—3 mg–40 mg qd in divided doses	To treat mild to moderate hypertension	*CNS:* headache, drowsiness, lethargy, nervousness, depression, fainting, vertigo, paresthesias, blurred vision, tinnitus *GI:* constipation, abdominal pain, dry mouth *Others:* edema, dyspnea, rash and itching, urinary frequency, impotence, nosebleeds, increased sweating	Monitor I&O. Check weight daily. Instruct patients to sit or lie down as soon as they feel weak or dizzy. Evaluate mental status. Check skin for rash, itch, and flushing. Assess visual acuity. Note dry mouth and moist skin.
propranolol HCl + hydrochlorothiazide (Inderide)	PO—1–2 tablets bid (dosage is determined by individual titration)	To treat hypertension	See propranolol and hydrochlorothiazide.	See propranolol and hydrochlorothiazide.
reserpine (Serpasil)	PO—For hypertension—0.5 mg qd for 1–2 weeks; then 0.1 mg–0.25 mg qd For psychiatric disorders—0.1 mg–1 mg qd	To treat mild essential hypertension; used in combination with other drugs to treat more severe forms of hypertension; used to treat agitated psychotic states; parenteral form may be used in hypertensive emergency situations	*CNS:* drowsiness, depression, nervousness, anxiety, nightmares, deafness, dizziness, headache, parkinsonism *Cardiovascular:* angina-like syndrome, arrhythmias, bradycardia *Endocrine:* impotence, decreased sex drive, breast enlargement *Respiratory:* nasal congestion, dyspnea *GI:* anorexia, nausea, vomiting, diarrhea, increased GI secretions, dry mouth, weight gain *Others:* rash and itch, muscular aches, dysuria syncope, epistaxis	Assess appetite. Keep stool chart. Assist with activities as necessary. Evaluate mental status. Evaluate hearing and visual acuity. Note any complaints of chest pain. Monitor BP and pulse. Note any difficulty with breathing. Check skin for rash or itch. Warn males of possible impotence. Inform patients of possible changes in sexual drive. Record I&O. Check weight daily. Note any abnormal muscle movements or complaints of muscle aches. Watch for nosebleed.
reserpine + hydralazine + hydrochlorothiazide (Ser-Ap-Es)	PO—1–2 tablets tid	To treat hypertension	See reserpine, hydralazine, and Table 20-1.	See reserpine, hydralazine, and Table 20-1.

tropic drugs have replaced them as tranquilizers, and today they are used chiefly to treat mild to moderate hypertension.

NURSING IMPLICATIONS

Response to antihypertensives may vary greatly from patient to patient, and the dosage must often be altered until the best response with minimal adverse effects is obtained. Treatment is usually started with a low dose, and the dose is increased gradually until the desired effect is achieved.

Vital signs, especially blood pressure, need to be checked frequently. At the beginning of therapy blood pressure may fluctuate from hour to hour. After a few weeks, the blood pressure in most cases is stablilized, and it is no longer necessary to check vital signs as often. Patients can be taught to take their own blood pressure at home.

With a fall in blood pressure, the patient will often experience a type of postural hypotension called *orthostatic* hypotension. This occurs when the patient gets up out of bed or changes position suddenly. He may complain of feeling dizzy or lightheaded, and if the blood pressure falls too low, he may faint. Encourage the patient to get out of bed slowly to avoid orthostatic hypotension. First, he should sit on the edge of the bed with his legs dangling over the side. After a few minutes in this position, he should stand quietly until any lightheadedness disappears. After these gradual changes, he may then walk around safely. While in the hospital, patients should have their blood pressure taken while lying, sitting, and standing to assess postural change.

Tell the patient not to walk about if he feels dizzy. He should return to bed and lie flat with his legs positioned slightly higher than his head. If getting back into bed is impossible, the patient may remain standing, but he should flex the calf muscles to keep blood from pooling in the lower extremities.

The patient should be cautioned against standing for long periods.

Patient teaching should include the following:

1. Heat increases blood flow, and this may cause a rise in blood pressure. Be careful about exposure to the sun on hot days and at the beach.
2. Some antihypertensives can cause impotence. Notify the physician if this occurs, since it may sometimes be overcome by skipping a dose or decreasing the dosage.
3. Carry an identification card or Medic-Alert tag with your name, your physician's name and telephone number, and the name and dosage of the drug being taken.
4. Salty foods and those containing tyramine (see Chapter 6) need to be eliminated from the diet.
5. Antihypertensives should never be discontinued abruptly, because blood pressure may rise to levels even higher than before drug therapy was begun (called *rebound*).

The *Rauwolfia* alkaloids have a cumulative action. Maximum response to these drugs may not occur until 2 weeks after the drug therapy is begun; and after it has been discontinued, its effects may last for up to 4 weeks. Both *Rauwolfia* alkaloids and methyldopa can produce sedation. Depending on the degree of sedation, the patient may need assistance with getting into and out of bed. He should not walk alone. Potentially hazardous activities, such as shaving, smoking, driving a car, or working around machinery, should not be attempted. The patient should be observed frequently for changes in mental status.

Some antihypertensives cause sodium and water retention. Diuretics may need to be given along with these medications. Diazoxide may also cause hyperglycemia, so urine tests for sugar should be done daily. Although this type of hyperglycemia is mild, it may necessitate administration of oral hypoglycemics or insulin. Many antihypertensives cause impotence, and patients need to be warned of this possible effect.

PRACTICE PROBLEMS—ANTIHYPERTENSIVES

1. The physician orders hydralazine (Apresoline) 20 mg IM q6h prn systolic blood pressure above 210. Hydralazine is dispensed in ampules of 20 mg/ml. How many milliliters of hydralazine will be given?

    $$\frac{D}{H} \times A = G$$

    $$1 \frac{20 \text{ mg}}{1 \text{ 20 mg}} \times 1 \text{ ml} = G$$

    $$1 \times 1 \text{ ml} = 1 \text{ ml}$$

    Thus, 1 ml of hydralazine (Apresoline) will be given.

2. The order reads: methyldopa (Aldomet) 500 mg PO tid.
    The label reads: methyldopa 250 mg/tablet.
    How many tablets will be given?

    $$\frac{D}{H} = G$$

    $$2 \frac{500 \text{ mg}}{1 \text{ 250 mg}} = 2$$

    Two tablets of methyldopa (Aldomet) will be given.

Work the following problems:
1. The order reads: metolazone (Zaroxolyn) 15 mg PO daily.
    The label reads: metolazone 5 mg/tablet.
    How many tablets will be given?

2. Guanethidine (Ismelin) 20 mg daily is ordered for the hypertensive patient. Guanethidine comes in 10-mg tablets. How many tablets will be given?

3. The order reads: labetalol (Normodyne) 300 mg PO bid.
    The label reads: labetalol 300 mg/tablet
    How many tablets will be given?

Answers are given on p. 284.

PART 6
Drugs used to help meet patients' needs for the maintenance of regulatory mechanisms and functions

CHAPTER 34
Hormones

Hormones are substances produced by the endocrine (ductless) glands. The endocrine glands include the pituitary, thyroid, parathyroids, adrenal, pancreas, and the gonads (sex organs). These glands empty their secretions directly into the bloodstream and thus have widespread effects on body function. Although the quantity of hormones produced and released into the circulation is small, the hormones control most body functions. For example, growth, development, and energy production are all under hormonal regulation. Hormones regulate secretion and motility within the gastrointestinal tract and the volume and composition of the extracellular fluid. Reproduction and, in the female, milk production, could not take place without hormonal secretion. General adaptation to the environment is also dependent on hormone secretion.

The blood level of each hormone is automatically regulated. Endocrine disorders are of two types, hypo- and hypersecretion. In *hyposecretion* not enough hormone, or none, is being produced. The treatment is administration of the hormone that is lacking. The other type of disorder, *hypersecretion*, means that there is overproduction of a hormone. This condition is treated either by surgical removal of all or part of the gland or by administration of medications that block the action of the specific hormone.

THE PITUITARY GLAND

The pituitary gland (also called the hypophysis), about the size of a pea, is located at the base of the brain. It is divided into anterior and posterior lobes. With the nervous system, the pituitary maintains internal homeostasis.

The secretions of the *anterior lobe* are called *trophic** hormones. They do not regulate body processes, but they stimulate other organs to do *their* work. The names, abbreviations for, and general functions of each of the anterior pituitary hormones are listed in Table 34-1.

ACTH, or adrenocorticotropic hormone, stimulates the adrenal cortex to produce its hormones, the adrenocorticosteriods. If ACTH is lacking in the body, it must be replaced. Administration of ACTH as a medication then promotes normal adrenal function. ACTH is especially useful in the treatment of allergic reactions, dermatologic disorders, certain eye disorders, and rheumatism. It may also be used to treat neurologic diseases, such as myasthenia gravis and multiple sclerosis.

Another anterior pituitary hormone preparation used medicinally is a combination drug that contains LH and FSH. It is used to treat infertility in females who are unable to ovulate. This drug is

* From the Greek word meaning "nourishment."

TABLE 34-1   ANTERIOR PITUITARY HORMONES

HORMONE	OTHER NAME BY WHICH KNOWN AND ABBREVIATION	FUNCTIONS
Somatotropic	STH Growth Hormone (GH)	Promotion of organ, skeletal and general body growth
Thyroid-stimulating	TSH	Development of the thyroid gland
Follicle-stimulating	FSH	Ovulation Menstruation Sperm production
Luteinizing	LH	Ovulation Menstruation Production of sex hormones
Prolactin	Lactogenic factor (LTH)	Milk production in the pregnant and postpartum female
Adrenocortico-trophic	ACTH	Stimulation of the adrenal cortex
Melanocyte-stimulating	MSH (Intermedin)	Darkens skin (in lower mammals)

called menotropins (Pergonal) or human menopausal gonadotropin (HMG).

The secretions of the *posterior lobe* of the pituitary gland are oxytocin and vasopressin. Oxytocin affects the uterus and plays an important part in childbirth and milk ejection. It is discussed in Chapter 39. Vasopressin is also called the antidiuretic hormone (ADH). Its function is to retain water in the body and thereby maintain a state of normal hydration. Preparations of vasopressin are available for injection or as nasal sprays. They are used to treat the polyuria associated with diabetes insipidus and to test kidney function.

THE THYROID GLAND

The thyroid gland is located in the neck, on either side of the larynx. Its hormones have widespread effects. They influence growth and development (both physical and mental), metabolism, and adaptation.

Natural preparations of thyroid hormones are made from the thyroid glands of animals. Synthetic thyroid preparations are also available. Thyroid hormone preparations are used to treat hypothyroidism and enlarged thyroid gland (goiter).

If the body manufactures too much thyroid hormone, the condition is called hyperthyroidism. It can be treated by surgical removal of thyroid tissue or administration of antithyroid drugs. These preparations interfere with the formation or release of thyroid hormones. Iodine is the oldest antithyroid drug. It is usually administered by mouth in solutions such as strong iodine solution (Lugol's solution) or potassium iodide solution (SSKI). Radioactive iodine (^{131}I) and thiouracil drugs are other effective antithyroid medications.

THE PARATHYROID GLANDS

There are usually four parathyroid glands located in or on top of the thyroid gland. Their hormone, parathormone, regulates the levels of calcium and phosphorus in the circulating blood.

THE ADRENAL GLANDS

There are two adrenal glands, one above each kidney. Their inner portion (medulla) produces the catecholamines epinephrine and norepinephrine, which are discussed in Chapter 34. The outer portion (cortex) of the adrenal gland produces the adrenocorticosteroids.*

The adrenocorticosteroids have many important actions, their main use being anti-inflammatory agents. They interfere with the body's natural immune response by causing a decrease in white blood cells. It is believed that they may also block histamine release, which would explain their effectiveness as antiallergic medications. Adrenocorticosteroids also have antipyretic action and help maintain blood pressure and increase energy production when the body is stressed (antistress action).

Although adrenocorticosteroids are very effective as anti-inflammatory agents, they are used only in cases that cannot be controlled by safer, less radical measures. Rheumatoid arthritis, collagen diseases, allergic reactions, inflammatory diseases of the skin, eye, bowel, or respiratory tract, blood disorders, cerebral edema, and cancer are conditions for which these drugs may be prescribed. Ad-

* Also called corticosteroids, or simply steroids.

renocorticosteroids are used to suppress the symptoms of the disease—they are not curative.

THE PANCREAS

The pancreas is an endocrine gland that lies behind the stomach. The secreting cells of the pancreas, the islets of Langerhans, produce two hormones, *glucagon* and *insulin*. Glucagon raises the blood sugar level and, therefore, is used in the treatment of hypoglycemia (a dangerously low blood sugar level). When the pancreas fails to release insulin or releases too little insulin, diabetes mellitus develops. In such cases, insulin must be administered to counteract this deficiency. Most insulin is obtained from the pancreas of sheep, hogs, and cattle. Through genetic engineering techniques it is now possible to manufacture *human* insulin, as well. These preparations (Humulin, Novalin) are given to those allergic to animal insulin. All insulin must be administered by injection because it is destroyed by stomach enzymes. Insulin preparations differ in their times of onset, peak action, and duration of effect. They are categorized as rapid-acting, intermediate-acting, or long-acting (Table 34-2).

TABLE 34-2 INSULIN PREPARATIONS

	ONSET OF ACTION	PEAK	DURATION
RAPID-ACTING			
crystalline zinc insulin injection (Iletin, CZI, Regular)	½–1 hr	2–4 hr	6–8 hr
prompt insulin zinc suspension (Semilente)	½–1 hr	2–8 hr	8–16 hr
INTERMEDIATE-ACTING			
isophane insulin suspension (NPH)	1–2 hr	6–12 hr	12–28 hr
insulin zinc suspension (Lente)	1–2 hr	8–12 hr	14–28 hr
LONG-ACTING			
extended insulin zinc suspension (Ultralente)	4–8 hr	18–24 hr	24–36 hr
protamine zinc insulin suspension (PZI)	4–8 hr	14–20 hr	24–36 hr

In addition to insulin, there are oral hypoglycemic agents used to treat some forms of diabetes mellitus. These drugs act only to stimulate the pancreas to secrete more insulin; thus, if the pancreas is unable to secrete any insulin, the oral hypoglycemics will have no effect.

THE GONADS

The ovaries

The gonads are the primary sex glands. The female gonads are called the *ovaries*. The ovaries are located in the lower abdomen, one on either side of the uterus. They produce two types of hormones, estrogen and progesterone. Estrogens play a role in regulating changes that occur in the reproductive organs during the first part of the menstrual cycle. They also influence development of female secondary sex characteristics at puberty. Progesterone prepares the lining of the uterus for implantation of a fertilized egg. It also helps to maintain pregnancy by inhibiting ovulation and menstruation and by keeping the uterus in a quiet state.

Estrogens are given as replacement therapy during and after menopause, when the body no longer produces them. They are also effective in treating genital atrophy, functional uterine bleeding, and certain menstrual problems. Some types of cancer (in the male, metastatic cancer of the prostate; in the postmenopausal female, metastatic cancer of the breast) may be treated palliatively with estrogens.

Progesterone is used to treat disorders of menstruation, abnormal uterine bleeding caused by hormonal imbalance, threatened abortion, and endometriosis. Combinations of estrogen and progesterone are given as oral contraceptives.

Oral contraceptives. Ovulation depends on levels of progesterone and estrogen. During the 28-day cycle, there is a normal increase in their secretion, which brings about ovulation. Later in the cycle, there is a normal decrease in secretion, which brings about menstrual bleeding. Oral contraceptives that contain estrogen and progestins (progesterone and its derivatives) suppress ovulation without interfering with menstruation. These combination-type birth control pills are considered nearly 100% effective when used exactly as directed. There are also oral contraceptives that contain only progestins in low doses. They do not usually interfere with normal ovulation but seem to inhibit implanatation of the sperm, thereby preventing pregnancy.

There are many oral contraceptive preparations in use today, each differing from the others in the type and amount of estrogen and progestins (see Table 34-3).

Diethylstilbestrol (DES) is given in emergency situations, such as rape or incest, as a postcoital contraceptive. If given within 72 hours of intercourse, it prevents the fertilized egg from implanting in the uterine wall.

Drugs used to stimulate ovulation. Women who have not been able to conceive may be given medications that promote conception. In a normal pregnant woman, the placenta produces human chorionic gonadotropin (HCG). To stimulate ovulation, preparations of HCG (Follutein, Pregnyl) may be given. Clomiphene citrate (Clomid) is a synthetic agent used to stimulate ovulation. With the use of these drugs, the incidence of multiple births, premature births, and spontaneous abortion is greatly increased.

TABLE 34-3 ORAL CONTRACEPTIVES

TYPES	TRADE NAME(S)
COMBINATION-TYPE (PROGESTINS + ESTROGEN)	
ethynodiol + ethinyl estradiol	Demulen
ethynodiol + mestranol	Ovulen
levonorgestrel + ethinyl estradiol	Nordette Triphasil
norethindrone + ethinyl estradiol	Brevicon Loestrin Modicon Norinyl Norlestrin Ortho-Novum Ovcon Tri-Norinyl
norethindrone + mestranol	Norinyl 2mg Ortho-Novum 2mg
norethynodrel + mestranol	Enovid
norgestrel + ethinyl estradiol	Lo/Ovral Ovral
PROGESTINS ALONE	
norethindrone	Micronor Nor-Q.D.
norgestrel	Ovrette

The testes

The male gonads are called the testes. They are located in the scrotal sac. Under stimulation by anterior pituitary gonadotropins (FSH and LH), the testes produce androgens, the male sex hormones. There are several androgens, the most potent being *testosterone.*

The androgens promote normal development of male secondary sexual characteristics including deep voice, body and facial hair, growth of the penis, and development of the reproductive organs. They play an important role in normal muscle development and achievement of normal weight.

Males whose sex organs are underdeveloped or who have been castrated are given androgens as replacement therapy. They also relieve symptoms associated with the male climacteric when gonadal function ceases. Other situations in which androgens are prescribed include surgery, severe trauma due to burns, infection, and muscle-wasting diseases, such as cancer and tuberculosis. Occasionally, androgens are given to obstetric patients to suppress lactation and breast engorgement, as discussed in Chapter 39. They are also prescribed for palliation in postmenopausal women with inoperable cancer of the breast.

More information on specific hormones is given in Table 34-4.

NURSING IMPLICATIONS

Hormonal therapy is, in most cases, a lifelong matter. Therefore, you need to be sure the patient understands the importance of taking his medication regularly, on schedule, and in the amount prescribed. Remember that these are potent drugs— very small amounts produce dramatic effects. Hormones that are still available only from animal sources are very expensive. The patient may need financial assistance.

Pituitary Hormones

Pituitary hormones are proteins. As medications, they cannot be given by mouth because they will be digested by the stomach enzymes, and thus they are available only in parenteral form. Because they are proteins, the pituitary hormones may act like foreign substances, triggering antibody production and allergic reactions.

(Text continues on p. 240.)

TABLE 34-4 HORMONES

DRUG	ROUTE AND DOSAGE RANGE	USE	ADVERSE EFFECTS	NURSING IMPLICATIONS
PITUITARY				
ACTH or corticotropin (Acthar, Acthar Gel)	SC, IM—Individualized doses (to a maximum of 80 U qd) IV—(for diagnostic purposes) 10 U–25 U	For diagnostic testing of adrenocortical function, to treat endocrine and rheumatic disorders; to treat collagen diseases, dermatologic diseases, allergic states, ophthalmic and respiratory diseases, blood disorders, neoplastic diseases, edema, GI diseases, tuberculous meningitis, and trichinosis	*CNS:* increased intracranial pressure, convulsions, headache, vertigo *Cardiovascular:* hypertension, angina, CHF *Fluid and electrolyte:* sodium retention, fluid retention, loss of potassium and calcium, alkalosis *Musculoskeletal:* muscle weakness, loss of muscle mass, osteoporosis, pathologic fractures of long bones *GI:* peptic ulcers, vomiting, nausea, pancreatitis, increased appetite, GI bleeding, abdominal distention, ulcerative esophagitis *Skin:* poor wound healing, thin and fragile skin, petechiae and ecchymotic areas, reddened face, acne, increased sweating, darkening of skin color, rashes *Eyes:* cataracts, glaucoma, damage to the optic nerve, exophthalmos *Endocrine:* menstrual irregularities, cushingoid state, poor adrenal response to stress, failure of children to grow, decreased carbohydrate tolerance, signs and symptoms of diabetes mellitus, hirsutism *Metabolic:* protein loss leading to negative nitrogen balance *Others:* mood swings, mental depression, decreased resistance to infection	Electrolyte levels should be checked frequently. Watch for signs of edema. Check weight daily. Keep accurate I&O records. Ambulate with assistance if necessary. Assess appetite. Test all stool and vomitus samples for the presence of blood. Always give steroids with an antacid, milk, or a meal. Evaluate wound healing. Check skin for rashes, change in color, and the presence of petechiae. Monitor vital signs. Warn females of possible menstrual irregularities. Be sure patients are told of possible changes in their appearance *before* they occur. Test urine for sugar and acetone. Evaluate mental status. Assess visual acuity. Encourage patients taking steroids to avoid persons with obvious infections and colds. Warn patients never to stop medications without a physician's order.
menotropins (Pergonal)	IM—Contents of 1–2 ampules qd for 9–12 days; followed by 10,000 U HCG 1 day after last dose of menotropins	To induce ovulation and pregnancy in anovulatory, infertile women when there is no ovarian failure	*GU:* enlarged ovaries, multiple births *Circulatory:* pleural effusion, blood concentration, arterial thromboembolism, ascites *Other:* febrile reactions	Couples should have thorough counseling about timing and frequency of intercourse during drug therapy. Ovaries should be checked for change in size at least every 2 days. Monitor I&O. Weigh patient daily. Blood tests should be done at frequent intervals.

(continued on page 234)

233

TABLE 34-4 (continued)

DRUG	ROUTE AND DOSAGE RANGE	USE	ADVERSE EFFECTS	NURSING IMPLICATIONS
human chorionic gonadotropin or HCG (A.P.L., Pregnyl, Profasi HP)	IM—Dosage and schedule vary from 500 U–5000 U 3 times a week	See menotropins, plus: prepubertal cryptorchidism, hypogonadotropic hypogonadism in males	See menotropins.	See menotropins.
clomiphene (Clomid, Serophene)	PO—50 mg–100 mg qd for 5 days	To induce ovulation in anovulatory women who desire pregnancy	CNS: nervousness, depression, headache, restlessness, insomnia, dizziness, fatigue GI: nausea, vomiting, bloating, constipation, increased appetite, weight gain GU: abdominal and pelvic discomfort, heavy menses, enlarged ovaries, urinary frequency Skin: rash or hives, hair loss Eyes: blurred and double vision, photophobia, visual changes Others: early abortion, multiple births, congenital abnormalities, hydatidiform mole, mild hot flashes, breast discomfort	Assess weight and appetite daily. Keep stool chart. Keep I&O record. Warn patient of possible heavy menses. Encourage frequent internal examinations. Evaluate visual acuity. Evaluate mental status. Assist with activity as necessary. Evaluate sleeping pattern. Check skin for rash, hives, and hair loss. Be sure patient has been told about adverse effects.
vasopressin (Pitressin, Pitressin Tannate in Oil)	SC, IM, Intranasal—5 U–10 U q3–4h IM—1.5 U–5 U q24–48h	To prevent and treat postoperative abdominal distention; to rid the abdomen of gas shadows when x-rays are taken; to treat diabetes insipidus	GI: abdominal cramps, gas, nausea, vomiting Skin: sweating, pallor around the mouth, rashes, hives Others: tremor, "pounding" in the head, vertigo, bronchial constriction, water intoxication (can lead to convulsions and coma), anaphylaxis, possible cardiac arrest	Note any abnormal muscle movements. Note whitish color around the mouth. Keep accurate I&O records. Check skin for reactions. Note respirations for rate and quality. Monitor vital signs. Do specific gravity on all urines. Watch for early signs of water intoxication (drowsiness, lethargy, headache).
THYROID				
thyroid	PO—Highly individualized doses Usual range—gr ¼–gr 4 a day (15 mg–260 mg)	To treat thyroid deficiency states, especially cretinism and myxedema; Also use along with thyroid-inhibiting agents to decrease the release of thyrotropic hormones	With overdose: CNS: headache, nervousness, tremors, insomnia Cardiovascular: tachycardia, cardiac arrhythmias, palpitations, increased pulse pressure, angina GI: changes in appetite, nausea, diarrhea Skin: increased sweating Others: fever, intolerance to heat, menstrual irregularities	Evaluate mental status. Note any tremor. Assess sleep pattern. Monitor apical pulse. Note any complaints of chest pain. Monitor BP, and note any changes in pulse pressure. Assess appetite. Keep stool chart. Monitor temperature. Note increased perspiration.

(continued on page 235)

TABLE 34-4 (continued)

DRUG	ROUTE AND DOSAGE RANGE	USE	ADVERSE EFFECTS	NURSING IMPLICATIONS
thyroglobulin (Proloid)	PO—gr 0.5–gr 3 (32 mg–200 mg) qd	Used as thyroid replacement therapy for conditions of inadequate endogenous thyroid; used to reduce the size of simple (nontoxic) goiters	See thyroid.	See thyroid.
levothyroxine (Synthroid, Levothroid)	PO, IM, IV—0.025 mg–0.4 mg qd	Replacement therapy for reduced or absent thyroid function of any etiology	See thyroid.	See thyroid, *plus:* Be sure diet contains iodine. Watch for signs of thyrotoxicosis (mainly an increased pulse rate).
ANTITHYROID DRUGS				
propylthiouracil	PO—100 mg–900 mg qd in 3 equally divided doses	To treat hyperthyroidism; to improve hyperthyroidism in preparation for subtotal thyroidectomy or radioactive iodine therapy	*GI:* nausea, vomiting, epigastric distress, loss of taste, disease of salivary and lymph glands, liver disease *Skin:* rash, itch, hives, hair loss, darkening skin color, jaundice *Musculoskeletal:* muscle and joint pain, lupus-like syndrome *Circulatory:* edema, blood disorders, periarteritis, bleeding *CNS:* paresthesias, headache, drowsiness, vertigo *Other:* drug fever	Observe skin for signs of rash, hives, or change in color. Note complaints of muscle discomfort or changes in sensation. Evaluate sense of taste. Warn patients of possible hair loss. Assist with ambulation and other activities as needed. Keep record of I&O. Blood tests should be done to check bleeding time. Monitor temperature.
methimazole (Tapazole)	PO—5 mg–60 mg qd divided into 3 equal doses given q8h	See propylthiouracil.	See propylthiouracil.	See propylthiouracil.
ADRENAL				
cortisone	PO—25 mg–300 mg qd IM—20 mg–300 mg qd (in divided doses)	See corticotropin, *except:* diagnosis of adrenocortical dysfunction	See corticotropin.	See corticotropin.
dexamethasone (Decadron, Hexadrol)	PO—0.75 mg–9 mg qd IM, IV—0.5 mg–16 mg qd (In divided doses) Topical—Many forms	See corticotropin, *plus:* parenteral use for cerebral edema associated with primary or metastatic brain tumor, craniotomy or head injury	See corticotropin, *plus:* possible blindness with parenteral use	See corticotropin, *plus:* Evaluate visual acuity.
fludrocortisone (Florinef)	PO—0.05 mg–0.2 mg qd	As partial replacement therapy for primary and secondary adrenocortical insufficiency in Addison's disease; to treat salt-losing adrenogenital syndrome	See corticotropin.	See corticotropin.

(continued on page 236)

TABLE 34-4 (continued)

DRUG	ROUTE AND DOSAGE RANGE	USE	ADVERSE EFFECTS	NURSING IMPLICATIONS
hydrocortisone (Cortef, Solu-Cortef)	PO—20 mg–240 mg qd in divided doses Topical—Many forms IM, IV—2 g–24 g qd in divided doses	See cortisone.	See corticotropin.	See corticotropin.
methylprednisolone (Medrol, Solu-Medrol)	PO—4 mg–48 mg qd in divided doses IM, IV—400 mg–1.5 g qd in divided doses Topical—Many forms	See prednisolone.	See corticotropin.	See corticotropin.
prednisone (Deltasone, Meticorten)	PO—5 mg–60 mg qd in single or divided doses Topical—Many forms	See cortisone.	See corticotropin.	See corticotropin.
prednisolone (Delta-Cortef, Sterane, Meticortelone)	PO, IM, IV—4 mg–60 mg qd in single or divided doses Topical—Many forms	See cortisone, *plus:* to treat systemic dermatomyositis (polymyositis)	See corticotropin.	See corticotropin.
triamcinolone (Artistocort, Kenalog)	PO—4 mg–48 mg qd IM—40 mg every week Topical—Many forms	See cortisone.	See corticotropin.	See corticotropin.

PANCREAS

Rapid-Acting Insulin Preparations

DRUG	ROUTE AND DOSAGE RANGE	USE	ADVERSE EFFECTS	NURSING IMPLICATIONS
crystalline zinc insulin injection (Iletin, CZI, Regular)	SC—Highly individualized dose	To treat diabetes mellitus	Hypoglycemic reactions: fatigue, headache, sweating, anxiety, drowsiness, nausea, tremors, weakness	Be sure patient fully understands and is able to follow his prescribed diet. Notify the physician if a meal is skipped. Teach patients to test their urine for sugar every 3 to 4 hours. Insulin suspensions should be resuspended by gently rolling or turning the vial, never by shaking it. If any symptoms of hypoglycemia appear, give the patient a carbohydrate, such as a lump of sugar or some candy.
prompt insulin zinc suspension (Semilente)	SC—Highly individualized dose	See crystalline zinc.	See crystalline zinc.	See crystalline zinc.

Intermediate-Acting Insulin Preparations

DRUG	ROUTE AND DOSAGE RANGE	USE	ADVERSE EFFECTS	NURSING IMPLICATIONS
isophane insulin suspension (NPH)	SC—Highly individualized dose	See crystalline zinc.	See crystalline zinc.	See crystalline zinc.

(continued on page 237)

TABLE 34-4 (continued)

DRUG	ROUTE AND DOSAGE RANGE	USE	ADVERSE EFFECTS	NURSING IMPLICATIONS
insulin zinc suspension (Lente)	SC—Highly individualized dose	See crystalline zinc.	See crystalline zinc.	See crystalline zinc.
Long-Acting Insulin Preparations				
extended insulin zinc suspension (Ultralente)	SC—Highly individualized dose	See crystalline zinc.	See crystalline zinc.	See crystalline zinc.
protamine zinc insulin suspension (PZI)	SC—Highly individualized dose	See crystalline zinc.	See crystalline zinc, *plus:* local sensitivity reactions	See crystalline zinc, *plus:* Check skin for signs of local reactions (rash, itch, or redness).
Oral Hypoglycemics				
tolbutamide (Orinase)	PO—0.25 g–3 g qd	To treat patients whose non-insulin-dependent diabetes cannot be controlled by diet alone	Severe hypoglycemia, photosensitivity, disulfiramlike reaction if alcohol is taken, GI upset, headache, allergic skin reactions	To avoid GI upset, give total daily dose in divided portions *after* meals. Teach patients signs and symptoms of hypoglycemia and how and when to test urine for sugar and acetone. Warn patients *not* to drink alcoholic beverages or take medications containing alcohol. Check skin for any reaction.
acetohexamide (Dymelor)	PO—250 mg–1.5 g in daily or divided doses	See tolbutamide.	See tolbutamide.	See tolbutamide.
chlorpropamide (Diabinese)	PO—100 mg–500 mg qd	See tolbutamide.	Jaundice, rash, blood disorders, fever, diarrhea, GI bleeding, anorexia, nausea, vomiting, weakness, paresthesias	Check skin for color change or rash. Keep stool chart. Test all stool and vomitus samples for the presence of blood. Monitor temperature. Blood tests should be done at regular intervals. Assess appetite. Note any complaints of abnormal sensations.
glipizide (Glucotrol)	PO—2.5 mg–40 mg/day (Doses greater than 15 mg/day should be given in 2 divided doses)	See tolbutamide.	See tolbutamide.	See tolbutamide.
glyburide (DiaBeta, Micronase)	PO—1.25 mg–20 mg/day in single or 2 divided doses	See tolbutamide.	See tolbutamide.	See tolbutamide.
tolazamide (Tolinase)	PO—100 mg–1000 mg qd in single or divided doses	See tolbutamide.	See tolbutamide.	See tolbutamide.

(continued on page 238)

TABLE 34-4 (continued)

DRUG	ROUTE AND DOSAGE RANGE	USE	ADVERSE EFFECTS	NURSING IMPLICATIONS
GONADS				
Estrogens				
conjugated estrogens (Premarin)	PO—0.3 mg–7.5 mg qd IM, IV—25 mg q6–12h Topical—Vaginal cream	See estradiol, *plus:* Use for palliation of breast cancer in certain men and women with metastatic disease and cancer of the prostate; to treat postpartum breast engorgement and abnormal uterine bleeding due to hormonal imbalance	See estradiol.	See estradiol.
diethylstilbestrol (DES)	PO, PV—0.2 mg–3 mg qd (to a maximum of 15 mg qd in breast cancer)	To treat vasomotor symptoms associated with menopause, atrophic vaginitis, kraurosis vulvae, female hypogonadism, female castration, primary ovarian failure, palliative treatment of breast and prostatic cancer in selected men and postmenopausal women	See estradiol.	See estradiol.
estradiol (Estrace)	PO—1 mg–2 mg qd	To treat moderate to severe vasomotor symptoms associated with the menopause, atrophic vaginitis, kraurosis vulvae, female hypogonadism, female castration, and primary-ovarian failure	*GU:* menstrual irregularities, increase in size of uterine fibroids, vaginal candidiasis, changes in cervical eversion and secretions, cystitislike syndrome *Endocrine:* breast tenderness, enlargement, or secretion *GI:* nausea, vomiting, abdominal cramps, bloating, gallbladder and liver disease *Skin:* discolorations and inflammations, scalp hair loss, hirsutism *Eyes:* visual changes *CNS:* headache, dizziness, mental depression, muscle twitching *Others:* increase or decrease in weight, edema, hypertension, increase in blood levels of calcium, decreased glucose tolerance, changes in libido, thromboembolic disease, increased incidence of cancer of the breast, cervix, vagina, endometrium, and liver	Warn patient about changes in menstrual cycle and possible change in sex drive. Encourage females to practice breast self-examination at regular intervals and to have internal examinations regularly. Note unusual frequency of voiding, pain on urination, or blood in the urine. Test all urine samples for the presence of blood. Warn patient about changes in breasts that may occur. Check skin for rash, inflammation, color changes. Note hair loss or new growth (especially on face). Assess visual acuity. Evaluate mental status. Note any abnormal muscle movements. Weigh patient daily. Note signs of fluid accumulation. Monitor BP. Blood tests should be done to test electrolytes, sugar, liver, and kidney function. Watch for redness, tenderness, and swelling in calfs.

(continued on page 239)

TABLE 34-4 (continued)

DRUG	ROUTE AND DOSAGE RANGE	USE	ADVERSE EFFECTS	NURSING IMPLICATIONS
Progestins medroxypro-gesterone (Amen, Curre-tab, Depo-Provera, Pro-vera)	PO—5 mg–10 mg qd for 5–10 days IM—400 mg–1000 mg every week to 400 mg every month	To treat secondary amenorrhea, abnormal uterine bleeding due to hormonal imbalance in the absence of organic diseases, such as fibroids or uterine cancer Given along with other therapy and palliative treatment for inoperable, recurrent and metastatic endometrial or renal cancer	*CNS:* nervousness, insomnia, depression, fatigue, dizziness *Cardiovascular:* thromboembolic disorders *Endocrine:* breast tenderness, galactorrhea, changes in menstrual flow and regularity, breakthrough bleeding, changes in cervical secretions and erosion *GI:* nausea, jaundice *Skin:* generalized rash, hives, itching, acne, hair loss, hirsutism *Others:* weight gain or loss, edema, fever, anaphylaxis	Evaluate mental status. Assist with activities as necessary. Assess sleep pattern. Warn patient to be aware of any calf tenderness or swelling. Warn patient about possible changes in breasts, menstrual cycle, and cervical secretions. Observe skin for rash, hives, color change, or other disorders. Be sure patient is aware of possible hair loss or growth. Check weight daily. Monitor temperature.
norethindrone (Norlutate, Norlutin)	PO—2.5 mg–30 mg qd	To treat amenorrhea, abnormal uterine bleeding due to hormonal imbalance (when no organic disease is present), and endometriosis	See medroxyprogesterone.	See medroxyprogesterone.
progesterone	IM—5 mg–50 mg qd Intravaginal—25 mg–400 mg qd	To treat functional uterine bleeding associated with a hyperplastic, nonsecretory endometrium, and the absence of genital malignancy; to treat primary and secondary amenorrhea in the presence of estrogen; to treat infertility when inadequate corpus luteum function is suspected, use to treat premenstrual tension, dysmenorrhea, threatened and habitual abortion, toxemia of pregnancy and after pains; used to prevent conception	Spotting, irregular menses, nausea, lethargy, possible aggravation of asthma, epilepsy, and migraine *Prolonged use at high doses can lead to:* *GI:* gastric upset, jaundice, liver damage *CNS:* headache, dizziness *Endocrine:* decreased libido, androgenic effects, breast congestion *Others:* edema, weight gain	Warn female patients that their periods will be irregular. Watch for symptoms of latent diseases. Weigh the patient at regular intervals. Warn patients about possible changes in sexual drive and the appearance of masculine effects. Assist with activities if necessary. Note any hair loss or unusual growth (especially on the face). Check skin for rash or itch.
Androgens danazol (Danocrine)	PO—200 mg–800 mg/day in 2 divided doses	To treat endometriosis in women who cannot tolerate other drug therapy, in whom other drugs are contraindicated, or in those who fail to respond to other drugs	*CNS:* nervousness, labile emotions *Endocrine:* decrease in breast size, mild hirsutism, deepening voice, clitoral hypertrophy (rare) *GU:* vaginitis with itching, drying and bleeding	Note mood swings, and reassure patient this is to be expected. Warn patient about possible changes in secondary sex characteristics and masculinization. Note complaints of vaginal discomfort.

(continued on page 240)

TABLE 34-4   (continued)

DRUG	ROUTE AND DOSAGE RANGE	USE	ADVERSE EFFECTS	NURSING IMPLICATIONS
danazol (*continued*)			*Skin:* acne, oily skin and hair, flushing, increased perspiration *Other:* weight gain	Observe skin for changes in color, oiliness, and perspiration. Check weight daily.
methyltestosterone (Oreton Methyl)	PO—10 mg–40 mg qd Buccal—5 mg–20 mg qd IM—100 mg–400 mg q4 weeks	*Males:* to treat eunuchoidism and eunuchism, male climacteric symptoms and impotence secondary to androgen deficiency, oligospermia and postpubertal cryptorchidism with evidence of hypogonadism *Females:* to prevent postpartum breast engorgement and pain; use in palliative treatment of inoperable, androgen-responsive, advancing breast cancer in women 1 to 5 years post menopause or with a proved hormone-dependent tumor	*Males:* decreased sperm and volume of ejaculation, testicular atrophy, epididymitis, priapism, gynecomastia *Females:* hoarseness, deepening voice, oily skin, acne, hirsutism, enlarged clitoris, increased libido, menstrual irregularities *Both:* bladder irritability, rashes, increased calcium levels, sodium and water retention, increased or decreased libido, flushed skin, acne, sleeplessness, chills, blood disorders, hives at the injection site	Buccal tablets must be placed under the tongue or between the gum and the cheek. Tell the patient *not to swallow* them and to avoid eating, drinking, chewing, and smoking until they dissolve. Watch for manifestations of virilization in females and feminization in males. Be sure patients know what to expect in the way of body changes. Both the patient and his sexual partner should be aware of the possible changes in sexual desire and ability. Check skin for signs of rash, flushing, or acne. Monitor temperature and BP. Record I&O. Check electrolyte levels regularly. Blood tests should be done at regular intervals.
testosterone cypionate (Depo-Testosterone)	IM—50 mg–200 mg q2–4 wk	See methyltestosterone.	See methyltestosterone.	See methyltestosterone.

Vasopressin can cause severe water retention (water intoxication). A patient with diabetes insipidus who is receiving this drug is probably restricting his intake of water. Careful recording of intake, output, and urine specific gravity is necessary to monitor fluid balance and kidney function.

Thyroid Hormones

Problems related to the use of thyroid hormones appear only after prolonged use and may not be noticed in the early stages. The first sign of thyrotoxicosis (overdose) is a more rapid pulse. The pulse should, therefore, be taken before each dose of hormone is given. Withhold the medication if the pulse rate exceeds 100 beats per minute, and notify the head nurse. Patients should be taught to check their own pulse if they will be taking thyroid drugs at home.

When radioactive iodine is prescribed, follow the same precautions as with other sources of radiation. With liquid iodide preparations, be sure to measure accurately; the amount prescribed is usually very small. The unpleasant taste may be disguised by mixing the drops with fruit juices or milk.

The most serious complication associated with the use of antithyroid medications is agranulocytosis, a condition characterized by a sharp decrease in the number of white blood cells. When this happens, the patient is vulnerable to infection. It is most commonly seen during long-term therapy. Instruct the patient to be alert to the first signs of infection (sore throat, fever, malaise) and to report them so prompt countermeasures may be taken.

Adrenal Hormones

Adrenocorticosteroids are associated with many potential adverse effects, which call for specific nursing action. *Fluid and electrolyte disturbances* are common because most steroids cause sodium and water retention while promoting loss of potassium. Calcium is also lost from the bones. Hypertension or congestive heart failure may result from long-term therapy. The blood pressure should be checked regularly. Salt and fluid restrictions may be ordered. Be observant of edema and other signs that may point to fluid retention such as tight clothes, rings, and shoes. Daily weights and strict intake and output records are essential. Laboratory electrolyte reports should be checked frequently. If the potassium level is low, supplemental potassium may be ordered.

Gastrointestinal disturbances related to steroids include nausea, abdominal distention, stomach ulcers, and bleeding. Therefore, steroids should always be taken with an antacid, milk, or food. Stools and emesis should be tested for traces of blood. Watch for and report tarry stools and complaints of abdominal pain.

Skin changes are possible with steroids. The skin may become thin and reddened, or it may darken. *Ecchymoses* (bruised areas) and *petechiae* (tiny red spots) may appear. Allergy to the medication may be manifested by a rash. Reassure the patient that changes in skin color are not unusual.

Hormonal imbalance is a common consequence of steroid medications. A woman may notice menstrual irregularities and abnormal growth of facial and body hair (hirsutism). In both sexes there may be decreased sex drive.

A round "moon" face, abnormal fat distribution on the back and abdomen, edema, weight gain, oily skin, and acne are common with long-term steroid therapy. Because these features resemble the signs of Cushing's syndrome (hypersecretion of the adrenal glands), they have been given the name of cushingoid features. Warn the patient about such body changes before they occur, so that their impact will be less upsetting.

Metabolic effects of steroid use include increased appetite and alterations in digestion. Protein metabolism is disrupted, leading to a state of negative nitrogen balance that causes delayed wound healing. Steroids cause fat deposits to move from storage areas to various parts of the body (cheeks, abdomen, back), and this brings changes

in body contour. Disruption of carbohydrate metabolism may lead to hyperglycemia and glycosuria. Latent diabetes mellitus may emerge at this time, necessitating dietary modifications. The urine should be tested each day for sugar and acetone.

Fluid retention causes the intraocular pressure to rise. If the patient receiving steroids has a family history of glaucoma or cataracts, he is a candidate for *eye disorders.* Be sure you inquire about the family history during your initial assessment.

Various *musculoskeletal* defects may be noted. There is a loss of muscle mass leading to weakness and lethargy. Calcium loss from the bones may give rise to osteoporosis and fractures (especially in the long bones). Patients must guard against placing themselves in hazardous situations that require great strength, as well as doing everything possible to avoid trauma to bone.

Mental changes are common in patients who take steroids for more than a short while. The patient may be depressed or euphoric, and his mood may fluctuate widely from day to day. The "steroid high" that is sometimes seen may make it difficult to deal with the patient on long-term therapy. Drastic changes in body image related to steroid use may cause a patient to feel so depressed that he may attempt suicide.

Extensive use of steroids may result in both physical and psychological dependence. They must never be discontinued abruptly because this may cause an acute flareup of the underlying disorder and because the adrenal glands, which have been rendered inactive by the extended use of the steroid, may be totally unable to function. Muscle weakness and exhaustion point to acute adrenal insufficiency, so be sure to follow the ordered schedule for tapering off the medication.

Steroids mask the signs and symptoms of disease by suppressing the normal inflammatory response. Although this often makes the patient more comfortable, it may also lead to a superimposed infection due to the lowered resistance to infection. Thus, the steroid may exacerbate (worsen) an infectious disease. Anyone who has an upper respiratory infection, such as a cold or a sore throat, should not care for the patient. Follow thorough handwashing and sterile techniques when indicated to prevent the transfer of infectious organisms.

Anyone taking steroids for long periods of time must report any new illness, infection, or emotionally stressful situation to his physician. The internal stress may in turn impair adrenal function. The dose of the steroid can be increased temporarily to deal with such problems. The patient needs to understand the importance of taking every dose on time, as well as the importance of appearing for laboratory tests and medical appointments at the specified intervals. He should also be encouraged to wear a Medic-Alert tag so the physician can be quickly notified in the event of accident or injury.

Pancreatic Hormones

Insulin preparations must be refrigerated, and the expiration date must be checked. All types of insulin (except Regular) need to be resuspended before being drawn up into the syringe. The vial should never be shaken but should be rolled between the palms or gently turned upside down a few times to distribute the suspended particles evenly.

Doses of insulin are ordered in *units*, not in milligrams. A special insulin syringe, which is calibrated in units, must be used (see Fig. 5-3). As with other hormones, small errors in dosage can cause serious problems because of the potency of the medicine.

Sometimes two different types of insulin are ordered for the same patient. In these cases, both types may be mixed in the same syringe (see Chapter 5) with the following precaution: Air is always injected into the vial with the *longer*-acting insulin first. The *shorter*-acting insulin is then withdrawn, followed by the longer-acting insulin. If the shorter-acting insulin is accidently injected into the vial containing the longer-acting insulin, it will be absorbed. The longer-acting insulin cannot be absorbed by the shorter-acting insulin.

Insulin must be given by the subcutaneous route because it is destroyed by stomach enzymes and poorly absorbed from muscle tissue. Be sure to rotate the injection sites (see Fig. 5-5) to prevent trauma to tissues and to increase absorption of the medication. There are many visual aids available to illustrate rotation schedules. Urine must be tested for sugar and acetone at regular intervals (usually before meals and at bedtime) and insulin given if sugar is present. When testing the urine with Clinitest tablets, be aware that some medications, cephalosporins, for example, will produce inaccurate results; in these cases, use Tes-tape.

Diet therapy is an important aspect of therapy with insulin, since daily doses are calculated according to usual food intake, among other things.

The patient must be taught to eat at regular intervals and to follow his diet plan closely. Doses of insulin may have to be changed if dietary intake is increased or decreased. Other conditions and circumstances that may call for a change in the insulin dose are an increase or decrease in activity, the presence of infection, use of anesthesia, and situations of stress.

If too much insulin is taken, meals are skipped, or activity is excessive, symptoms of *hypoglycemia* may appear. The first signs are weakness, tremors, and increased perspiration. The patient complains of feeling nervous, hungry, and vaguely apprehensive. He may look pale, but his vital signs are usually within normal limits. At the first suspicion of hypoglycemia, you should give the patient a soluble carbohydrate, such as a sugar lump, piece of hard candy, or a glassful of orange juice. If the patient is unconscious, he will need intravenous dextrose.

If his insulin dosage is insufficient, if he overeats, if he has an infection, or if he does not get the needed exercise, the opposite condition, called *hyperglycemia*, will develop. Signs and symptoms include fatigue, dull headache, abdominal pain, nausea, vomiting, fever, increased respiratory rate and depth, and low blood pressure. The patient complains of thirst and appears flushed. His skin is hot and dry. His breath has the sweet odor of acetone. Insulin and fluids must be administered, because if the hyperglycemia is not brought under control, it can lead to diabetic coma and death.

The patient's family should be included in teaching sessions whenever possible. Although the patient should take responsibility for his own care to the extent possible, there may be instances when a family member will be called on to test urine and administer injections.

Patients on oral hypoglycemics rarely experience adverse effects; however, they must adhere to the prescribed diet, just as patients on insulin do.

Sex Hormones

A patient with sexual dysfunction or a disorder of the reproductive organs is bound to be emotionally stressed, because of the importance society places on sex roles. Such a patient needs much psychological support, so he can retain and maintain his self-esteem. This is especially true should hormone therapy cause bodily changes.

Sex hormones cause few adverse effects when given in usual doses for short periods of time, but with long-term therapy, body changes may appear. These are most pronounced in the male who becomes feminized due to therapy with female hormones or the female who receives androgens and is masculinized. Thus, the benefits of treatment must be weighed against the impact of bodily changes. The patient must be informed of this possibility beforehand.

Sex hormones can also cause changes in sex drive in both sexes. The patient's spouse or significant other person should be told of this possibility.

Women taking estrogens may face an increased risk of thromboembolism. Instruct them to inform their physician should calf tenderness, redness, or swelling develop. A woman who smokes while using oral contraceptives is inviting even greater risk of thromboembolism.

Some investigators believe that estrogens are carcinogenic in women with a hereditary predisposition to cancer of the reproductive tract. These women should be taught the importance of monthly self-breast examination and should have regular internal examinations.

Many combinations of contraceptives available today make it difficult to generalize about their effects. The patient needs to know that problems of mood changes, changes in sexual desire, and weight gain are common. Encourage the patient to read the label on her prescription carefully and follow instructions to the letter. Oral contraceptives are close to 100% effective, provided they are taken in the correct dose and according to schedule. Help the patient to establish a routine so she will remember to take her pills correctly. Initial nausea usually disappears within a few weeks. Taking pills with food or after meals may help.

Broad-spectrum antibiotics such as the tetracyclines may cause failure of oral contraceptives. Birth control pills may interfere with the action of anticonvulsants, tricyclic antidepressants, antihypertensives, vitamins, and antidiabetic agents.

Androgens can upset the electrolyte balance and produce edema. A change in diet along with a diuretic may be necessary. Electrolyte levels should be monitored closely and intake and output charted.

Virilism—a deepening voice, increased body hair, and acne—may develop in a woman taking androgens. There may also be other manifestations such as a reduction in the size of the breasts and enlargement of the clitoris. The desire for sexual intercourse may increase. All these changes are upsetting to most patients, and they need much emotional support along with informed explanations.

PRACTICE PROBLEMS—HORMONES

1. The physician orders 25 units NPH insulin and 6 units of regular insulin to be given before breakfast. The two insulins are to be mixed in the same syringe. If both insulins come in a concentration of 100 U/ml, how would the procedure be done?

First, 25 units of air is drawn into the syringe. The air is injected into the NPH insulin vial. The needle and syringe are removed from the vial without any solution.

Second, 6 units of air is drawn into the syringe. The air is injected into the regular insulin vial and 6 units of regular insulin is drawn into the syringe. The needle and syringe are removed from the vial.

The needle is then inserted into the NPH insulin vial. The 25 units of NPH insulin is removed. There is now a total of 31 units of insulin (25U + 6U) in the syringe.

2. The order reads: methimazole (Tapazole) 20 mg PO q8h.
The label reads: methimazole 10 mg/tablet.
How many tablets will be given?

$$\frac{D}{H} = G$$

$$\frac{2\ \cancel{20}\ \cancel{mg}}{1\ \cancel{10}\ \cancel{mg}} = 2$$

Two tablets of methimazole (Tapazole) will be given.

Work the following problems:
1. The order reads: NPH 18 units and regular insulin 10 units before breakfast.
The labels read: NPH 100 U/ml. Regular insulin 100 U/ml.

If mixing the two insulins in the same syringe, what will be the total volume?
What volume will the NPH be?
What volume will the regular insulin be?
Which insulin will actually be drawn into the syringe first?

2. The order reads: vasopression (Pitressin) 5 units SC tid.

The label reads: 10 U/0.5 ml.
What volume will be given?

3. The order reads: prednisone 15 mg PO daily in the AM.
The label reads: prednisone 5 mg/tablet.
How many tablets will be given?

Answers are given on p. 284.

CHAPTER 35
Antineoplastic drugs

The word *cancer* is a general term that describes a malignant tumor (neoplasm) anywhere in the body. The drugs used to treat neoplasms are called antineoplastic agents. Malignant cells grow and reproduce very rapidly. Antineoplastic drugs are especially toxic to rapidly growing cells. By interfering with cellular metabolism, they prevent cell reproduction. The aim of cancer chemotherapy (treatment with drugs) is to destroy the cancer cells without doing serious harm to normal cells. Chemotherapy is generally done along with radiation or surgery. The goal of this combined treatment is to remove the mass tumor surgically, and then destroy the remaining cancer cells with radiation or drugs.

Treatment with antineoplastic drugs is generally considered palliative—relieving symptoms and slowing the disease process but not affecting the final outcome. There are, however, a few types of cancer that are now considered curable because they respond so well to chemotherapy. In these, long-term remissions (the period of time when the patient is symptom free) of 5 years or more are possible.

CLASSIFICATION OF ANTINEOPLASTIC DRUGS

Many different types of drugs are used to treat cancer, and each has a specific destructive action on the cancerous cells (see Table 35-1). Consequently, drugs have been developed that are expressly designed to act on a particular type of cancer.

Alkylating agents, such as mustard gas and drugs with similar action, are used to treat cancers of the bone marrow and lymph tissue. *Antimetabolites* disrupt normal metabolism and destroy growing cells, both normal and cancerous. Some *natural substances*, like antibiotics, also have an antineoplastic effect in that they block the malignant cells' ability to grow. *Adrenocorticosteroid hormones* (see Chapter 34) are known to suppress lymphocyte growth, which is the basis of their anti-inflammatory action. They are also useful in treating such cancers as childhood acute leukemia. Sex hormones are sometimes prescribed in cancer of the reproductive organs.

RADIOACTIVE ISOTOPES

One advantage of radiation therapy is that a high concentration of radiation can be aimed at a specific target area. The result is selective destruction of mainly the malignant cells, rather than the widespread destruction of normal cells along with the malignant ones.

Radiation can be administered by x-ray or by radioactive rods or seeds implanted directly in the tumor. The radioactive isotopes currently in use are cobalt 60, iodine 131, phosphorus 32, and radium 226.

(*Text continues on p. 252.*)

TABLE 35-1 ANTINEOPLASTIC DRUGS

DRUG	ROUTE AND DOSAGE RANGE	USE	ADVERSE EFFECTS	NURSING IMPLICATIONS
ALKYLATING AGENTS				
busulfan (Myleran)	PO—4 mg–8 mg qd	To treat chronic myelocytic leukemia	*Endocrine:* impotence, sterility, amenorrhea, gynecomastia *GI:* GI upset, nausea, vomiting, diarrhea, weight loss *Skin:* inflammation of the lips and tongue, increased skin pigmentation, decreased perspiration, hair loss *Others:* blood disorders (may lead to hemorrhage), increased uric acid in the blood (can cause kidney damage), pulmonary fibrosis, muscular weakness	Blood tests should be done frequently to check on bone marrow function. Uric acid levels need to be checked periodically. Assess condition of lips and tongue. Check weight daily. Warn patients about the possibility of sexual difficulties. Women should be warned about changes in menstrual cycle that are likely to occur. Check skin for color change. Note changes in male breast tissue, and reassure him this is not unusual. Note hair loss. Note any respiratory difficulty. Keep stool chart. Antiemetics given before medicating the patient may lessen nausea and vomiting.
carmustine (BCNU, BiCNU)	IV—200 mg/M² every 6 weeks	For palliative treatment of brain tumors, multiple myelomas, Hodgkin's disease and non-Hodgkin's lymphomas	Delayed bone marrow depression (4–6 weeks after drug is given), anemia, nausea, vomiting, liver damage, burning at injection site	Frequent complete blood cell counts need to be checked, as well as tests of liver function. Check for reaction at injection site. Give antiemetics prn.
chlorambucil (Leukeran)	PO—4 mg–10 mg qd for 3–6 weeks Maintenance—2 mg–4 mg qd (or less)	To treat chronic lymphocytic leukemia and malignant lymphomas, including lymphosarcoma, giant follicular lymphoma, Hodgkin's disease	*Endocrine:* problems with menstruation, sterility (may be permanent) *GI:* anorexia, nausea, vomiting, diarrhea, jaundice *Skin:* hair loss *Others:* severe bone marrow depression, immunosuppression, chromosomal abnormalities, increased uric acid	Blood tests should be done frequently to check on bone marrow function. Assess appetite. Keep stool chart. Give antiemetics prn. Check skin and sclera for yellowish color. Evaluate hearing and balance. Encourage genetic counseling to patients anticipating childbirth. Warn patient of possible changes in menstruation and sterility. Have patient avoid persons with obvious infections or colds.
cisplatin (Platinol)	IV—Testicular tumors—20 mg/M² qd for 5 days; then repeat after 3 weeks and again after another 3 weeks Ovarian tumor—50 mg/M² once every 3 weeks	Used in combination therapy to treat metastatic testicular and ovarian tumors and advanced cancer of the bladder	Nausea, vomiting, renal and ototoxicity, myelosuppression, anaphylaxis, neurotoxicity, hyperuricemia	Evaluate hearing and urinary output. Record I&O. Frequent blood tests and liver function tests should be done. Evaluate mental status. Give antiemetics prn. Keep stool chart. **(continued on page 247)**

TABLE 35-1 (continued)

DRUG	ROUTE AND DOSAGE RANGE	USE	ADVERSE EFFECTS	NURSING IMPLICATIONS
cisplatin (*continued*)	Bladder cancer—50 mg–75 mg/M² every 3–4 weeks			Observe for any sign of anaphylaxis. Be sure patient is well hydrated 8–12 hours before treatment.
cyclophosphamide (Cytoxan, Neosar)	*Initially:* PO—1 mg–5 mg/kg qd IV—40 mg–50 mg/kg in divided doses over 2–5 days *Maintenance:* PO—1 mg–5 mg/kg qd IV—10 mg–15 mg/kg q 7–10 days or 3 mg–5 mg/kg twice weekly	To treat malignant lymphomas, multiple myeloma, leukemias, mycosis fungoides, neuroblastoma, adenocarcinoma of the ovary, carcinoma of the breast, malignant neoplasms of the lung	*Endocrine:* amenorrhea, sterility *GI:* anorexia, nausea, vomiting *GU:* sterile hemorrhagic cystitis, kidney damage *Skin:* hair loss, darkening of the skin and fingernails, dermatitis *Others:* secondary malignancies, bone marrow suppression, anemia, delayed wound healing, ovarian fibrosis, interstitial pulmonary fibrosis	Blood tests should be done frequently to check on bone marrow function. Evaluate appetite. Force fluids and encourage the patient to void frequently. Test all urine for blood. Warn patients of changes in menstruation and the possibility of sterility. Encourage female patients to have regular gynecologic examinations. Watch for change in color of skin and nails. Note any respiratory difficulty. Warn patients of hair loss. Give antiemetics prn.
lomustine (CCNU, CeeNU)	PO—100 mg–130 mg/M² qd every 6 weeks	Use in palliative treatment of brain tumors and Hodgkin's disease	*CNS:* disorientation, lethargy, ataxia, dysarthria *GI:* nausea, vomiting, stomatitis, liver damage *Others:* hair loss, anemia, bone marrow depression	Give antiemetics prn. Inspect mouth for sores. Warn patient of hair loss. Blood tests should be done regularly (until 6 weeks after treatment ends) to check on bone marrow and liver function. Assist with ambulation and activities as necessary. Evaluate mental status. Note any difficulty with speech.
mechlorethamine (Mustargen, Nitrogen Mustard)	IV—0.1 mg–0.2 mg/kg qd until total dose of 0.4 mg/kg is reached; may repeat after 3 weeks	Use in palliative treatment of Hodgkin's disease, lymphosarcoma, chronic myelocytic and chronic lymphocytic leukemias, polycythemia vera, mycosis fungoides, bronchogenic cancer	See chlorambucil, *plus:* painful inflammation and tissue sloughing if extravasation occurs	See chlorambucil, *plus:* Watch intravenous infusions carefully to prevent any leakage of medication into surrounding tissue.
melphalan (Alkeran)	PO—Multiple myeloma—6 mg qd as a single dose for 2 to 3 weeks; after a rest period of up to 4 weeks, maintenance dose of 2 mg qd Ovarian cancer—0.2 mg/kg qd for 5 days; may be repeated every 4–5 weeks	Use in palliative treatment of multiple myeloma and nonresectable epithelial cancer of the ovary	Bone marrow depression, nausea, vomiting, rash, fibrotic changes in lung tissue	Blood tests should be done at regular intervals. Give antiemetics prn. Note any difficulty with respirations. Observe skin for rash.

(continued on page 248)

TABLE 35-1 (continued)

DRUG	ROUTE AND DOSAGE RANGE	USE	ADVERSE EFFECTS	NURSING IMPLICATIONS
procarbazine (Matulane)	PO—2 mg–4 mg/kg qd in a single or divided doses for 1 week; then 4 mg–6 mg/kg qd until maximum response Maintenance—1 mg–2 mg/kg qd	To treat Hodgkin's disease	*CNS:* weakness, fatigue, drowsiness, paresthesias, headache, dizziness, depression, apprehension, insomnia, nightmares, hallucinations, decreased reflexes, footdrop, tremors, confusion, coma, convulsions, nystagmus *Cardiovascular:* tachycardia, hypotension *Respiratory:* cough, pneumonia *GI:* anorexia, dry mouth, nausea and vomiting, dysphagia, diarrhea, and constipation *Skin:* dermatitis, herpes, increased skin pigmentation, flushing *Others:* muscle and joint pain, chills, fever, sweating, hoarseness, bleeding tendencies, secondary infections, edema, photophobia, retinal hemorrhage, difficulties with urination	See lomustine, *plus:* Assess appetite. Note any difficulty with swallowing. Keep stool chart. Monitor temperature, pulse, and respirations. Warn patient to avoid dangerous activities. Warn patient to avoid persons with obvious infections or colds. Keep record of I&O. Check weight daily. Check skin for reactions (rash, inflammations, changes in color). Evaluate sleep patterns. Encourage exercise of the ankle muscles. Note any unusual muscle movements. Observe the eyeball for any bleeding or unusual movements. Tell patient to avoid brightly lit rooms and direct sunlight.
streptozocin (Zanosar)	IV—500 mg/M² qd for 5 days, repeated every 6 weeks or 1000 mg–1500 mg/M² weekly for 2–5 weeks	To treat metastatic islet cell cancer of the pancreas	*CNS:* confusion, lethargy, depression *GI:* nausea, vomiting, diarrhea, liver damage *GU:* azotemia, anuria, hypophosphatemia, glycosuria, renal tubular acidosis *Other:* bone marrow depression	Evaluate mental status. Keep stool chart. Keep strict I&O records. Check urine for sugar and acetone. Blood and urine tests should be done at regular intervals to check on liver and kidney function. Give antiemetics prn.
thiotepa	IV—Initial dose—0.3 mg–0.4 mg/kg Maintenance—repeat initial dose every 1–4 weeks Intratumor—0.6 mg–0.8 mg/kg Maintenance—0.07 mg–0.8 mg/kg every 1–4 weeks Intracavity—0.6 mg–0.8 mg/kg Intrabladder—60 mg in 30 ml–60 ml distilled water (retained 2 hr) every week for 4 weeks. Course may be repeated prn	Use in palliative treatment of adenocarcinoma of the breast, ovary, and bladder; to control intracavity effusions secondary to diffuse or localized neoplastic disease of various serosal cavities; also effective against lymphomas	*CNS:* dizziness, headache *Endocrine:* amenorrhea, male sterility *GI:* anorexia, nausea, vomiting *Skin:* rash, hives *Others:* fever, bone marrow depression, pain at injection site	Give antiemetics prn. Assist with activities as necessary. Warn females of changes in menstruation and males of possible sterility. Check skin for rash or hives. Monitor temperature. Blood tests should be done regularly to check bone marrow function. Check injection site for reaction.

(continued on page 249)

TABLE 35-1 (continued)

DRUG	ROUTE AND DOSAGE RANGE	USE	ADVERSE EFFECTS	NURSING IMPLICATIONS
ANTIMETABOLITES				
cytarabine (Ara-C, Cytosar-U)	SC—1 mg/kg every week IV—200 mg/M² qd (by continuous infusion) for 5 days; repeat every 2 weeks Intrathecal—30 mg/ M² every 4 days	To induce remission in acute granulocytic leukemia of adults and for other acute leukemias of adults and children	Bone marrow depression, nausea, vomiting, anemia, diarrhea, inflammation of the mouth or mouth ulcers, thrombophlebitis, liver dysfunction, fever	Blood tests should be done frequently to check liver and bone marrow function. Give antiemetics prn. Keep stool chart. Check mouth for lesions. Note complaints of calf tenderness, pain, or swelling. Monitor temperature.
fluorouracil (5-FU, Adrucil)	IV—12 mg/kg qd for 4 days (daily dose not to exceed 800 mg); if tolerated, 6 mg/kg on 6th, 8th, 10th, 12th day In poor-risk or poorly nourished patients—6 mg/kg qd for 3 days (daily dose not to exceed 400 mg); if tolerated, 3 mg/kg on 5th, 7th, 9th day Maintenance—repeat first course 30 days after last one ends or 10 mg–15 mg/kg every week (not to exceed 1 g/wk)	Use in palliative treatment of cancer of the colon, rectum, breast, stomach, and pancreas in patients who are considered incurable by surgery or other means	*CNS:* euphoria, ataxia *GI:* anorexia, nausea, vomiting, diarrhea, sloughing of mucosa in the upper GI tract (as a complication of inflammation) *Skin:* hair loss, rash, dry skin, photosensitivity, increased tearing, darkening of the skin, loss of nails *Others:* low white blood cell count, nosebleeds	Check mouth for sores. Test all stool and vomitus samples for the presence of blood. Assess appetite. Give antiemetics prn. Blood tests should be done frequently to check bone marrow and liver function. Warn patient of possible hair loss. Check skin for hydration, rash, or changes in color. Tell patient to avoid brightly lit rooms and direct sunlight. Note excessive tears and loss of fingernails and toenails. Evaluate mental status. Assist with activities as necessary. Watch for nosebleeds.
methotrexate (Folex, Mexate)	PO, IM, IV, Intrathecal—Dosage is highly individualized, depending on the condition being treated	To treat gestational choriocarcinoma, chorioadenoma destruens, hydatiditorm mole, acute lymphocytic leukemia, meningeal leukemia, alymphoblastic leukemia, breast cancer, epidermoid cancer of the head and neck, and lung cancer; used to treat advanced stages of lymphosarcoma and mycosis fungoides; used to control symptoms of severe, recalcitrant, disabling psoriasis that does not respond to other therapy	*CNS:* headache, drowsiness, blurred vision, aphasia, hemiparesis, convulsions, dizziness *Endocrine:* sterility, menstrual irregularities, abortion *GI:* abdominal distress, anorexia, inflamed GI tract, GI bleeding *GU:* cystitis, renal failure *Skin:* rash, itching, photosensitivity, depigmentation, ecchymosis, acne, boils, hemorrhage *Others:* chills, fever, decreased resistance to infection, pneumonia	See lomustine, *plus:* Monitor temperature. Warn patients to avoid those with obvious infections. Check skin for rash or itch. Caution patients to avoid brightly lit rooms and direct sunlight. Note changes in skin color. Note any increased acne or boils. Assess appetite. Note any bruising. Test all stool, urine, and vomitus samples for the presence of blood. Encourage high fluid intake and frequent voiding. Record all I&O. Warn male patient of possible sterility and females of changes in menstruation and possible abortion. Evaluate visual acuity. Note any difficulty with movements on one side of the body.

(continued on page 250)

TABLE 35-1   (continued)

DRUG	ROUTE AND DOSAGE RANGE	USE	ADVERSE EFFECTS	NURSING IMPLICATIONS
NATURAL SUBSTANCES				
bleomycin (Blenoxane)	IM, IV, SC—10 U–20 U/M^2 once or twice a week	To treat squamous cell cancer of the head and neck; Hodgkin's disease, lymphosarcoma, testicular and penile cancer, and cancer of the cervix and vulva	*Respiratory:* pulmonary fibrosis, pneumonia *GI:* vomiting, anorexia *Skin:* hair loss, rash, darkening of the skin, changes in the nails *Others:* fever, chills	See dactinomycin.
dactinomycin (Cosmegen, Actinomycin D)	IV—0.5 mg qd for a maximum of 5 days	To treat Wilms' tumor, rhabdomyosarcoma, cancer of the testis and uterus, Ewing's sarcoma, sarcoma botryoides	*Cardiovascular:* decreased calcium levels, blood disorders *GI:* anorexia, nausea, vomiting, diarrhea, abdominal pain, GI bleeding, inflammation of the upper GI mucosa, rectal discomfort *Skin:* hair loss, rash, acne, darkening of the skin, tissue necrosis if extravasation occurs *Others:* malaise, fever, muscle aches	Assess appetite. Give antiemetics prn. Keep stool chart. Test all stool, urine, and vomitus samples for the presence of blood. Monitor temperature. Note complaints of rectal and muscular discomfort. Check mouth for sores. Blood tests should be done at regular intervals. Warn patient of hair loss. Check skin for rash and changes in color. Watch intravenous infusions closely to avoid leakage of medication into surrounding tissue. Check calcium levels.
doxorubicin (Adriamycin)	IV—60 mg–75 mg/ M^2 (as a single injection) every 21 days or 30 mg/M^2 on 3 successive days; repeat every 4 weeks (total cumulative dose should not exceed 550 mg/M^2)	To produce remissions in acute lymphoblastic and acute myeloblastic leukemias, Wilms' tumor, neuroblastoma, soft tissue and bone sarcomas, cancer of the breast, ovary and thyroid, transitional cell bladder cancer, lymphomas, and bronchogenic cancer	*GI:* acute and often severe nausea and vomiting, inflammation of the upper GI mucosa, anorexia, diarrhea *Skin:* complete hair loss, hives, severe local tissue necrosis if extravasation occurs *Others:* bone marrow depression, fever, chills, cardiac failure, possible anaphylaxis	See dactinomycin, *plus:* Watch for hives. Monitor pulse. Warn patient about possibility that urine may be red.
etoposide (VePesid)	IV—50 mg–100 mg/ M^2/day for 5 days or 100 mg/M^2/day on days 1, 3, and 5. Repeat every 3–4 weeks	To treat refractory testicular tumors	*CNS:* sleepiness, fatigue, peripheral neuropathy *Cardiovascular:* hypotension, ECG changes *GI:* nausea, vomiting, anorexia, diarrhea, stomatitis, liver damage *Others:* alopecia, bone marrow depression, anaphylactic-like reactions	See dactinomycin, *plus:* Observe patient for chills, fever, tachycardia, dyspnea caused by anaphylactic-like reactions.

(continued on page 251)

TABLE 35-1 (continued)

DRUG	ROUTE AND DOSAGE RANGE	USE	ADVERSE EFFECTS	NURSING IMPLICATIONS
mitomycin (Mitomycin-C, Mutamycin)	IV—20 mg/M² as a single dose or 2 mg/M² for 5 days, then skip 2 days, then 2 mg/M² for 5 days. Repeat every 6–8 weeks Intravesical—40 mg instilled into the bladder	To treat cancer of the stomach and pancreas and superficial bladder cancer	*CNS:* headache, blurred vision, confusion, drowsiness, syncope, fatigue *Respiratory:* dyspnea, nonproductive cough, lung infiltrates *GI:* nausea, vomiting, anorexia, stomatitis *Others:* bone marrow damage, cellulitis at injection site	See dactinomycin.
vinblastine (Velban)	IV—3.7–18.5 mg/M²/day; repeat every 7 days	Use in palliative treatment of generalized Hodgkin's disease, lymphocytic lymphoma, histiocytic lymphoma, advanced mycosis fungoides, advanced cancer of the testis, resistant choriocarcinoma and cancer of the breast	See dactinomycin, *plus:* *CNS:* numbness and paresthesias, mental depression, loss of deep tendon reflexes, headache, convulsions *GI:* constipation, ileus *Others:* pain in tumor site, skin blistering	See dactinomycin, *plus:* Note any complaints of abnormal sensations. Evaluate mental status. Check deep tendon reflexes. Institute seizure precautions. Give gentle skin care and note any blistering.
vincristine (Oncovin)	IV—1.4 mg/M² every week	To treat acute leukemia, Hodgkin's disease, lymphosarcoma, reticulum cell sarcoma, rhabdomyosarcoma, neuroblastoma and Wilms' tumor	See vinblastine, *plus:* *CNS:* difficulty walking ("slapping gait"), muscle wasting, dropfoot, cranial nerve involvement *GU:* polyuria, dysuria *Others:* weight loss, fever	See vinblastine, *plus:* Evaluate walking and note any unusual gait. Watch for muscle deterioration and footdrop. Check weight daily. Monitor temperature. Note any change in senses, facial movements, chewing, or swallowing. Assess voiding pattern, and keep record of I&O.
MISCELLANEOUS AGENTS				
asparaginase (Elspar)	IM—6000 IU/M² qd IV—200 IU–1000 IU/kg qd (doses are repeated at intervals that depend on the protocol being followed)	To treat acute lymphocytic leukemia, especially in children	*CNS:* hyperthermia (can be fatal), mental depression, lethargy, confusion, agitation, hallucinations, coma, parkinsonism, headache, irritability *Cardiovascular:* increased blood sugar, depression of the clotting mechanism, increased or decreased blood lipids, increased albumin levels, peripheral edema, bone marrow depression *GI:* anorexia, nausea, vomiting, abdominal cramps, liver damage, pancreatitis	Check skin for any rash or hives. Assess appetite. Check weight daily. Monitor temperature and respirations. Keep record of I&O. Test all urine for sugar and albumin. Blood tests should be done frequently to check on bone marrow function and levels of lipid, albumin, and sugar. Evaluate mental status. Assist with activities as necessary. Note any abnormal muscle movements. Give antiemetics prn.

(continued on page 252)

TABLE 35-1 (continued)

DRUG	ROUTE AND DOSAGE RANGE	USE	ADVERSE EFFECTS	NURSING IMPLICATIONS
asparaginase (continued)			GU: polyuria, glyco- suria, kidney damage Skin: rash, hives Others: fever, joint aches, respiratory dis- tress, allergic reac- tions (may lead to an- aphylaxis and death)	
hydroxyurea (Hydrea)	PO—Intermittent— 80 mg/kg qd as a single dose every 3 days Continuous—20 mg–30 mg/kg as a single dose qd	To treat melanoma, re- sistant chronic mye- locytic leukemia and recurrent, metastatic or inoperable can- cer of the ovary; use with radiation in the treatment of squa- mous cell carci- noma of the head (except the lip) and neck	GI: stomatitis, anorexia, nausea, vomiting, diarrhea and consti- pation GU: temporary kidney impairment, dysuria Skin: rash, facial ery- thema, hair loss Others: bone marrow depression, fever, chills	Blood tests should be done frequently to check on bone marrow function. Keep record of I&O. Check mouth for sores. Assess appetite. Keep stool chart. Check skin for rash. Warn patients about the pos- sibility of hair loss and change in face color. Give antiemetics prn.

COMBINED CHEMOTHERAPY

Several antineoplastic drugs may be given to the patient in an effort to balance toxic and therapeutic effects. It is believed that combinations are more potent, for longer periods of time, than single drugs.

NURSING IMPLICATIONS

Most patients receiving chemotherapy are aware that they may be facing death and may be in great need of emotional support. The treatment is highly stressful. Therefore, the nurse should be aware of what and how much the patient knows about his disease and prognosis and how he is coping with that knowledge. Patients and families need complete teaching regarding the drugs, their actions, and the related problems.

Cancer chemotherapy is long and drawn-out. Progress may be slow, and the patient may feel worse as time goes on. The patient's hope for a cure should not be reinforced unless this is a definite possibility; hopes for remission are more realistic.

The major drawback to cancer chemotherapy is that high doses of drugs are required and their action is not selective. As a result, not only cancer cells but all rapidly growing cells are damaged. Hair follicles, the mucous membranes lining the mouth and gastrointestinal tract, the gonads, and the bone marrow are among the structures that may be damaged. It is this type of damage that gives rise to the anorexia, nausea, vomiting, hair loss, mouth sores, sterility, and bone marrow depression associated with chemotherapy.

Alopecia, or hair loss, will obviously cause an alteration in body image. How deeply the patient will be disturbed will depend largely on his previous self-image and the significant relationships that give him emotional support. A woman who has lost her hair needs constant reassurance that she has not lost her femininity too. Scarfs, wigs, and make-up can all help if she feels she is unattractive.

Stomatitis (mouth sores) interferes with nutrition because almost any food will irritate the inflamed tissues. Inflammation of the pharynx may also cause difficulty in swallowing. Make sure the patient knows about special mouthwashes that can be used before meals to soothe the membranes. Recommend bland, soft foods. The first signs of stomatitis are reddened membranes and white patches that can lead to ulceration and bleeding. Be sure to check the patient's mouth frequently so these early signs will be noted. Use a flashlight, so you can have a clear view of the membranes.

Severe nausea, vomiting, and anorexia are common during treatment with antineoplastic drugs. These can sometimes be avoided by giving antiemetic drugs ahead of the antineoplastic medication, or by giving the antineoplastic drug late in the day, followed by nighttime sedation. Antiemetics are available in timed-release capsules for prolonged effect. The active ingredient in marijuana (THC) has been reported to decrease nausea and vomiting, and prescriptions may now be written for it, but only for investigational purposes.

Menstrual irregularities are common for several months after antineoplastics have been used. Sterility may result from antineoplastic therapy. Remember that with hormones given to treat cancer of the reproductive organs, masculinization in females and feminization in males are possible (see Chapter 34). Be sure the patient is aware of these possibilities before the chemotherapy is begun.

Bone marrow depression is perhaps the most serious complication of treatment with antineoplastic drugs. With diminished production of white blood cells in the bone marrow, the body's normal immune mechanism is severely damaged. This phenomenon is called immunosuppression. The end result may be an infection that overwhelms body defenses and causes death.

When giving certain types of care to this patient, as when drawing blood, follow strict aseptic technique, and keep anyone with an infectious disease away from the patient. Frequent blood tests are necessary to measure the white blood cell count. Platelets are also formed in the bone marrow, and their function is to promote clotting. With bone marrow depression due to chemotherapy, platelets decrease in number (thrombocytopenia), and this can cause hemorrhage from ulcerated tissues or trauma; such hemorrhage may be fatal because the clotting mechanism has been destroyed.

The patient must avoid doing anything that could cause bruising or bleeding. A male patient should shave with great care. Teeth must be brushed very gently. The use of a plain rinse may be advisable instead of a toothbrush, since the oral mucosa may be irritated and sore, and bleed readily. Straining at stools can cause rectal bleeding; prevent this by using stool softeners. If the patient is unsteady, he will need assistance so as to avoid bumps and falls. If he is confused or agitated, be sure the siderails are padded so he will not injure himself. After blood is drawn, apply pressure at the site long enough to be certain that there will be no bleeding into the tissues. If possible, give all medications by mouth, rather than by injection.

Be sure irritating medications do not come in contact with the patient's skin. This may necessitate wearing protective glasses or gloves. If these drugs are given intravenously, they must be carefully monitored to ensure that no medication leaks into the tissues.

Skin reactions are common following radiation. These so-called radiation burns are areas of highly reddened or darkened skin that are extremely painful and may blister or peel, like a severe sunburn. Never tape bandages to these sensitive, irritated areas. Rather, encourage the patient to wear loose clothing made of a soft, absorbent material.

Some chemotherapeutic agents cause cystitis, and this can lead to hemorrhagic complications. The patient should be encouraged to drink at least three liters of fluid every day to keep the bladder flushed.

PRACTICE PROBLEMS—ANTINEOPLASTIC DRUGS

1. The order reads: busulfan (Myleran) 6 mg PO daily.
   The label reads: busulfan 2 mg/tablet.
   How many tablets will you give?

$$\frac{D}{H} = G$$

$$\frac{3 \; \cancel{6} \; \cancel{mg}}{1 \; \cancel{2} \; \cancel{mg}} = 3$$

Thus, 3 tablets of busulfan (Myleran) will be given.

Work the following problems:
1. The order reads: chlorambucil (Leukeran) 10 mg daily.
   The label reads: chlorambucil 2 mg/tablet.
   How many tablets will be given?

2. The physician orders melphalon (Alkeran) 6 mg daily for 2 weeks. The drug comes in 2-mg tablets. How many tablets will you give?

3. The order reads: cyclophosphamide (Cytoxan) 125 mg daily.

The label reads: cyclophosphamide 50 mg/tablet.
How many tablets will be given?

Answers are given on p. 284.

PART 7
Drugs used to help meet patients' needs for the maintenance of sensory and motor mechanisms and functions

CHAPTER 36
Anticonvulsants

Epilepsy is a disorder characterized by abnormal brain activity that causes attacks of altered consciousness or motor activity called seizures. It affects more than 2 million Americans, making it the most common nervous system disorder in this country.

A person with epilepsy may or may not have convulsions. Convulsions are involuntary contractions of a muscle or a group of muscles. If all muscles contract, the person becomes rigid and the activity is termed *tonic*. In a *clonic* convulsion the opposing muscle groups alternately contract and relax, causing rhythmic or jerking muscle movements.

Seizures are classified by their pattern of onset and the body parts involved (see International Classification of Epileptic Seizures on p. 261). In *generalized* seizures, both consciousness and motor activity are affected. A *partial* seizure may involve specific motor or sensory areas in the brain, causing specific symptoms. *Unilateral* seizures are those that occur on only one side of the body. The *grand mal* is a type of generalized seizure involving loss of consciousness, falling, and tonic and clonic contractions of the muscles. An *absence* attack, or *petit mal* seizure, is a brief generalized seizure in which consciousness may be lost for a period of a few seconds. It usually occurs in children and involves no convulsions. *Status epilepticus* is a state of continuous seizure activity with no recovery between episodes. It can be life threatening and must be treated with emergency measures.

CLASSIFICATION OF ANTICONVULSANT DRUGS

The purpose of therapy with anticonvulsant drugs is to prevent seizures or reduce their frequency. The ideal anticonvulsant has a minimum of adverse effects and is effective in decreasing seizure activity. There are a great number of anticonvulsant drugs in use today. They are usually effective in a particular type of seizure and are ordered according to the individual patient's seizure type (see Table 36-1).

In addition to specific anticonvulsant drugs, phenobarbital (see Chapter 15) is often prescribed. Although it is one of the safest anticonvulsants, it is also a sedative and may cause the patient to be sleepy and lethargic.

A patient in status epilepticus requires intravenous administration of an anticonvulsant as a lifesaving measure. Medications used in these cases are diazepam (Valium) and phenytoin (Dilantin).

NURSING IMPLICATIONS

The dose schedule for anticonvulsants must be regulated in each individual case, since dosage varies with the person's requirements and his tolerance of the drug. During the adjustment phase, the patient should be warned that he may have further seizures

(*Text continues on p. 260.*)

TABLE 36-1 ANTICONVULSANTS

DRUG	ROUTE AND DOSAGE RANGE	USE	ADVERSE EFFECTS	NURSING IMPLICATIONS
carbamazepine (Tegretol)	PO—200 mg–1600 mg qd in divided doses	To treat partial seizures with complex symptomatology (psychomotor, temporal lobe); to treat generalized tonic-clonic seizures (grand mal) and mixed seizure patterns; used after other anticonvulsants have been tried; to treat trigeminal neuralgia	*CNS:* dizziness, speech and hearing disturbances, abnormal involuntary movements, paresthesias, mental depression and agitation, talkativeness, confusion, headache, blurred vision, hallucinations *Cardiovascular:* blood disorders, hypertension, hypotension, CHF, collapse, edema, thrombophlebitis *GI:* diarrhea or constipation, abdominal pain, dry mouth, stomatitis, glossitis, liver damage, jaundice *GU:* urinary frequency or retention, oliguria, blood and albumin in urine *Skin:* itching, hives, photosensitivity, changes in skin color, hair loss, increased perspiration *Musculoskeletal:* aching joints and muscles, leg cramps *Others:* fever, chills, Stevens-Johnson syndrome	Evaluate hearing and speech. Note any unusual muscle movements or changes in sensation. Blood tests should be done frequently to check function of bone marrow, liver, and kidneys. Monitor BP and temperature. Check weight daily. Keep record of I&O. Watch for signs of thrombophlebitis (pain, redness, swelling). Keep a stool chart. Assess mucosa of mouth and the tongue for inflammation. Note skin color. Check for blood in urine with Hemastix. Check skin for rash, hives, or itching. Note any increased perspiration. Note any hair loss. Note any complaints of sore muscles or joints.
clonazepam (Clonopin)	PO—1.5 mg–20 mg qd in 2–3 divided doses	To treat Lennox-Gastaut syndrome (petit mal variant), akinetic and myoclonic seizures; used in patients with absence seizures who have not responded to other drugs	*CNS:* drowsiness, ataxia, abnormal eye movements, double vision, speech disorders, headache, muscle twitching, hemiparesis, confusion, depression, memory loss, hallucinations, hysteria, insomnia, increased sex drive, suicidal attempts *Cardiovascular:* palpitations, ankle and face edema, dehydration, blood disorders *Respiratory:* chest congestion, runny nose, shortness of breath, increased respiratory tract secretions, decreased respiratory rate *GI:* anorexia, constipation, coated tongue, dry mouth, increased appetite, nausea, sore gums	Assist with activities as necessary. Caution patients not to perform dangerous activities. Assess visual acuity and speech. Note any abnormal muscle movements. Evaluate mental status. Note one-sided weakness. Assess sleep pattern. Alert patient and significant others to possible changes in sex drive. Take apical pulses. Note swelling in face and ankles. Keep record of I&O. Note respiratory difficulty and any decrease in rate. Assess appetite. Check weight daily. Keep a stool chart. Evaluate gums. Note hair loss or unusual new growth. Check skin for rash. Monitor temperature.

(continued on page 259)

TABLE 36-1 (continued)

DRUG	ROUTE AND DOSAGE RANGE	USE	ADVERSE EFFECTS	NURSING IMPLICATIONS
clonazepam (*continued*)			*GU:* bed wetting, dysuria, urinary retention *Skin:* hair loss, rash, increased growth of hair (especially on the face) *Others:* muscle pains and weakness, fever, weight loss or gain, liver damage	
ethosuximide (Zarontin)	PO—250 mg–1.5 g qd in divided doses	To control absence seizures	*CNS:* drowsiness, headache, dizziness, euphoria, hiccoughs, irritability, hyperactivity, fatigue, lethargy, ataxia, insomnia, night terrors, inability to concentrate, aggressiveness, increased suicidal thoughts, paranoia *Endocrine:* increased sex drive, vaginal bleeding, hirsutism *GI:* anorexia, nausea, vomiting, diarrhea, abdominal cramps, weight loss, swelling of the tongue, overgrowth of the gums (gingival hyperplasia), abnormal liver function *Skin:* hives, rash, itching Stevens-Johnson syndrome, lupuslike syndrome *Others:* myopia, alopecia, muscle weakness, hirsutism	Caution patients not to perform dangerous activities. Assist with activity as necessary. Evaluate mental status. Note activity level. Assess sleep pattern. Warn patient about possible changes in sex drive and menstruation. Note any abnormal hair growth, especially on the face. Evaluate appetite. Keep stool chart. Check weight daily. Note any abnormality in tongue or gums. Check skin for reactions. Frequent blood tests should be done to check liver function.
phenytoin (Dilantin)	PO—100 mg–600 mg qd in divided doses IM—100 mg–200 mg q4h IV—150 mg–250 mg; then 100 mg–150 mg after 30 min if needed	To control grand mal and psychomotor seizures; to control status epilepticus of the grand mal type and to prevent and treat seizures occurring during neurosurgery	*CNS:* nystagmus, ataxia, slurred speech, mental confusion, dizziness, nervousness, insomnia, headache, muscle twitching *GI:* nausea, vomiting, constipation *Skin:* measlelike rash (with or without fever), Stevens-Johnson syndrome *Circulatory:* anemia, other blood disorders *Others:* overgrowth of the gums, hirsutism, hyperglycemia, liver damage	Observe pupils for unusual movements. Evaluate speech. Evaluate mental status. Assist with activities as necessary. Assess sleep pattern. Note any abnormal muscle movements. Give after meals to avoid GI upset. Keep stool chart. Check skin for rash or hives. Monitor temperature. Blood tests should be done at regular intervals. Encourage good mouth care, including frequent brushing and gum massage. Note unusual hair growth on face. Caution patients never to discontinue medication abruptly.

(continued on page 260)

TABLE 36-1   (continued)

DRUG	ROUTE AND DOSAGE RANGE	USE	ADVERSE EFFECTS	NURSING IMPLICATIONS
primidone (Mysoline)	PO—0.75 g–2 g qd in divided doses	To control grand mal, psychomotor, and focal epileptic seizures	*CNS:* ataxia, vertigo, irritability, emotional disturbances, drowsiness, nystagmus, fatigue *GI:* anorexia, nausea, vomiting *Others:* double vision, impotence, rash	Assist with activities as necessary. Evaluate mental status. Observe unusual pupil movement. Caution patient not to engage in dangerous activities. Assess appetite. Assess visual acuity. Warn male of possible impotence. Check skin for rash.
valproic acid (Depakene, Depakote)	PO—15 mg/kg/day increasing by 5 mg–10 mg/kg/day at 1-wk intervals until seizures are controlled or to a maximum of 60 mg/kg/day Doses over 250 mg should be divided.	To treat simple and complex absence seizures; to treat patients with multiple seizure types (including absence seizures)	*CNS:* sedation, ataxia, headache, nystagmus, double vision, jerking movements of the wrist, tongue, or foot, spots before eyes, muscle tremor, changes in speech, dizziness, incoordination, depression, emotional upset, psychosis, aggression, hyperactivity, behavioral changes, muscle weakness *Cardiovascular:* altered bleeding time, blood disorders *GI:* anorexia, weight loss, nausea, vomiting, constipation or diarrhea, indigestion, increased appetite with weight gain, liver disorders *Skin:* hair loss, petechiae, rash	Caution patient not to perform dangerous activities. Assist with activity as necessary. Note any unusual eye movements. Assess visual acuity. Note any muscle tremor or jerking movements. Evaluate speech. Evaluate mental status. Note activity level. Blood tests should be done at regular intervals. Assess appetite. Check weight daily. Keep stool chart. Note any hair loss. Check skin for any reaction.

and that a period of weeks may be needed to achieve the proper dosage. Blood testing will be necessary to see that medication is in a therapeutic range.

Seizure activity needs to be reported to the physician so he can adjust the dose. Nursing observations should include the hour of the day that the seizure started and ended, whether the patient felt a warning (called an *aura*), whether he lost consciousness, and the type of muscle movements observed. Other important facts to note include the presence of urinary or fecal incontinence and changes in vital signs, color, or sweating.

Initially, many patients complain that anticonvulsant drugs make them apathetic and sleepy. This lethargy usually passes after a period of time. If drowsiness or ataxia is a problem, be sure the patient is assisted with ambulation and cautioned against performing acts that may present safety hazards to himself and others.

Skin reactions are common. Usually these are mild and may be mistaken for measles or acne. Occasionally, however, they may progress to serious reactions, such as Stevens-Johnson syndrome (see Chapter 7) or exfoliative dermatitis. Inspect the skin daily and report any rash immediately.

Some anticonvulsants can cause bone marrow depression (see Chapter 35 for a discussion of bone marrow depression). Anemia may develop gradually. Agranulocytosis and thrombocytopenia are other potentially serious problems. Thus, the patient's blood should be tested regularly.

If phenytoin is used over a long period, gingival hyperplasia will appear. In this condition, the gums grow over the teeth. Excellent oral hygiene including thorough, regular brushing of the teeth and daily gum massage may prevent its development; surgery to remove excess gum tissue may be necessary from time to time.

Another problem related to phenytoin therapy is hirsutism, characterized by an increase in the growth of body hair, especially on the face. It is, obviously, extremely distressing to women. Various methods of hair removal may be suggested.

Once a diagnosis of epilepsy has been made, the patient may require life-long medication. It is important that patients understand the necessity of strict adherence to the medication schedule if they are to remain seizure free—the most common cause of seizures in epileptic patients is failure to take medication as ordered. It is important that the patient

continue to take his medication even if he has been seizure free for a year. In the event a seizure does occur, the medication should not be increased without an order from the physician. If two anticonvulsants are ordered, it is important that both be taken regularly. If medications are discontinued abruptly for any reason, a seizure is likely to occur. All patients with epilepsy should wear Medic-Alert tags that specify what medications they are taking.

These patients need much psychological support. The public must be educated to dispel the myths related to epilepsy. It should be stressed that a person with epilepsy is normal in all other respects. Epilepsy is not rare, disfiguring, or painful, nor does it cause mental illness or deficient mentation. A person with epilepsy can lead a normal life.

INTERNATIONAL CLASSIFICATION OF EPILEPTIC SEIZURES

I. PARTIAL SEIZURES (seizures beginning locally)
  A. Partial seizures with elementary symptomatology (generally without impairment of consciousness)
    1. With motor symptoms (*including seizures formerly called jacksonian*)
    2. With special sensory or somatosensory symptoms
    3. With autonomic symptoms
    4. Compound forms
  B. Partial seizures with complex symptomatology (generally with impairment of consciousness)
    1. With impairment of consciousness only
    2. With cognitive symptomatology   *formerly called*
    3. With affective symptomatology   *temporal lobe*
    4. With "psychosensory" symptomatology   *or*
    5. With "psychomotor" symptomatology (automatisms)   *psychomotor*
    6. Compound forms   *seizures*
  C. Partial seizures secondarily generalized
II. GENERALIZED SEIZURES (bilaterally symmetrical and without local onset)
  A. Absences (*formerly called petit mal*)
  B. Bilateral massive epileptic myoclonus
  C. Infantile spasms (*formerly referred to as hypsarrhythmia*)
  D. Clonic seizures
  E. Tonic seizures
  F. Tonic-clonic seizures (*formerly called grand mal*)
  G. Atonic seizures
  H. Akinetic seizures
III. UNILATERAL SEIZURES (or predominantly)
IV. UNCLASSIFIED EPILEPTIC SEIZURES (due to incomplete data)
(Gastaut H: Clinical and electroencephalographical classification of epileptic seizures. Epilepsia 11:102–113, 1970)

PRACTICE PROBLEMS—ANTICONVULSANTS

1. The order reads: phenytoin (Dilantin) suspension 200 mg PO tid.
The label reads: phenytoin 125 mg/5 ml.
How many milliliters will be given?

$$\frac{D}{H} \times A = G$$

$$\frac{\overset{8}{\cancel{200}\ \cancel{mg}}}{\underset{5}{\cancel{125}\ \cancel{mg}}} \times 5\ ml = G$$

$$\frac{8}{5} \times 5\ ml = 8\ ml.$$

Thus, 8 ml of phenytoin (Dilantin) will be given.

Work the following problems:

1. The order reads: primidone (Mysoline) 250 mg PO bid.
The label reads: primidone 250 mg/tablet.
How many tablets will you give?

2. The physician orders phenytoin (Dilantin) 100 mg IM stat. Phenytoin comes 50 mg/ml. How much will you give?

3. The order reads: carbamazepine (Tegretal) 400 mg PO q6h.
The label reads: carbamazepine 200 mg/tablet.
How many tablets will be given?

Answers are given on p. 284.

CHAPTER 37
Eye and ear medications

EYE MEDICATIONS

Eye or ophthalmic medications have three main effects on the eye and visual function. *Miotics* are drugs that cause constriction of the pupil or miosis. Drugs that cause dilation of the pupil (mydriasis) are called *mydriatics*. Finally, the *cycloplegic* drugs paralyze the ciliary muscle; it is that muscle that accommodates for near and far vision.

Classification of drugs used as eye medications

Most of the drugs used to diagnose and treat eye disorders belong to groups that have already been discussed. In this chapter, their specific effects on the eye and the nursing implications involved in administration of ophthalmic preparations are described. The adverse effects and general nursing implications of the general categories that are described in previous chapters should be reviewed.

The groups of drugs that are useful in treatment of disorders of the eye include autonomic drugs (cholinergics, anticholinesteraselike drugs, adrenergics, and anticholinergics), topical anesthetics, diuretics (carbonic anhydrase inhibitors and osmotic agents), lubricants, anti-inflammatory, and anti-infective drugs (see Table 37-1).

Autonomic drugs (see Chapters 18 and 34). *Cholinergic* and *anticholinesteraselike* drugs work in slightly different ways but produce the same end result. They promote the release of acetylcholine for a parasympathetic effect. These drugs are used to treat glaucoma, a condition characterized by increased pressure within the eyeball. This increased intraocular pressure (IOP) may be due to overproduction of aqueous humor or to decreased drainage of the fluid. If untreated, glaucoma can lead to permanent blindness by causing damage to the optic nerve. Drugs used to treat glaucoma cause miosis, as well as vasodilation of the vessels draining the eye, and both these actions lower the intraocular pressure.

Adrenergic drugs produce mydriasis and decrease congestion in ocular blood vessels by their vasoconstrictive action. They also cause slight relaxation of the ciliary muscle and decreased production of aqueous humor. They are given during eye examinations, to treat glaucoma, and to relieve congestion in the ocular blood vessels.

Anticholinergic drugs produce both mydriasis and cycloplegia. They are used during eye examinations, pre- and postoperatively in eye surgery, and to treat inflammatory diseases of the eye such as keratitis. In these cases they relieve eye pain by relaxing the ciliary muscles and allowing the eye to rest.

Topical anesthetics (see Chapter 11). Topical anesthetics are applied to the eye to decrease pain during eye examinations and surgery. Cocaine is an old drug used for this purpose that has now been replaced by the newer drugs like tetracaine (Pon-

TABLE 37-1 EYE MEDICATIONS

DRUG	ROUTE AND DOSAGE RANGE	USE	ADVERSE EFFECTS	NURSING IMPLICATIONS
atropine	Topical Ointment Solution—1 gtt–2 gtt q8h	To produce mydriasis and cycloplegia for refraction and for iris dilation and relaxation of ciliary muscle in treatment of acute inflammatory conditions of the anterior uveal tract	*With prolonged use:* local irritation, reddened or swollen eyes, conjunctivitis, dermatitis	Check eyes for any signs of irritation or inflammation.
cyclopentolate (Cyclogyl)	Topical Solution—(0.5%–2%) 1 gtt in each eye followed by another gtt in 5 min if necessary	For mydriasis and cycloplegia in diagnostic procedures	*CNS:* (in children) behavioral changes, psychotic reactions, ataxia, incoherent speech, restlessness, hallucinations, disorientation, seizures *Cardiovascular:* tachycardia, vasodilation *ANS:* decreased GI motility, urinary retention, decreased saliva and sweat production *Others:* fever, increased IOP	After drops are instilled, apply pressure over nasolacrimal sac for 2 to 3 minutes to keep medication from entering systemic circulation. Watch patient closely for approximately 30 minutes for CNS effects. Evaluate mental status. Monitor pulse, BP, and temperature. Keep record of I&O. Note decrease in saliva and sweat.
echothiophate (Phospholine)	Topical Solution—(0.03%–0.25%)—1 gtt qd bid	To treat open-angle glaucoma; to treat conditions obstructing aqueous humor outflow; to treat accommodative esotropia	Stinging, burning, tearing, twitching of eyelids, redness, brow ache, headache, myopia, visual blurring, iris cysts, cataracts, occasional retinal detachment, activation of latent eye infections	Eyes should be examined at regular intervals. Avoid systemic absorption (see cyclopentolate). Assess visual acuity. Assist with activities as necessary. Observe for abnormal muscle movements (lids).
homatropine	Topical Solution—(2%, 5%)—1 gtt–2 gtt as directed	To produce mydriasis and cycloplegia	See atropine.	See atropine.
methylcellulose (Tearisol)	Topical Solution (0.5%)—3 gtt–4 gtt q8–12h	To replace tears when eyes are dry; used as a lubricant for artificial eyes and contact lenses; used as an alkaline eye bath	None	
natamycin (Natacyn)	Topical Suspension—(5%)—Initially—1 gtt q1–2h for 3–4 days; then 1 gtt q3–4h (usual treatment lasts 14–21 days)	To treat fungal blepharitis, conjunctivitis, and keratitis	None, usually	

(continued on page 265)

TABLE 37-1   (continued)

DRUG	ROUTE AND DOSAGE RANGE	USE	ADVERSE EFFECTS	NURSING IMPLICATIONS
pilocarpine (Isopto Carpine)	Topical Solution—(0.25%–10%) 2 gtt q4–6h	To decrease elevated IOP in the treatment of glaucoma and other conditions that obstruct the outflow of aqueous humor; used after iridectomy; to treat certain types of strabismus; used especially in emergency situations prior to surgery	Painful eye muscle spasms, blurred vision, poor vision in dim light, local irritation, photophobia, increased incidence of "floaters," cataracts	Caution patients not to drive at night. Avoid systemic absorption of medication (see cyclopentolate). Encourage patients to avoid direct sunlight and brightly lit rooms. Check for any local irritation.
polyvinyl alcohol (Liquifilm Wetting Solution, Liquifilm Tears)	Topical—1 gtt prn	To soothe and lubricate the dry eye for comfort and to allow longer wearing of hard contact lenses	Eye irritation	Check for any irritation.
timolol (Timoptic)	Topical Solution—(0.25%–0.5%)—1 gtt qd bid	To reduce elevated intraocular pressure in glaucoma and ocular hypertension	Mild sensitivity reactions (rash, eye irritation), occasional mild bradycardia and bronchospasm	Watch for any hypersensitivity reactions. Monitor apical pulse and respirations.
trifluridine (Viroptic)	Topical Solution (1%)—1 gtt onto cornea q2h while awake (maximum 9 gtt per day) until ulcer reepithelializes, then 1 gtt q4h while awake for 7 days (minimum dose of 5 gtt/day)	To treat eye infections due to herpes simplex virus, types 1 and 2	Mild, transient burning or stinging after installation, edema of the eyelid, increased ocular pressure	Store medication under refrigeration. Note any swelling of eyelid.
tropicamide (Mydriacyl)	Topical Solution—(0.5%–1%)—1 gtt–2 gtt; repeat in 5 min and again after another 30 min if necessary	See cyclopentolate.	See cyclopentolate, *plus:* transient stinging, dry mouth, blurred vision, photophobia, headache, allergic reactions	See cyclopentolate, *plus:* Assess visual acuity. Caution patient to avoid direct sunlight and brightly lit rooms. Check skin for allergic manifestations. Note any complaints of stinging.

tocaine) and proparacaine (Ophthaine). The newer drugs have fewer systemic effects. Since all topical anesthetics will interfere with healing, they are never used for long-term therapy.

Diuretics (see Chapter 20).   Carbonic anhydrase is an enzyme necessary for the production of aqueous humor. When drugs that inhibit its action (carbonic anhydrase inhibitors [CAI]) are given, less aqueous humor is produced and the intraocular pressure drops. Carbonic anhydrase inhibitors, such as acetazolamide (Diamox), were originally used as diuretics but have generally been replaced by newer preparations. Their main use now is to treat eye disorders characterized by production of excessive aqueous humor.

Osmotic diuretics decrease intraocular pressure by moving fluid from the intraocular vessels into the general circulation. Glycerin (Glyrol, Osmoglyn) can be administered by mouth or as eye drops. It will cause a fall in intraocular pressure within 10 minutes. Mannitol (Osmitrol) and urea (Ureaphil) are osmotic diuretics given intravenously in more critical situations.

Lubricants. Eye lubricants, or "artificial tears," are necessary when normal tear production is absent or insufficient. Their purpose is to lubricate eye prostheses and contact lenses and to protect the cornea during eye examinations. Comatose patients who have lost their blink reflex may also need artificial tears to prevent corneal abrasion.

Anti-inflammatory drugs (see Chapter 13). *Corticosteroids* are used for short-term treatment of eye disorders caused by severe trauma, allergic reactions, or inflammations not associated with the production of pus. If pus is present, steroids are not used because of the possibility that the disease may spread. Long-term use is also avoided, since it can contribute to the development of glaucoma and cataracts. Steroids used as eye medications are cortisone, dexamethasone, fludrocortisone, hydrocortisone, methylprednisolone, prednisolone, and triamcinolone.

Anti-infectives (see Chapter 7). Anti-infectives in solution or ointment form are used to treat eye infections, such as conjunctivitis, keratitis (inflamed cornea), and blepharitis (inflamed eyelids). Cysts and styes may also respond to anti-infective therapy. Almost any anti-infective, in topical form, can be used.

Eye inflammation due to viral infection is difficult to treat because so few drugs are available. Idoxuridine (Stoxil, Herplex) is effective in viral disease caused by herpes simplex or vaccinia virus. Newer medications with similar action are vidarabine (Vira-A) and trifluridine (Viroptic) (see Chapter 7).

NURSING IMPLICATIONS

Ophthalmic medications are available in topical forms such as solutions and ointments. Although solutions are easy to administer (as drops) and usually do not interfere with vision, they may cause burning. They are also quickly diluted and washed away by tears and, therefore, are in contact with the eye only briefly.

Ointments are more comfortable on instillation and stay on the eye longer. They tend to create a thin film, however, that temporarily interferes with vision. There is also greater likelihood of skin reactions when the medication is in the form of an ointment.

All solutions, ointments, and equipment (droppers, tubes) used in administration of eye medications must be kept sterile. The tip of a dropper or tube must never touch the eye. Cloudy or discolored solutions should never be used.

When administering eye drops or ointment, ask the patient to assume a comfortable position, with his head tilted; for instance, he might be lying in bed or sitting in a chair with his head tilted back. Ask the patient to look up, while you gently hold his lids apart. Steady the hand holding the medication by resting it on the patient's forehead. Approach the eye slowly and carefully. Drop the solution into the lower conjunctival sac from a height of no more than 1 inch. Squeeze the ointment in a thin ribbon from the inner to the outer part of the lower conjunctival sac.

Some eye medications should be followed by a gentle massage to speed absorption, whereas others should be prevented from getting into the systemic circulation. To do the latter, apply slight pressure over the inner corner of the eyelid. This blocks the tear ducts, which would normally drain fluids from the eye into the bloodstream. Apply pressure immediately after the medication has been administered and maintain it for about 2 minutes. Check the nursing implications for each eye medication so you know whether systemic absorption is to be encouraged or avoided.

The autonomic drugs cause many adverse effects if systemically absorbed. Cycloplegics, in particular, may cause serious adverse reactions. The patient's face becomes flushed, and he cannot focus on near objects, so necessary safety precautions must be taken. Extreme sensitivity to light (called *photophobia*) is likely, so encourage the patient to wear sunglasses when in sunlight or brightly lit areas.

Drugs having miotic action can cause blurred distant vision as well as local irritation. The initial burning sensation disappears after a few seconds, but blurred vision persists for hours. Patients may also complain of darkened vision, owing to the decrease in light coming through the constricted pupil.

When diuretics are given, strict records of fluid intake and output must be kept. Monitor electrolyte levels and vital signs, because diuretics can cause electrolyte imbalance and disturbances of fluid balance. The result may be pulmonary edema or congestive heart failure.

Headaches due to cerebral dehydration may be a problem following administration of glycerin. To help prevent this, have the patient remain lying down during and after administration of the eye medication. Glycerin causes acidosis when metabolized, and this may lead to hyperglycemia. If a diabetic patient receives glycerin, frequent urine and blood tests for sugar should be carried out. Glycerin is a clear, thick, oily liquid that can cause nausea and vomiting when given by mouth. Mask the flavor by mixing it with fruit juices. Pour it over cracked ice and have the patient sip it through a straw to make it more palatable.

Ointments used to treat eye inflammations and infections can cause allergic reactions. Watch for any signs of reaction, such as rash, itching, reddened skin, or increased temperature.

EAR MEDICATIONS

Ear (otic) medications are those given to treat infection, inflammation, and pain associated with external, middle, and inner ear disorders and for surgery on the ear. Disorders of the external ear include impacted wax, otitis externa or "swimmer's ear," and infections. Otitis media is infection of the middle ear. Motion sickness is the most frequent inner ear disorder.

Classification of ear medications

Anti-infectives, corticosteroids, and local anesthetics are widely used in ear disorders (see Table 37-2). The general actions of these drugs have al-ready been discussed. Their special use in treating ear disorders will be discussed here. Ceruminolytic drugs and those for motion sickness are especially effective in ear disorders.

Anti-infectives inhibit the growth of or destroy organisms in the ear canal. It is important that ear infections be treated quickly and effectively to prevent their spread into areas such as the mastoid bone (causing mastoiditis) and the coverings of the brain (causing meningitis).

Corticosteroids will lessen the inflammation, redness, edema, and itching (pruritus) associated with some ear disorders.

Local anesthetics ease the discomfort of diagnostic and surgical procedures to the ear. Benzocaine, for example, is used when impacted ear wax is removed. *Ceruminolytic* drugs soften and emulsify accumulated hardened ear wax (cerumen) so it can then be easily removed. These drugs are administered in liquid form at prescribed intervals, followed by ear irrigations to flush the wax away.

Motion sickness is probably due to an inner ear disturbance involving the labyrinth, brought on by continuous body motion as is experienced in a moving automobile, train, airplane, or ship. Motion sickness drugs apparently act by depressing the central nervous system, which in turn decreases inner ear sensitivity to motion. Barbiturates (Chapter 15) and tranquilizers (Chapter 6) are useful for this purpose. Most effective, however, are antihistamines, such as cyclizine (Marezine), dimenhydrinate (Dramamine), and meclizine (Antivert or Bonine). In most cases, these drugs prevent the nausea and vomiting that would occur without treatment.

TABLE 37-2 EAR MEDICATIONS

DRUG	ROUTE AND DOSAGE RANGE	USE	ADVERSE EFFECTS	NURSING IMPLICATIONS
carbamide peroxide (Debrox Drops, Murine Ear Drops)	Topical—5 gtt–10 gtt bid	To prevent and treat ear wax buildup	None	None
triethanolamine (Cerumenex)	Topical—gtt to fill ear canals prn (Fill ear canal, insert cotton plug, allow to remain 15–30 min; then flush ear.)	To remove impacted ear wax prior to ear examination, therapy, or audiometry	Local skin reactions (mild redness and itching to severe eczemalike reaction)	Watch for any signs of local irritation.

NURSING IMPLICATIONS

Otic medications are available in solution or suspension form. Most act locally with only small amounts being absorbed into the general circulation. Many agents are combinations of two or more drugs.

These drugs must be carefully administered to avoid damaging the delicate membranes of the ear. Solutions should be warmed to room temperature or slightly above, since solutions that are too hot or too cold can adversely stimulate the central nervous system. Moreover, certain medications will be rendered ineffective by high heat and may burn tissue if heated beyond the comfort range.

To administer ear drops, have the patient lie down with the affected ear toward you. Straighten the external ear canal by gently pulling the pinna upward and back in adults, down and back in children. The medication dropper should never touch the ear. Instill the drops, and instruct the patient to remain in the same position for a few minutes. He may then roll to the other side or get up.

Motion sickness medications should be taken about an hour before the trip. Antihistamines such as cyclizine and dimenhydrinate will cause drowsiness, so safety precautions should be taken.

If the eardrum is perforated, do not administer medication. Symptoms of perforation include a decrease in hearing acuity, and pain.

PART 8
Drugs used in special circumstances

CHAPTER 38
Drugs used in pediatrics

Pediatrics is the branch of medicine that deals with the specialized care of children, a group that includes infants (from birth to about 2 years of age), children, and adolescents. When the nurse administers medications to children, many considerations must be taken into account. It is possible in this chapter to provide only an overview of pediatric medication administration. A pediatric textbook should be consulted for a more detailed discussion of pediatric pharmacology.

As with adults, drug action in a child is influenced by age, weight, fluid and electrolyte balance, the drug's properties, and the child's physical state (presence of disease and organ maturity).

DOSAGE CALCULATION

When giving medications to infants and children, the dose is less than the average dose for an adult. The dosage of medication ordered is based on weight, age, or body surface of the pediatric patient.

The following are guides to follow when in doubt as to which category the patient is placed:

0–24 months is an infant
2–12 years is a child
Over 12 years is considered an adult

The amount of medication is always ordered by the physician. The following rules for dosage cal-

culation are just guidelines to be certain that the dose of medication is within correct limits.

There are four formulas used to calculate dosage for the pediatric patient:

Young's rule is used for calculation of dosage for a child. It states:

$$\frac{\text{age in years}}{\text{age in years} + 12} \times \text{adult dose} = \text{child's dose}$$

For example: The adult dose of tetracycline is 500 mg q6h. The dose for a 4-year-old would be what?

$$\frac{\text{age in years}}{\text{age in years} + 12} \times \text{adult dose} = G$$

$$\frac{4 \text{ years old}}{4 \text{ years} + 12} \times 500 \text{ mg} = G$$

$$\frac{1 \; \cancel{4}}{4 \; \cancel{16}} \times 500 \text{ mg} = G$$

$$\frac{1}{4} \times 500 \text{ mg} = 125 \text{ mg}$$

Thus, 125 mg of tetracycline will be given to a 4-year-old child every 6 hours.

Fried's rule is used to calculate dosage for an infant. It is based on age in months in relation to 150 months, which is $12\frac{1}{2}$ years (the adult age).

$$\frac{\text{age in months}}{150 \text{ months}} \times \text{adult dose} = \text{infant dose}$$

For example: Streptomycin is ordered for a 15-month-old infant. If the adult dose is 0.5 g every 2 hours, what would the dose be for a 15-month-old infant?

$$\frac{\text{age in months}}{150 \text{ months}} \times \text{adult dose} = \text{infant dose}$$

$$\frac{1}{10} \frac{\cancel{15 \text{ months}}}{\cancel{150 \text{ months}}} \times 0.5 \text{ g} = \text{infant dose}$$

$$\frac{1}{10} \times 0.5 \text{ g} = 0.05 \text{ g} = 50 \text{ mg}$$

Thus 50 mg of streptomycin will be given to a 15-month-old infant every 12 hours.

Clark's rule is based on the relation of body weight of the child and the weight of the average adult, which is considered to be 150 pounds. The rule states:

$$\frac{\text{weight in pounds}}{150 \text{ pounds}} \times \text{adult dose} = \text{child dose}$$

For example: A child weighs 75 pounds. He is to receive acetaminophen (Tylenol). The adult dose is gr X. How much will he receive?

$$\frac{\text{weight in pounds}}{150 \text{ pounds}} \times \text{adult dose} = \text{child's dose}$$

$$\frac{1}{2} \frac{\cancel{75 \text{ lb}}}{\cancel{150 \text{ lb}}} \times \text{gr} \ 10 = \text{child's dose}$$

$$\frac{1}{2} \times \text{gr} \ 10 = \text{gr} \ 5$$

The 75-pound child will receive gr V of acetaminophen (Tylenol).

The fourth way of determining dosage for the pediatric patient is with *nomograms*. The basis for determining dosage is the body surface area (BSA) of the infant or child on the nomogram chart (see Fig. 38-1).

To determine the BSA with the nomogram:

1. The child's height and weight are plotted on the left and right vertical columns.
2. A straight edge is placed on the vertical height and weight lines.

3. The BSA is the point where the line crosses the surface area (SA) scale.

For example, if the height is 30 inches and the weight is 35 pounds, the BSA is 0.6. The usual adult dosage of digoxin (Lanoxin) is 0.25. What would the dose be for a child with a BSA of 0.6?

The formula for calculating drug dosage based on BSA is:

$$\frac{\text{surface area}}{1.7} \times \text{adult dose} = \text{child dose}$$

Thus,

$$\frac{0.6}{1.7} \times 0.25 \text{ mg} = \text{child's dose}$$

$$0.35 \times 0.25 = 0.09 \text{ mg}$$

You would give 0.09 mg of digoxin (Lanoxin) to a child whose BSA is 0.6.

In many drug reference books, the dosage for medication for the pediatric patient is given per kilogram of body weight. To convert pounds to kilograms, the pounds are divided by 2.2. There are 2.2 pounds (lb) in one kilogram (kg).

If the order reads ASA 5 mg/kg q4h and the child weighs 75 lb, how much ASA will he receive?

First, convert pounds to kilograms:

$$\frac{75 \text{ lb}}{x} = \frac{2.2 \text{ lb}}{1 \text{ kg}}$$

$$2.2x = 75$$

$$x = 34.1$$

Then proceed with the calculation of drug dosage:

$$5 \text{ mg of ASA} \times 34.1 \text{ kg} = 170.5 \text{ mg}$$

Thus, 170.5 mg ASA will be given to the child whose weight is 75 lb.

DRUG ADMINISTRATION ROUTES

An infant with a good sucking and swallowing reflex may receive medication by mouth. The best time to medicate an infant is just before a feeding, when he is hungry and will swallow readily. For an older child, the medication may be crushed or

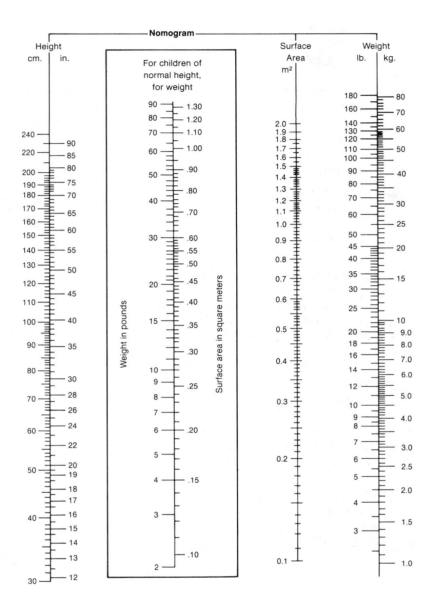

Figure 38-1. The West nomogram for body surface area (BSA). (After Shirkey HC: Drug therapy. In Vaughn VC, III, McKay RJ [eds]: Nelson's Textbook of Pediatrics, 11th ed. Philadelphia, WB Saunders, 1979)

mixed with fruit juice or another pleasant-tasting substance.

When intramuscular administration is indicated, nursing actions will vary according to the child's age. The safest site for an intramuscular injection in children is the anterior midlateral thigh—the vastus lateralis muscle. Other sites carry a danger of accidental penetration of major nerves and blood vessels.

It is thought that a young infant will not retain a memory of any previous painful injections. But after the age of about 16 months, the infant may cry when he sees the syringe, and it may be necessary to restrain him. Distract him as much as possible, and spend a few minutes with him afterward to offer comfort and reassurance.

Intravenous medications are administered much as in adults. A pediatric intravenous catheter may be inserted into the scalp if veins elsewhere are too small.

DRUGS USED FOR PEDIATRIC PATIENTS

Most of the drugs already discussed in this text may be given to children, as well as to adults. However, there are some drugs that are prescribed primarily for children, including anthelmintics, vaccines, infant formulas, silver nitrate, and vitamins. (Anthelmintics and immunizations are discussed in Part 2.)

Special infant formulas are prescribed for various congenital disorders of metabolism. Infants with these disorders lack an enzyme needed for normal fat or carbohydrate metabolism, and the missing enzyme is supplied in the formula. Examples of such disorders are pancreatic enzyme deficiency, celiac disease, cystic fibrosis, phenylketonuria (PKU), milk allergy, and galactosemia.

Silver nitrate is given routinely to most newborns. Its purpose is to prevent or control blindness or infection in the eyes of the newborn due to maternal gonorrhea. A 1% to 2% solution of silver nitrate is instilled into the newborn's eyes, followed by a normal saline flush. Many states have laws requiring that this medication be given to every newborn.

The vitamins most frequently given to children are vitamin K and multivitamin preparations. Vitamin K is prescribed for a child who is in danger of hemorrhaging due to a low prothrombin level. The prothrombin level is extremely low in newborns until about the fifth day of life, at which point intestinal bacteria and milk in the intestine begin to produce vitamin K. Vitamin K preparations, such as AquaMEPHYTON, are administered as part of routine newborn care. There are many multiple-vitamin preparations especially formulated for pediatric use. Some common trade names are Poly-Vi-Sol, Tri-Vi-Sol, and Vi-Daylin.

PRACTICE PROBLEMS—DRUGS USED IN PEDIATRICS

1. The adult dose of dexamethasone (Decadron) is 2 mg daily. What would be the dose for an infant 15 months old?

2. The adult dose of hydralazine (Apresoline) is 100 mg qid. What is the dose for a 10-year-old child?

3. The adult dose of meperidine (Demerol) is 50 mg q4h prn. Using the nomogram what would be the dose for a child weighing 82 lb and 54 inches tall?

4. The adult dose of morphine is 10 mg. What would be the dose for a child weighing 45 kg?

5. The adult dose of vancomycin (Vancocin) is 2 g daily. What would be the dose for an infant of 18 months?

6. The adult dose of erythromycin is 1 g daily. Using the nomogram what would be the dose for a child 47 inches tall who weighs 47 pounds?

Answers are given on p. 284.

CHAPTER 39
Drugs used in obstetrics

The specialized medical and nursing care of the woman during pregnancy, labor, and the postpartum period is called *obstetrics*. In this chapter, drugs commonly given to women during pregnancy and immediately following childbirth will be discussed briefly. For a more detailed discussion, it is suggested that an obstetrics textbook be consulted.

The uterus is the hollow organ in which the fertilized egg develops, first as an embryo, then as a fetus. The uterine smooth muscle (myometrium) is extremely responsive to many drugs, and there are a few drugs that act specifically on the myometrium. Their purpose is to intensify muscle contractions and step up their number (oxytocics) or to diminish uterine contractions (uterine relaxants) (see Table 39-1).

OXYTOCICS

The word "oxytocic" means rapid labor; thus drugs that intensify uterine contractions are called *oxytocics*. They are used during the latter part of pregnancy and especially during and immediately following labor to restart a labor that has slowed down or stopped, to cause expulsion of the placenta, and to prevent postpartum bleeding. There are three categories of oxytocic drugs: synthetic oxytocics, ergot alkaloids, and prostaglandins.

In Chapter 34 the hormone oxytocin is mentioned as being one of two hormones secreted by the posterior pituitary gland. It initiates labor by causing contractions of the myometrium. Oxytocin also helps to release milk from the mother's breasts after delivery. *Synthetic oxytocin* (Pitocin or Syntocinon) is given to induce labor or increase uterine contractions during delivery. It also helps to decrease bleeding after the placenta is delivered. Like the natural oxytocin, the synthetic preparations promote milk ejection from the mother's breasts.

The *ergot alkaloids* cause constriction of all blood vessels and contraction of smooth muscle. Ergot preparations have been discussed as analgesics for migraine headache. Their use in obstetrics is to promote effective uterine contractions and to stop uterine bleeding by promoting general vasoconstriction. These preparations are quickly absorbed from the gastrointestinal tract and, therefore, rapid acting—within 5 minutes of either oral or parenteral administration. The intravenous route is seldom used.

Prostaglandins are chemicals naturally present in many parts of the body. Although research is in progress to discover their many functions, it is already known that prostaglandins influence platelet clumping, the inflammatory response, and smooth muscle action. Their main use is in the therapeutic termination of pregnancy. They are injected directly into the amniotic fluid surrounding the developing embryo or fetus, or into a dead fetus, which then is aborted. Prostaglandins are also available as vaginal suppositories.

TABLE 39-1 DRUGS USED IN OBSTETRICS

DRUG	ROUTE AND DOSAGE RANGE	USE	ADVERSE EFFECTS	NURSING IMPLICATIONS
dinoprost tromethamine (Prostin F₂ Alpha)	Intra-amniotic instillation by a physician	To terminate pregnancy during the second trimester	*CNS:* headache, drowsiness, dizziness, convulsions, paresthesias, anxiety, double vision, hiccoughs *Endocrine:* lactation, breast tenderness, "hot flash" *Cardiovascular:* bradycardia, hypertension, secondary heart block *Respiratory:* dyspnea, coughing, bronchospasm *GI:* nausea, vomiting, abdominal cramps, diarrhea *GU:* uterine pain, cervical perforation, endometritis, urinary retention, hematuria *Others:* flushing, backache, chills, increased sweating	Caution patient not to perform any dangerous activities. Assist with activity as necessary. Assess visual acuity. Note any complaints of unusual sensations. Evaluate mental status. Warn patient about breast tenderness and possible milk production. Monitor pulse and BP at regular intervals. Note any respiratory distress or difficulty. Keep a stool chart. Report immediately any complaints of uterine pain. Keep accurate I&O. Test for blood in the urine. Note increased sweating and flushed skin.
ergonovine maleate (Ergotrate Maleate)	PO—0.2 mg–0.4 mg q6–12h for 48 hr IM, IV—0.2 mg; repeat in 2–4 hr if needed	To prevent and treat postpartum and postabortal hemorrhage and death due to uterine atony	Hypertension, nausea, vomiting, abdominal cramping, allergic reactions	Monitor BP. Observe color and amount of vaginal bleeding. Check skin for reactions. Evaluate uterine response.
methylergonovine (Methergine)	PO—0.2 mg q6–8h IM, IV—0.2 mg q2–4h	For routine management after delivery of the placenta; to treat postpartum hemorrhage, atony, and subinvolution	*CNS:* headache, dizziness, tinnitus *Cardiovascular:* transient hypertension, palpitations, temporary chest pain *Others:* nausea, vomiting, diaphoresis, dyspnea	Assist patient with ambulation and other activities as needed. Monitor BP and apical pulse. Note any complaints of chest pain. Note increased perspiration.
oxytocin (Pitocin, Syntocinon)	IV—10 U–40 U in 1000 ml D₅W Spray—One spray into one or both nostrils 2 to 3 min before nursing or pumping of breasts	To initiate or improve uterine contractions during the third stage of labor or when it is in the best interest of mother and fetus; to control postpartum bleeding or hemorrhage; use for initial milk letdown	Fetal bradycardia, anaphylaxis, cardiac arrhythmias, pelvic hematoma, postpartum hemorrhage	Monitor vital signs of both mother and fetus frequently. Check perineum for bleeding or hematoma. Watch for allergic reactions.
ritodrine (Yutopar)	PO—10 mg q2h for 24 hours then 10 mg–20 mg q4–6h IV—0.1 mg–0.35 mg/min for at least 12 hr after uterine contractions cease	For the management of preterm labor in suitable patients	*CNS:* nervousness, restlessness, emotional upset, anxiety, headache, malaise *Cardiovascular:* tachycardia (in both mother and fetus), palpitations, hypertension, angina *GI:* nausea, vomiting, diarrhea, bloating, constipation *Others:* rash, dyspnea, sweating, chills, weakness	Frequent monitoring of mother's uterine contractions, heart rate and BP; fetal heart rate. Keep accurate I&O records. Keep stool chart. Evaluate mental status. Note any behavioral changes. Evaluate appetite. Avoid fluid overload—keep mother in left lateral position during IV infusion. Note rate and character of maternal respirations. Note any chills or sweating.
testosterone + estradiol (Deladumone OB)	IM—2 ml	To prevent postpartum breast engorgement	See Table 34-3, *plus:* virilization (see testosterone) and acne	See Table 34-3, *plus:* Warn patient about possible masculinization and skin changes.

UTERINE RELAXANTS

When labor begins earlier than it should or uterine contractions are too frequent and uncoordinated, drugs may be given that relax the myometrium. *CNS depressants*, such as alcohol (given intravenously), and some *adrenergic drugs* are occasionally given to relax the myometrium. Analgesics and sedatives also cause uterine activity to diminish, as do opiates, general anesthetics, and barbiturates.

Prostaglandin inhibitors block the normal action of prostaglandins. Besides their use in labor, they may also relieve dysmenorrhea.

NURSING IMPLICATIONS

Observe and report carefully when giving oxytocic drugs. If contractions are too strong or frequent, blood flow to the fetus may be reduced, causing fetal hypoxia. For this reason, it is important to monitor both the fetal heart tone and the mother's heart rate, assessing both strength and timing of contractions. Remember that contractions that are too strong may damage the fetus.

Ergot alkaloids may cause a severe rise in blood pressure (hypertensive crisis), which, if untreated, can lead to cardiac and circulatory problems. Be sure to measure the mother's blood pressure frequently while she receives oxytocic drugs.

The prostaglandins almost always cause nausea and vomiting. Abdominal cramps, diarrhea; uterine pain, and lactation may also result from prostaglandin use. Try to make the mother as comfortable as possible and encourage only quiet activities.

DRUGS GIVEN TO PREVENT BREAST ENGORGEMENT

Drugs are given to suppress lactation when a woman chooses to feed her baby by bottle rather than by breast. Estrogens and progestins (female hormones), androgens (male hormones), and ergot alkaloid preparations are effective for this purpose. To avoid the problems related to androgen use, estrogen preparations are commonly administered (see Chapter 34). Combinations of estrogens and androgens are also available. Examples are methyltestosterone plus estrogens (Estratest) and testosterone enanthate plus estradiol valerate (Deladumone). Bromocriptine (Parlodel) is an ergot preparation that prevents lactation by inhibiting prolactin secretion (see Table 14-1).

NURSING IMPLICATIONS

Breast engorgement is extremely uncomfortable, and analgesics may be necessary for relief. The breasts should be supported by a brassiere. Hot packs or cold applications sometimes help to relieve the discomfort. Engorgement is only a temporary condition, and the woman may be reassured that the discomfort will end within 2 or 3 days.

CHAPTER 40
Diagnostic agents

Diagnostic agents are administered by the physician or a member of the nursing staff when a diagnostic test is to be done. Regardless of who gives the drug, the nurse must deal with any adverse effects or severe reactions that may result from its use. In this chapter the commonly used diagnostic agents are described. Specialized texts are available for a more detailed discussion of laboratory tests.

Histamine stimulates the secretion of HCl in the stomach, therefore it is often given to test for gastric acid secretion.

Dyes have many applications in laboratory tests of organ function. Their purpose is to allow visualization of certain organs or structures. Examples of such dyes are fluorescein, indocyanine green (Cardio-Green), phenolsulfonphthalein (Pheno-Red), and sulfobromophthalein (Bromsulphalein). These dyes are usually injected, after which their presence is watched for in body fluids, such as urine, blood, and mucus.

Radiopaque materials cannot be penetrated by x-rays. Thus, they are used as contrast media to make visible various internal structures (see Table 40-1). The gastrointestinal tract, gallbladder, kidneys, lungs, and other organs may all be studied in this way.

Barium sulfate is the contrast medium used most often. It is given by mouth in the form of a thick liquid to outline the upper part of the gastrointestinal tract and by enema to outline the lower tract.

Compounds containing iodine are used for examinations of the liver, gallbladder, and bile ducts. These medications may be given the night before the test is to be done or immediately before the test. When subsequent radiographic films are taken, the structure being studied will be visible because it will be outlined by the contrast medium. The emptying and filling of the gallbladder, for instance, may be studied. Any stones present in the gallbladder will be outlined as well.

Iodine compounds are also used to study the urinary tract. These are given intravenously.

Hollow organs, such as the fallopian tubes and the uterus, are visualized when a contrast medium such as ethiodized oil (Ethiodol) is used.

A *radioactive isotope*, or a radioisotope, as it is more commonly called, is a radioactive form of an element. The isotope consists of unstable atoms that emit rays of energy. Radioactive isotopes are widely used in diagnostic studies because they are readily detected even when distributed throughout the body. They are injected intravenously and detected externally by instruments that pick up the rays emitted from the organs where the isotope is concentrated. The isotope most frequently used as a diagnostic agent is radioactive iodine.

NURSING IMPLICATIONS

Patients undergoing diagnostic testing feel apprehensive and anxious, both about the procedure itself

TABLE 40-1 DIAGNOSTIC AGENT

DRUG	ROUTE AND DOSAGE RANGE	USE	ADVERSE EFFECTS	NURSING IMPLICATIONS
iopanoic acid (Telepaque)	PO—6–12 tablets with water in the evening after a fat-free dinner, about 14 hours before the test	For oral studies of the gallbladder and bile ducts	*Usually mild:* nausea, vomiting, abdominal cramps, diarrhea, stinging on urination *Rare:* rash, hives, redness, edema	Observe skin for any signs of reaction. Keep stool chart.

and about the possible outcome. The patient should receive a careful and thorough explanation. Make time available for the patient to ask questions. Since the test results may not be known for several days, you need to be especially supportive to the patient during this trying time.

Check to see whether special dietary restrictions are called for before the test. For some tests, only clear liquids can be taken for a few days beforehand. For some others, a specific diet or a test meal may be ordered.

Be sure to follow orders carefully as to specific times for administration of the medication. Timing is also important when follow-up x-ray studies or urine or blood samples are ordered.

Dyes or diagnostic agents given intravenously are more likely to cause adverse reactions than when other routes are used. Before the test, check to make sure that the patient has no known history of sensitivity to iodine or other agents that may be specified. Careful observations must be made during the first 15 to 30 minutes after the dye is injected, since this is the period when a histaminelike reaction or early anaphylaxis is likely to occur. Other adverse reactions to dye are tachycardia and extreme hypotension; therefore, temperature, blood pressure, pulse, and respiratory rate should be carefully and frequently monitored.

Barium is not absorbed into the systemic circulation and is not irritating to the mucosa. There is, therefore, no danger that it will be toxic to the patient. However, there is a possibility of constipation and impaction if all the barium is not completely evacuated after the test. To guard against this, a cleansing enema or a cathartic is ordered. Be sure to note and record the number and appearance of stools. The patient should be informed that stools will be very light in color until all the barium has been eliminated.

When a radioactive isotope such as iodine 131 is used for diagnostic purposes only, no special precautions are necessary. Reassure the patient that he is not radioactive and that the isotope will gradually be eliminated from his body, with no ill effects.

CHAPTER 41
Heavy metal antagonists

Heavy metal poisoning occurs when metals, such as arsenic, copper, gold, iron, lead, or mercury, are ingested in amounts the body cannot metabolize. The metal may have been ingested accidentally or with suicidal intent. Symptoms range from abdominal discomfort, anorexia, nausea, vomiting, and weight loss to nervous system involvement. There may eventually be circulatory collapse and death. There are specific antagonist drugs to treat each type of poisoning (see Table 41-1).

specific schedule be followed for optimum effect.

Hypersensitivity reactions, ranging from a mild rash to anaphylaxis, are possible with these drugs. Careful observation of all adverse reactions is essential.

Since these drugs rid the body of poisons by increasing heavy metal excretion through the kidneys, kidney damage is possible. The nurse should encourage the patient to drink fluids freely to flush out the kidneys.

NURSING IMPLICATIONS

Most heavy metal antagonists are given in specific doses over a period of days. It is important that the

TABLE 41-1   HEAVY METAL ANTAGONISTS

DRUG	ROUTE AND DOSAGE RANGE	USE	ADVERSE EFFECTS	NURSING IMPLICATIONS
deferoxamine mesylate (Desferal Mesylate)	IM, IV—1 g–0.5 g q4h (not to exceed 6 g per 24 hr IM or 15 mg/kg/hr IV) SC—1 g–2 g/day over 8–24 hr via continuous infusion	To facilitate the removal of iron in the treatment of acute iron intoxication and in chronic iron overload due to transfusion-dependent anemias	Hives, generalized reddened skin reaction, hypotension, pain at injection site With long-term use anaphylaxis, blurred vision, problems with urination, abdominal discomfort, diarrhea, leg cramps, tachycardia, fever	Observe for skin reactions. Monitor BP. With long-term use—Evaluate visual acuity. Record I&O. Keep a stool chart. Monitor pulse and temperature.

(continued on page 282)

TABLE 41-1   (continued)

DRUG	ROUTE AND DOSAGE RANGE	USE	ADVERSE EFFECTS	NURSING IMPLICATIONS
dimercaprol (BAL)	IM—2.5 mg–5 mg/kg qd–qid for up to 10 days	To treat poisoning from arsenic, gold, and mercury; use with calcium disodium edetate to treat acute lead poisoning	Fever, tachycardia, hypertension, nausea, vomiting, increased salivation and sweating, tearing of the eyes, runny nose, burning sensation in lips, mouth, throat, and penis, tight feeling in throat, chest, and hands, pain at injection site	Monitor vital signs. Note increased secretions. Note any complaints of tight or burning sensations.
calcium disodium edetate (CaEDTA, Calcium Disodium Versenate)	IM, IV—500 mg–1.5 g/M^2 qd (50 mg/ kg/day)	To treat acute and chronic lead poisoning and lead encephalopathy	*CNS:* headache, numbness, tingling, malaise, increased thirst *Cardiovascular:* thrombophlebitis, hypotension, arrhythmias, bone marrow depression *Respiratory:* sneezing, nasal congestion *GI:* anorexia, nausea, vomiting, diarrhea, abdominal cramps *GU:* renal tubular necrosis, protein and blood in the urine, urinary frequency and urgency *Musculoskeletal:* muscle and joint pain, leg cramps *Skin:* mucous membrane lesions, reddened, cracked lips *Others:* fever, chills, hypercalcemia, increased tearing, pain at injection site	Record I&O. Assist patient with ambulation and activity as needed. Monitor BP and apical pulse. Frequent blood tests should be done to check bone marrow and renal function. Note any respiratory difficulty. Evaluate appetite. Keep a stool chart. Daily urinalysis should be done to check for albumin or blood. Note any complaints of muscle or joint pains. Evaluate mucous membranes in mouth and lips for any lesion. Monitor temperature. Note increased tears.
penicillamine (Cuprimine, Depen Titratabs)	PO—125 mg–4 g qd	To treat Wilson's disease, cystinuria, and patients with severe, active rheumatoid arthritis who have not been helped by other therapy	*CNS:* tinnitus, inflammation of the optic nerve *Cardiovascular:* bone marrow depression, thrombophlebitis *GI:* anorexia, epigastric pain, nausea, vomiting, diarrhea, peptic ulcer, abnormal liver function, jaundice, pancreatitis, loss of sense of taste, mouth sores *GU:* protein and blood in the urine *Others:* muscle weakness, joint aches, hair loss, fever, enlarged breast tissue, lupus-like syndrome	Evaluate hearing and visual acuity. Blood tests should be done regularly to check function of bone marrow and liver. Assess appetite. Keep a stool chart. Note skin color. Check inside mouth for sores. Assess sense of taste. Regular urinalysis should be done to check for albumin or blood. Note complaints of muscle aches, pain. Note any hair loss. Warn patients about breast changes.

Answers to practice problems

CHAPTER 4

1. $\dfrac{2}{5}$
2. $\dfrac{1}{2}$
3. $\dfrac{1}{3}$
4. $1\dfrac{1}{3}$
5. $1\dfrac{3}{10}$
6. $\dfrac{43}{11}$
7. $\dfrac{47}{3}$
8. $1\dfrac{13}{24}$
9. $\dfrac{5}{6}$
10. $\dfrac{5}{9}$
11. $7\dfrac{1}{12}$
12. 1
13. $\dfrac{1}{28}$
14. $24\dfrac{4}{15}$
15. $3\dfrac{5}{24}$
16. $7\dfrac{1}{16}$
17. 10.805
18. 1.335
19. 10.314
20. 8.25
21. 2.146
22. 1.762
23. 2484
24. 0.4375
25. $\dfrac{3}{8}$
26. 31.5
27. 0.072
28. 80%
29. 15
30. 21
31. $3\dfrac{1}{3}$ (or 3.33)
32. $6\dfrac{2}{3}$ (or 6.67)

CHAPTER 6

1. 12.5 ml
2. 1.5 ml
3. 25 ml
4. 3 tablets

CHAPTER 7

1. 0.8 ml
2. 2.5 ml
3. 20 ml
4. 4.5 ml

CHAPTER 11

1. 2 ml
2. 1½ tablets
3. 2 tablets

CHAPTER 12

1. 15 ml
2. 2½ tablets

CHAPTER 13

1. 1½ tablets
2. 2 tablets
3. 1 tablet
4. 4 tablets
5. 2.5 ml

CHAPTER 14

1. 1.5 ml
2. 4 capsules
3. 1 tablet

CHAPTER 15

1. 3 ml
2. 2 capsules
3. 7.5 ml

CHAPTER 16

1. 13 gtt/min; 13 hours
2. 25 gtt/min
3. 28 gtt/min
4. 25 gtt/min
5. 25 gtt/min
6. 6.26 hours, or approximately 1 hour, 15 minutes

CHAPTER 18

1. 1½ tablet
2. 0.5 ml

CHAPTER 19

1. 2 tablets
2. 0.5 ml
3. 1 capsule

CHAPTER 20

1. 2 ml
2. 1 tablet
3. ½ tablet

CHAPTER 24

1. ½ tablet
2. 2 tablets
3. 37.5 ml

CHAPTER 29

1. 0.8 ml

2.   2 tablets
3.   0.25 ml

CHAPTER 31

1.   2.5 ml
2.   ½ tablet
3.   2 tablets

CHAPTER 32

1.   1 tablet
2.   2 tablets
3.   0.8 ml

CHAPTER 33

1.   3 tablets
2.   2 tablets
3.   1 tablet

CHAPTER 34

1.   0.28 ml; 0.18 ml; 0.10 ml; the regular insulin would be drawn into the syringe first.

2.   0.25 ml
3.   3 tablets

CHAPTER 35

1.   5 tablets
2.   3 tablets
3.   2½ tablets

CHAPTER 36

1.   1 tablet
2.   2 ml
3.   2 tablets

CHAPTER 38

1.   0.2 mg
2.   45 mg
3.   35 mg
4.   6.6 mg
5.   0.24 g or 240 mg
6.   0.5 g or 500 mg

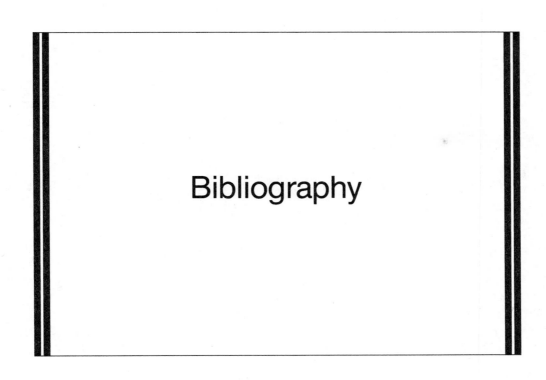

Bibliography

Abrams AC: Clinical Drug Therapy, Philadelphia, JB Lippincott, 1983

Asperheim MK: The Pharmacologic Basis of Patient Care, 5th ed. Philadelphia, WB Saunders, 1985

Hahn AB, Barkin RL, Oestreich SJK: Pharmacology in Nursing, 15th ed. St. Louis, CV Mosby, 1982

Gilman AG et al (eds): Goodman and Gilman's The Pharmacological Basis of Therapeutics, 6th ed. New York, Macmillan, 1980

Govoni L, Hayes JE: Drugs and Nursing Implications, 5th ed. New York, Appleton-Century-Crofts, 1985

Kozier B, Erb G: Techniques in Clinical Nursing. California, Addison-Wesley, 1982

Lipsey SI: Mathematics for Nursing Service: A Programmed Text, 2nd ed. New York, John Wiley and Sons, 1977

Martin EW: Hazards of Medication, 2nd ed. Philadelphia, JB Lippincott, 1978

Metheney NM, Snively WD: Nurses' Handbook of Fluid Balance, 4th ed. Philadelphia, JB Lippincott, 1983

Miller BF, Keane CB: Encyclopedia and Dictionary of Medicine, Nursing, and Allied Health, 3rd ed. Philadelphia, WB Saunders, 1983

Physician's Desk Reference, 39th ed. Oradell, Medical Economics, 1985

Rodman MJ, Smith D: Clinical Pharmacology in Nursing, 2nd ed. Philadelphia, JB Lippincott, 1984

Rodman MJ, Smith D: Pharmacology and Drug Therapy in Nursing, 3rd ed. Philadelphia, JB Lippincott, 1985

Scherer JC: Introductory Clinical Pharmacology, 2nd ed. Philadelphia, JB Lippincott, 1982

Scherer JC: Lippincott's Nurses' Drug Manual. Philadelphia, JB Lippincott, 1985

Squire JE, Clayton BD: Basic Pharmacology For Nurses, 7th ed. St. Louis, CV Mosby, 1982

Weaver M, Koehler V, Arcangelo V: Programmed Mathematics of Drugs and Solutions. Philadelphia, JB Lippincott, 1984

INDEX

Aarane, 180
absence seizure(s), 257
acacia gum, 146
acetaminophen (Tylenol, Phenaphen), 95, 97
    adverse effects, 97
    hypersensitivity reactions, 97–98
acetazolamide (Diamox), 160, 161, 265
acetohexamide (Dymelor), 237
    interaction with phenylbutazone, 9
acetophenazine maleate (Tindal), 43–44
acetylcholine, 117, 147, 150, 203, 263
acetylcysteine (Mucomyst), 184
acetylsalicylic acid. *See* aspirin
achlorhydria, 187
Achromycin, 63
acid–base balance, 136
acidosis, 136, 168
acid rebound, 143
Acidulin, 146
acquired immune deficiency syndrome, 191
ACTH. *See* adrenocorticotropic hormone
Acthar. *See* adrenocorticotropic hormone
Acthar Gel. *See* adrenocorticotropic hormone
Actifed, 187, 189
Actifed with codeine, 184
Actinomycin D, 250
activated charcoal, 146
acyclovir (Zovirax), 72
Adapin, 49
addiction. *See* drug dependence
additive effect, definition, 10
adrenal glands, 230–231
Adrenalin. *See* epinephrine
adrenergic-blocking agents, 204, 211, 219
adrenergic drug(s), 177, 203–205
    in eye treatment, 263
    in obstetrics, 277
adrenergic fibers, 204
adrenocorticosteroids, 230
    adverse effects, 241
    antineoplastic effect, 245
adrenocorticotropic hormone (ACTH, Acthar, Acthar Gel), 229, 230, 233

Adriamycin, 250
Adrucil, 249
adsorbent action, 146
adverse reaction(s), 8–10
Aerosporin. *See* polymyxin B
Afrin, 187, 216
Aftate, 79
agar, 167, 168
age of patient, effect on drug action, 5
agranulocytosis, 240, 260
AIDS, 191
albuterol (Proventil, Ventolin), 177, 178
alcohol, 43, 87–89
    interactants, 9, 128
    interaction
        with antimalarials, 75
        with MAO inhibitors, 9
        with narcotics, 97
        with tranquilizers, 9, 51
    local effect, 87
    as solvent, 88
    systemic effect, 87–88
alcohol abuse, 88–89
Alcoholics Anonymous, 89
alcoholism
    acute, 88
    chronic, 88–89
Aldactazide, 159
Aldactone, 159
Aldomet. *See* methyldopa
Aldoril, 222
alkalosis, 136–137, 168
Alka-Seltzer, 153
Alkeran, 247
alkylating agents, 245–248
allergies, 187
allopurinol (Lopurin, Zyloprim), 109, 133
alopecia, with chemotherapy, 252–253
alprazolam (Xanax), 44, 46
AlternaGel, 144
aluminum acetate (Burow's solution), 78
aluminum compounds
    as antacids, 143
    nursing implications, 145
aluminum hydroxide (AlternaGel, Amphogel), 144
aluminum hydroxide + magnesium hydroxide (Maalox), 144

aluminum hydroxide + magnesium hydroxide + simethicone (Digel, Gelusil, Maalox Plus, Mylanta), 144
Alupent, 177, 179
amantadine HCl (Symmetrel), 71–73, 123
amebiasis, 75
amebic dysentery, 75
Amen, 239
Amicar, 198, 199
amikacin (Amikin), 64
Amikin, 64
amiloride (Midamor), 159
amiloride + hydrochlorothiazide (Moduretic), 159
aminocaproic acid (Amicar), 198, 199
aminoglycosides, 64–65, 68
    adverse effects, 68
aminophylline, 178
aminosalicylic acid (PAS, Parasal), 62, 68
    interaction with isoniazid, 9
amitriptyline (Elavil), 52
    adverse effects, 48–49
    interaction
        with imipramine, 9
        with α-methyldopa, 9
    nursing implications, 48–49
    route and dosage range, 48
    use, 48
amitriptyline + perphenazine (Etrafon, Triavil), 49
ammonia, 173
amobarbital (Amytal), 126
amoxicillin (Amoxil, Polymox, Trimox, Wymox), 59
amoxicillin + potassium clavulanate (Augmentin), 59
Amoxil, 59
amphetamine(s), 105, 107
    interaction with MAO inhibitors, 9
Amphogel, 144
amphotericin B (Fungizone), 69, 70
ampicillin (Omnipen, Polycillin), 59
ampule(s), 6
amyl nitrite, 211, 212
amyotrophic lateral sclerosis, 117
Amytal, 126
anabolic steroids, interaction with coumarin anticoagulants, 9

analeptics, 105, 173
analgesics, 91–98, 102
  narcotic, 91–98
    adverse effects, 91–96
    allergic reactions, 96
    as antidiarrheals, 169
    antitussives, 186
    nursing implications, 96–97
  non-narcotic, 94–95, 97–98
    nursing implications, 98
  in obstetrics, 277
anaphylactic shock, 67, 133
anaphylaxis, definition, 8
Anaprox. See naproxen
Ancef, 61
androgen(s), 232, 239–240, 243
  for breast engorgement, 277
Anectine. See succinylcholine
anemia, 193, 260
  iron-deficiency, 193
  megaloblastic, 193
  pernicious, 193
anesthetic(s), 98–102
  general, 98–99, 117
    nursing implications, 101
  interaction
    with MAO inhibitors, 9
    with narcotics, 97
    with reserpine, 10
    with tranquilizers, 51
  local, 98–101, 117
    adverse effects, 101
    in ear treatment, 267
    para-aminobenzoic
      acid-containing, interaction
      with sulfonamides, 10
    toxicity, 101
  spinal, 117
  topical, in eye treatment,
    263–265
anorexia, with chemotherapy, 253
Anspor, 62
Antabuse. See disulfiram
antacid(s)
  classification, 143–145
  interaction with tetracyclines, 10
  nonsystemic, 143
  nursing implications, 145
  self-medication with, 145
  systemic, 143
  use, 143
antagonism, definition, 10
Antepar. See piperazine salts
anthelminthics, 73, 274
anthraquinones, 165
antianemics, 193–195
antianxiety drug(s). See
    tranquilizer(s), minor

antiarrhythmic drug(s), 205
antibacterial drug(s), 55–69
antibiotics, antineoplastic effect,
    245
antibodies, 83
anticholinergic drug(s), 98, 123,
    147–151, 153, 204
  adverse effects, 150
  as antidiarrheals, 169
  in eye treatment, 263
  nursing implications, 150–151
anticholinesteraselike drug(s), in
    eye treatment, 263
anticoagulant(s). See also coumarin
    anticoagulant(s)
  adverse effects, 199
  classification, 197–199
  definition, 197
  interactants, 9
  uses, 197
anticonvulsant(s), 257–262
  classification, 257
  nursing implications, 257–261
  and oral contraceptives, 243
antidepressant(s), 48–49, 51–52.
    See also tricyclic
    antidepressant(s)
  antihypertensive effect, 219
  definition, 43
  interaction with narcotics, 97
antidiarrheals, 169–170
  adsorbent, 170
  astringent, 170
  local effect, 170
  nursing implications, 170
  systemic, 169
antidiuretic hormone, 230
antiemetics, 153–156
  with chemotherapy, 253
  nursing implications, 156
antifungal agents, 69–71
  nursing implications, 71
antigen(s), 83
antihistamine(s), 187–189
  adverse effects, 187
  anticholinergic effects, 123
  antiemetic effect, 153
  interaction
    with MAO inhibitors, 9
    with tranquilizers, 51
  nursing implications, 187
antihypertensive(s), 219–225
  classification, 219–224
  interaction with narcotics, 97
  nursing implications, 224
  and oral contraceptives, 243
anti-infectives, 55–76
  allergic reactions to, 68

broad-spectrum, 55, 63–68
  definition, 55
  for diarrhea, 170
  dosing time, 69
  in ear treatment, 267
  in eye treatment, 266
  and food, 69
  loading dose, 55
  maintenance dose, 55
  narrow-spectrum, 55
  nursing implications, 68–69
anti-inflammatory agents, 110
  definition, 109
  in eye treatment, 266
antilipemics, 201–202
  nursing implications, 201
antimalarial drug(s), 75, 114
antimetabolites, 245
Antiminth. See pyrantel pamoate
anti-narcotics. See narcotic
    antagonist(s)
antineoplastic drug(s), 245–254
  adverse effects, 252–253
  classification, 245
  nursing implications, 252–253
antineurotic drug(s). See
    tranquilizer(s), minor
antiparasitic agents, 73–75
  nursing implications, 75
antiparkinsonian drug(s), 121–124
antiplatelet drug(s), 197
antipsychotics. See tranquilizer(s),
    major
antipyretic drug(s), definition, 109
antirheumatic drug(s), 111–112
  definition, 109
antispasmodics, 147–151
antithyroid drug(s), 235
  adverse effects, 240
antitoxin(s), 83
antitubercular drug(s), 55, 62–63,
    67–68
antitussives, 183–186
  classification, 185–186
  nursing implications, 186
  over-the-counter, 186
anti-ulcer drug(s), 143–145
Antivert. See meclizine
antiviral agents, 71–73
Anturane. See sulfinpyrazone
anxiety, 125
A.P.L. See human chorionic
    gonadotropin
apomorphine, 153, 154
apothecaries' system, 13, 15
Apresoline, 221
AquaMEPHYTON. See
    phytonadione

Aquasol A. *See* vitamin A
Ara-A. *See* vidarabine
Ara-C, 249
Aralen. *See* chloroquine
Aramine. *See* metaraminol
Aristocort. *See* triamcinolone;
    triamcinolone acetonide
aromatic spirits of ammonia, 173
arrhythmia(s), 203, 205, 208
Artane. *See* trihexyphenidyl
arthritis, 114, 117
artificial tears, 266
ascorbic acid. *See* vitamin C
Ascriptin. *See* aspirin +
    magnesium-aluminum
    hydroxide
asparaginase (Elspar), 251–252
aspirin (Empirin), 94, 97
    as anticoagulant, 197
    contraindications, 98
    interaction
        with anticoagulants, 9
        with methotrexate, 9
        with tranquilizers, 51
    toxicity, 98
aspirin + caffeine + orphenadrine
    citrate (Norgesic), 95
aspirin + magnesium-aluminum
    hydroxide (Ascriptin), 95, 98
asthma, bronchial, 177
AsthmaNefrin, 177
Atarax. *See* hydroxyzine
    hydrochloride
atenolol (Tenormin), 220
atherosclerosis, 201
Ativan. *See* lorazepam
atrial fibrillation, 203
atrial flutter, 203
Atromid S. *See* clofibrate
atropine sulfate, 148, 150, 208, 264
atropinism, 150
Augmentin, 59
aurothioglucose (Solganal), 111, 114
autonomic drugs, in eye treatment,
    263
autonomic nervous system, 147, 203
AVC, 57
Azo Gantrisin, 56
Azulfidine, 57

Baciguent. *See* bacitracin
bacitracin (Baciguent), 65
    interaction with muscle
    relaxants, 9
baclofen (Lioresal), 118, 122
Bactocill, 59

Bactrim, 56
Bactrim DS, 56
BAL, 282
barbiturate(s), 98, 125
    administration route, 129
    adverse effects, 129
    dependence, 128
    interaction
        with alcohol, 128
        with coumarin anticoagulants,
        9
        with narcotics, 97
        with tranquilizers, 51
    nursing implications, 125–129
    in obstetrics, 277
    toxicity, 129
    uses, 125
barium sulfate, 279, 280
BCNU. *See* carmustine
belladonna, 150
Benadryl. *See* diphenhydramine
Benemid. *See* probenecid
Bentyl, 149
Benylin, 186
benzalkonium chloride (Zephiran),
    78
benzocaine, in ear treatment, 267
benzodiazepines, 44
    paradoxical states with, 51
benzonatate (Tessalon), 185
benzquinamide (Emete-con), 154
benztropine (Cogentin), 121, 123
betamethasone valerate (Valisone),
    79
bethanechol chloride (Duvoid,
    Urecholine), 148, 150
Bicillin Long-Acting, 60
BiCNU. *See* carmustine
bile salts, 145
bisacodyl (Dulcolax), 165, 166
Blenoxane, 250
bleomycin (Blenoxane), 250
blepharitis, 266
blood clotting, drugs affecting,
    197–199
blood group incompatibility, 191
blood products, 191
blood transfusions, 191
body size, effect on drug action, 5
body surface area, determination, 272
bone marrow suppression, 253, 260
Bonine. *See* meclizine
boric acid, 78
bowel movement(s), 168
bradykinesia, 122
brand name, 4
breast engorgement, drugs that
    suppress, 277

Brethaire. *See* terbutaline
Brethine. *See* terbutaline
bretylium, interaction with
    sympathomimetics, 10
Brevicon, 232
Brevital, 99
Bricanyl. *See* terbutaline
British Pharmacopeia, 4
bromocriptine mesylate (Parlodel),
    121, 123
    for breast engorgement, 277
brompheniramine maleate
    (Dimetane), 188
brompheniramine maleate +
    phenylephrine +
    phenylpropanolamine
    (Dimetapp), 188
Bromsulphalein, 279
bronchitis, chronic, 177, 181
bronchodilators, 177–181
    classification, 177–180
    nursing implications, 180–181
Bronkosol. *See* isoetharine
bumetanide (Bumex), 160
Bumex, 160
bupivicaine (Marcaine,
    Sensorcaine), 100
Buretrols, 139
Burow's solution, 78
busulfan (Myleran), 246
butalbital + aspirin + caffeine
    (Fiorinal), 95
Butazolidin. *See* phenylbutazone
Butisol, 126
butorphanol (Stadol), 92, 97

CaEDTA, 282
Cafergot, 217
caffeine, 105, 177
Calan. *See* verapamil
calciferol. *See* vitamin D
calcium, 136, 241
calcium carbonate (Dicarbosil,
    Titralac), 143, 144
calcium channel blockers, 211
calcium disodium edetate
    (CaEDTA, Calcium Disodium
    Versenate), 282
Calcium Disodium Versenate, 282
calcium gluconate, interaction with
    digitalis, 9
Camphorated opium tincture, 169
cancer, 245
Capoten. *See* captopril

capsule(s), 6
    preparation for administration,
        30
captopril (Capoten), 219, 220
Carafate, 145
caramiphen +
        phenylpropanolamine
        (Tuss-Ornade), 185
carbamazepine (Tegretol), 258
carbamide peroxide (Debrox Drops,
        Murine Ear Drops), 267
carbenicillin (Geocillin, Geopen,
        Pyopen), 59
carbidopa + levodopa (Sinemet),
        122, 123
carbonic anhydrase, 265
carbonic anhydrase inhibitors, 160,
        161, 265
carboxymethylcellulose, 167
cardiac depressants, 205–209
    classification, 205–208
    emergency, 205–208
    nursing implications, 208
cardiac stimulants, 203–205
    classification, 203
Cardio-Green, 279
cardiotonics, 203
Cardizem. See diltiazem
carisoprodol (Rela, Soma), 117, 118
carminitives, 146
carmustine (BCNU, BiCNU), 246
cascara sagrada, 165, 166
castor oil, 165, 166, 168
Catapres, 220–221
catecholamines, 205, 215, 230
cathartics
    bulk, 167, 168
    classification, 165–168
    contraindications, 168
    definition, 165
    emollient, 167–168
    irritant, 165, 168
    lubricant, 167–168
    nursing implications, 168–169
    saline, 167, 168
    stimulant, 165
    uses, 165
CCNU. See lomustine
Ceclor, 60
CeeNU. See lomustine
cefaclor (Ceclor), 60
cefadroxil monohydrate (Duricef,
        Ultracef), 60
Cefadyl, 61
cefamandole (Mandol), 61
cefazolin (Ancef, Kefzol), 61
Cefizox, 61
Cefobid, 61

cefonicid (Monocid), 61
cefoperazone (Cefobid), 61
ceforanide (Precef), 61
cefotaxime (Claforan), 61
cefoxitin (Mefoxin), 61
ceftizoxime (Cefizox), 61
cefuroxime (Zinacef), 61
celiac disease, 274
central nervous system
        depressant(s). See also
        hypnotics; sedative(s)
    adverse effects, 129
    interaction
        with alcohol, 9
        with narcotics, 97
    in obstetrics, 277
central nervous system depression,
        with tranquilizers, 51
Centrax. See prazepam
cephalexin (Keflex), 61
cephalosporins, 55, 60–62, 67
    adverse effects, 67
cephalothin (Keflin, Seffin), 60
cephapirin (Cefadyl), 61
cephradine (Anspor, Velosef), 62
cerebral palsy, 117
cerebrovascular accident, 201
cerebrovascular disease, 197
Cerumenex, 267
ceruminolytic drug(s), 267
cestodes, 73
chalk, 143
chemotherapy, 245
    combined, 252
children
    dosage calculation for, 5, 271–272
    drug administration routes for,
        272–273
chloral hydrate (Noctec), 127, 129
    interaction with coumarin
        anticoagulants, 9
chlorambucil (Leukeran), 246
chloramphenicol (Chloromycetin),
        65
chlordiazepoxide (Libritabs,
        Librium), 44, 46
chlordiazepoxide + amitriptyline
        (Limbitrol), 49
chlordiazepoxide + clidinium
        (Librax), 46
chloride, 136
Chloromycetin, 65
chloroprocaine (Nesacaine), 100
chloroquine (Aralen), 73, 114
chlorothiazide (Diuril), 158
chlorphenesin carbamate (Maolate),
        117
chlorpheniramine maleate

        (Chlor-Trimeton, Teldrin),
        188
chlorpheniramine maleate +
        phenylpropanolamine
        (Ornade), 188
chlorpromazine (Thorazine), 43
    adverse effects, 45
    interactants, 9
    nursing implications, 45
    route and dosage range, 45
    use, 45
chlorpropamide (Diabinase), 237
chlorthalidone (Hygroton), 159
Chlor-Trimeton, 188
chlorzoxazone + acetaminophen
        (Parafon Forte), 95
Choledyl, 179
cholestyramine (Questran), 201,
        202
cholinergic-blocking agents, 147,
        150–151, 204
cholinergic drug(s), 147–150,
        203–204
    adverse effects, 150
    definition, 147
    in eye treatment, 263
    nursing implications, 150
    uses, 147
cholinergic fibers, 203
cholinesterase, 147
choreiform movement(s), 123
chromium, 136
chronic obstructive lung disease,
        177
chronic obstructive pulmonary
        disease, 177
Chronulac, 166
chrysotherapy, 114
cimetidine (Tagamet), 144, 145,
        187
cinchonism, 208
circulatory system
    parasympathetic effects, 204–205
    sympathetic effects, 204–205
cisplatin (Platinol), 246–247
Claforan, 61
Clark's rule, 272
Cleocin, 66
clindamycin (Cleocin), 66
Clinitest, effect of anti-infectives
        on, 69
Clinoril. See sulindac
clofibrate (Atromid S), 202
    interaction with coumarin
        anticoagulants, 9
Clomid. See clomiphene citrate
clomiphene citrate (Clomid,
        Serophene), 232, 234

clonazepam (Clonopin), 258–259
clonidine (Catapres), 220–221
Clonopin, 258–259
clorazepate dipotassium (Tranxene), 44, 46
clotrimazole (Gyne-Lotrimin, Lotrimin, Mycelex, Mycelex-G), 70
clotting factors, 197
coagulants, 197–199
coal tar, 78
cobalt, 136
cobalt 60, 245
cocaine, 100, 101, 263
codeine, 91, 92, 96
    antitussive effect, 186
codeine + triprolidine + pseudoephedrine (Actifed with codeine), 184
Cogentin. See benztropine
Colace. See docusate sodium
colchicine, 109, 110, 114
COLD. See chronic obstructive lung disease
Colestid, 202
colestipol (Colestid), 202
colistin, interaction with muscle relaxants, 9
Combid, 148
Compazine. See prochlorperazine
congestive heart failure, 157, 161, 197, 203
conjugated estrogens (Premarin), 238
conjunctivitis, 266
constipation, 165
contraindication(s), definition, 5
contrast media, 279
Controlled Substances Act, 3–4
convulsant(s), 105
convulsions, 257
COPD. See chronic obstructive pulmonary disease
copper, 136
Cordran, 79
coronary artery disease, 197
Cortef. See hydrocortisone
corticosteroid(s), 109, 114, 157. See also adrenocorticosteroids
    dependence, 241
    dermatologic use, 77
    in ear treatment, 267
    in eye treatment, 266
    interaction with diuretics, 163
    topical, 77–80
corticotropin. See adrenocorticotropic hormone

cortisone, 235
    in eye treatment, 266
Cosmegen, 250
Cotazym, 145–146
coughing, 183–186
Coumadin, 198
coumarin anticoagulant(s), 197
    interactants, 9
    interaction with phenytoin, 9
cream(s), 6
cromolyn (Aarane, Intal), 178, 180
crotamiton (Eurax), 75
crystalline zinc insulin injection (CZI, Iletin, Regular), 231, 236
Crysticillin, 60
Crystodigin, 204
Cuprimine, 282
curare, 122
Curretab, 239
Cushing's syndrome, 241
cyanocobalamin (vitamin B_{12}, Rubramin-PC), 134, 193, 194
    allergic reactions to, 194
cyclandelate (Cyclospasmol), 212
cyclizine (Marezine), 153, 267, 268
cyclobenzaprine (Flexeril), 118–119
Cyclogyl, 264
cyclopentolate (Cyclogyl), 264
cyclophosphamide (Cytoxan, Neosar), 247
cycloplegic drug(s), 263
Cyclospasmol, 212
cyproheptadine (Periactin), 188
cystic fibrosis, 274
cytarabine (Ara-C, Cytosar-U), 249
Cytosar-U, 249
Cytoxan, 247
CZI, 231, 236

dactinomycin (Actinomycin D, Cosmegen), 250
Dalmane, 127
danazol (Danocrine), 239–240
Danocrine, 239–240
danthron, 165
Dantrium. See dantrolene
dantrolene (Dantrium), 120, 122
dapsone (DDS), 56
Daraprim, 74
Darvocet-N, 94
Darvon. See propoxyphene HCl
Darvon compound, 94

DDS, 56
Debrox Drops, 267
Decadron. See dexamethasone
Decholin, 145
decimals, 21–24
    addition and subtraction of, 21–22
    changing to fractions, 23–24
    definition, 21
    division of, 22–23
    multiplication of, 22
Declomycin, 63
decongestant(s), 187
deferoxamine mesylate (Desferal Mesylate), 281
dehydration, 136, 162, 168
dehydrocholic acid (Decholin), 145
Deladumone, 277
Deladumone OB, 276
Delta-Cortef. See prednisolone
Deltasone, 236
demeclocycline (Declomycin), 63
Demerol. See meperidine
demulcents, 146, 170
    respiratory, 186
Demulen, 232
Depakene, 260
Depakote, 260
Depen Titratabs, 282
depilatories, 77
Depo-Provera, 239
Depo-Testosterone, 240
depression
    endogenous, 51–52
    exogenous, 51
    psychotic, 51
    reactive, 51–52
dermatologic drugs
    allergic reactions, 80
    nursing implications, 80–81
dermatology, 77
DES. See diethylstilbestrol
Desferal Mesylate, 281
desipramine (Norpramin, Pertofrane), 49, 52
Desoxyn, 107
Desyrel, 50
dexamethasone (Decadron, Hexadrol), 235
    in eye treatment, 266
dexbrompheniramine maleate + pseudoephedrine sulfate (Drixoral), 216
Dexedrine, 107
dextroamphetamine (Dexedrine), 107
dextromethorphan (Romilar), 186

DiaBeta, 237
diabetes, 231
  aspirin use in, 98
Diabinase, 237
diagnostic agents, 279–280
  nursing implications, 279–280
Diamox. *See* acetazolamide
diarrhea, 169, 170
diazepam (Valium), 44
  abuse, 51
  adverse effects, 47
  anticonvulsant effect, 257
  as muscle relaxant, 119, 122
  nursing implications, 47
  route and dosage range, 47
  use, 47
diazoxide, 224
dibucaine (Nupercainal), 100
Dicarbosil. *See* calcium carbonate
dicloxacillin (Dycill, Dynapen,
    Pathocil), 59
dicumarol, 198
dicyclomine (Bentyl), 149
diethylpropion (Tenuate, Tenuate
    Dospan, Tepanil, Tepanil
    Ten-Teb), 106
diethylstilbestrol, 232, 238
Digel, 144
digestants, 145–146
digitalis, 203
  interactants, 9
  nursing implications, 205
  toxicity, 163, 205, 208
  uses, 203
digitoxin (Crystodigin), 204
digoxin (Lanoxin), 204
dihydrocodeine + aspirin + caffeine
    (Synalgos-DC), 92
Dilantin. *See* phenytoin
Dilaudid. *See* hydromorphone
diltiazem (Cardizem), 211, 212
dimenhydrinate (Dramamine), 153,
    154, 187, 267, 268
dimercaprol (BAL), 282
Dimetane, 188
Dimetapp, 188
dimethyltubocurarine (Metubine
    Iodide), 122
dinoprost tromethamine (Prostin F$_2$
    Alpha), 276
diphenhydramine (Benadryl), 123,
    153, 154–155, 187
  interactants, 9
diphenhydramine + alcohol
    (Benylin), 186
diphenoxylate + atropine (Lomotil),
    169
diphtheria and tetanus toxoids and

pertussis vaccine, combined
    (DPT), 84, 85
dipyridamole (Persantine), 197,
    211, 212
disease, effect on drug action, 5
disk problems, 117
disopyramide (Norpace, Norpace
    CR), 206
disulfiram (Antabuse), 88–89
  interaction with alcohol, 9
Ditropan. *See* oxybutinin
Diulo. *See* metolazone
diuretics, 157–163, 219. *See also*
    carbonic anhydrase
    inhibitors; thiazide
    diuretic(s)
  acidotic, 162
  with antihypertensives, 224
  classification, 157, 161–162
  definition, 157
  in eye treatment, 265
  interactants, 163
  interaction
    with digitalis, 9
    with lithium, 51
    with narcotics, 97
  loop, 160–161, 161
  nursing implications, 162–163
  osmotic, 158, 161, 265
  potassium-sparing, 159–160, 161
  potent, 160–161
    adverse effects, 161–162
  xanthine, 161
Diuril, 158
docusate calcium (Surfak), 167
docusate sodium (Colace), 167–169
docusate sodium + casanthranol
    (Peri-Colace), 167
Dolophine. *See* methadone
Donnatal, 149
dopamine HCl (Intropin), 215
dopaminergic drug(s), 123
Dopar. *See* levodopa
dosage form(s), effect on drug
    action, 5–6
doxepin (Adapin, Sinequan), 49
doxorubicin (Adriamycin), 250
doxycycline (Vibramycin), 63
DPT. *See* diphtheria and tetanus
    toxoids and pertussis vaccine,
    combined
Dramamine. *See* dimenhydrinate
Drixoral, 216
droperidol (Inapsine), 100
droperidol + fentanyl citrate
    (Innovar), 100
drug(s)
  definition, 3

liquid, dose calculation, 38
local action, 6
oral, 6
patient response to, 8–10
rectal, 6
schedules, 4
solid, dose calculation, 36–38
sources, 3
sublingual, 6
systemic action, 6
drug abuse, 8
drug action
  factors affecting, 5–8
  after parenteral injection, 8
  and patient belief, 5
drug administration
  chart, 36
  maintenance dose, 55
  nurse's responsibilities, 29
  observing, 36–37
  parenteral, 6–8
  preparing patient for, 30
  procedure, 30–31
  recording, 36–37
  reporting, 36–37
  route, 6–8. *See also* injection(s)
    for children, 272–273
  stock system, 29
  unit dose system, 29
drug allergy, definition, 8
drug dependence
  definition, 8
  physical, 8
  psychological, 8
drug dosage
  calculation, 15, 36–39
    for children, 5, 271–272
  conversion, 38–39
Drug Enforcement Agency, 3
Drug Facts and Comparisons, 4
drug handbooks, 4
drug hangover, 129
drug idiosyncrasy, 8
drug information, sources of, 4
drug interaction(s), 9–10, 51
  definition, 10
drug names, 4
drug overdose, definition, 10
drug use, laws governing, 3–4
dry mouth, 150, 151
Dulcolax. *See* bisacodyl
Duracillin, 60
Duraquin, 207
Duricef, 60
Duvoid. *See* bethanechol chloride
Dyazide, 160
Dycill, 59
dye(s), 279, 280

adverse effects, 280
Dymelor, 237
Dynapen, 59
Dyrenium, 160
dysentery, amebic, 75
dyskinesia(s), 44, 123

ear drops, 268
eardrum, perforated, 268
ear medications, 267–268
    classification, 267
    nursing implications, 268
ear wax, impacted, 267
ecchymoses, 241
echothiophate (Phospholine), 264
Edecrin, 161
edema, 157, 161, 243
edrophonium (Tensilon), 120
EES. See erythromycin
Elavil. See amitriptyline
electroconvulsive therapy, 43, 122
electrolyte(s). See also fluids and
        electrolytes
    with androgen therapy, 243
    definition, 136
    monitoring, in diuretic therapy,
        163
electrolyte balance, with stomas,
    163
electrolyte imbalance, 136, 157, 161
    with cathartics, 168
elixir(s), 6, 88
Elixophyllin. See theophylline
Elspar. See asparaginase
embolus, definition, 197n
Emete-con, 154
emetics, 153, 154
emollient(s), 80
emphysema, 177
Empirin. See aspirin
E-Mycin. See erythromycin
endocrine disorders, 229
endocrine glands, 229
enemas, 168–169
enflurane (Ethrane), 99
Enovid, 232
enzyme(s)
    digestive, 145–146
    pancreatic, 145–146
ephedrine + phenylephrine
        (Neo-Synephrine), 187
epilepsy, 157, 161, 257, 260–261
    diagnosis, stimulants as aid in,
        105–107
epinephrine (Adrenalin,

Medihaler-Epi), 177, 178,
    187, 205, 215, 230
Equagesic, 95
Equanil. See meprobamate
equivalent(s), definition, 13
ergocalciferol. See vitamin D
Ergomar, 216
ergonovine maleate (Ergotrate
        Maleate), 276
Ergostat, 216
ergot alkaloids, 217
    for breast engorgement, 277
    nursing implications, 277
    in obstetrics, 275
ergotamine + caffeine (Cafergot),
    217
ergotamine tartrate (Ergomar,
        Ergostat), 216
Ergotrate Maleate, 276
Eryc. See erythromycin
Erythrocin. See erythromycin
erythromycin (EES, E-Mycin, Eryc,
        Erythrocin, Ilosone, Ilotycin),
        64, 68
erythromycin + sulfisoxazole
        (Pediazole), 64
Esidrix, 158
Eskalith. See lithium
Estrace, 238
estradiol (Estrace), 238
Estratest, 277
estrogen(s), 231, 238
    adverse effects, 243
    for breast engorgement, 277
ethacrynic acid (Edecrin), 161
ethambutol (Myambutol), 62
ethanol, 87
ethchlorvynol (Placidyl), 127
ethiodized oil (Ethiodol), 279
Ethiodol, 279
ethionamide, interaction with
        isoniazid, 9
ethosuximide (Zarontin), 259
Ethrane, 99
ethyl alcohol, 87, 211
    adverse effects, 88
    nursing implications, 88
    route and dosage range, 88
    as solvent, 88
    use, 88
ethynodiol + ethinyl estradiol
        (Demulen), 232
ethynodiol + mestranol (Ovulen),
    232
etoposide (VePesid), 251
Etrafon, 49
Eurax, 75
Ex-Lax, 165

expectorants, 183, 186
extrapyramidal symptoms, 44–51
extravasation, 140
eye disorders, with steroids, 241
eye drops, 266
eye lubricants, 266
eye medications, 263–267
    classification, 263–267
    nursing implications, 266–267

Fastin, 106
fats, dietary, 201
Federal Food, Drug and Cosmetic
        Act, 3
Feldene, 112–113
fenoprofen (Nalfon), 111
Feosol, 194
Feostat, 195
Fergon, 195
ferrous fumarate (Feostat, Ircon),
    195
ferrous gluconate (Fergon), 195
ferrous sulfate (Feosol), 194
Fiorinal, 95
Flagyl. See metronidazole
Fleet Enemas, 168
Fleet Phospho-Soda, 167
Flexeril, 118–119
Florinef. See fludrocortisone
fludrocortisone (Florinef), 235
    in eye treatment, 266
fluid extract(s), 6, 88
fluids and electrolytes, 136–140
    balance, 161
    imbalances, with corticosteroids,
        241
    replacement therapy, 136
        intravenous, 137–140
fluocinolone (Fluonid, Synalar), 79
fluocinonide (Lidex, Topsyn), 79
Fluonid, 79
fluorescein, 279
fluorine, 136
fluorouracil (5-FU, Adrucil), 249
Fluothane, 99
fluphenazine HCl (Prolixin), 43, 45
flurandrenolide (Cordran), 79
flurazepam (Dalmane), 127
Folex. See methotrexate
folic acid (Folvite), 194
    allergic reactions to, 194
    deficiency, 193
follicle-stimulating hormone, 230

Follutein, 232
Folvite, 194
food
    and anti-infectives, 69
    effect on drug action, 5
    interaction with MAO inhibitors,
        9, 51
fractions, 15–21
    addition of, 17–18
    changing to decimals, 23
    changing to percents, 24–25
    division of, 20
    improper, 16–17
    larger and smaller, 20–21
    multiplication of, 19
        with whole numbers, 19
    proper, 16
    reduced to lowest terms, 16
    subtraction of, 18
    types of, 16
Fried's rule, 271–272
5-FU. See fluorouracil
Fulvicin. See griseofulvin, microsize
Fulvicin P/G. See griseofulvin,
    ultramicrosize
Fungizone. See amphotericin B
Furadantin, 57
furazolidone, interaction with
    alcohol, 9
furosemide (Lasix), 160

galactorrhea, 51
galactosemia, 274
Gamimune. See immune serum
    globulin
gamma benzene hexachloride. See
    lindane
gamma globulin. See immune
    serum globulin
Gamma Globulin. See immune
    serum globulin
Gamulin-Rh. See Rh₀ immune
    globulin
Gantanol, 56
Gantrisin, 56
Garamycin. See gentamicin
gastrointestinal tract, autonomic
    nervous system effect in, 147
Gelusil, 144
generic name, 4
genitourinary tract, autonomic
    nervous system effect in, 147
gentamicin·(Garamycin), 64, 163
gentian violet, 79

Geocillin, 59
Geopen, 59
glacial acetic acid, 77
glaucoma, 157, 161, 263
glipizide (Glucotrol), 237
glucagon, 231
glucocorticosteroids, interaction
    with thiazide diuretics, 10
Glucotrol, 237
glutamic acid HCl (Acidulin), 146
glutethimide, interaction with
    coumarin anticoagulants, 9
glyburide (DiaBeta, Micronase), 237
glycerin (Glyrol, Osmoglyn), 166,
    168, 265
    demulcent, 146
    in eye treatment, adverse effects,
        267
glycosides, 203
Glyrol, 265
goiter, 230
gold salts, 114
gold sodium thiomalate
    (Myochrysine), 111, 114
gonads, 231–232
gout, 109, 114
grain alcohol, 87
Grifulvin V. See griseofulvin,
    microsize
griseofulvin, 69–71
    interaction
        with alcohol, 9
        with coumarin anticoagulants,
            9
    microsize (Fulvicin, Grifulvin V),
        70
    ultramicrosize (Fulvicin P/G,
        Gris–Peg), 70
Gris-Peg. See griseofulvin,
    ultramicrosize
guaifenesin (Robitussin), 183, 184,
    186
guanethidine (Ismelin), 219, 221
    interactants, 9
    interaction with
        sympathomimetics, 10
Gyne-Lotrimin, 70

habituation. See drug dependence
Halcion, 128
hallucinogen(s), 43
haloperidol (Haldol), 44
halothane (Fluothane), 99
Harrison Act, 3
H-BIG, 85

HCG. See human chorionic
    gonadotropin
heavy metal antagonists, 281–282
helminths, 73
hemostatic agents, 197
heparin, 197, 198
hepatitis, viral, 191
hepatitis B immune globulin
    (H–BIG, Hep-B-Gamma-gee,
    Hyper-hep), 85
Hep-B-Gamma-gee, 85
Herplex. See idoxuridine
Herplex Liquifilm. See idoxuridine
Hexadrol. See dexamethasone
Hiprex, 57
hirsutism, 241, 261
histamine, 187, 279
histamine antagonist(s), 145
HMG. See human menopausal
    gonadotropin
homatropine, 264
hormonal imbalance, with steroids,
    241
hormones, 229–244
    adrenal, 235–236
        nursing implications, 241–242
    anterior pituitary, 229, 230
    definition, 229
    gonadal, 238–239
    hypersecretion, 229
    hyposecretion, 229
    nursing implications, 232–243
    pancreas, 236–237
        nursing implications, 242
    pituitary, nursing implications,
        232–240
    posterior pituitary, 230
    thyroid, 230, 234–235
        nursing implications, 240
    trophic, 229
household measurement system, 13
human chorionic gonadotropin, 232
    preparations (A.P.L., Follutein,
        Pregnyl, Profasi HP), 232,
        234
Humulin, 231
Hu-Tet. See tetanus immune
    human globulin
hydralazine (Apresoline), 221
Hydrea, 252
hydrochloric acid
    deficiency, 145
    excess, 143
hydrochlorothiazide (Esidrix,
    Hydrodiuril, Oretic), 158
hydrocodone + phenyltoloxamine
    (Tussionex), 186

hydrocortisone (Cortef, Solu-Cortef), 236
in eye treatment, 266
Hydrodiuril, 158
hydrogen peroxide, 78, 80
hydromorphone (Dilaudid), 93, 96
hydroxychloroquine (Plaquenil), 114
hydroxyurea (Hydrea), 252
hydroxyzine hydrochloride (Atarax), 44, 47
hydroxyzine pamoate (Vistaril), 44
Hygroton, 159
Hyoscine. See scopolamine
hyperactive behavior disorder(s), 105
hyperalimentation, 140
definition, 136
hyperchlorhydria, 143
hyperglycemia, 157, 242
with hypertensives, 224
Hyper-hep, 85
hyperkalemia, 157, 161, 163
hyperkinetic behavior, 105
hyperlipidemia(s), 201
hypersecretion, 229
hypertension, 157, 161, 241
arterial, 219
essential, 219
malignant, 219
primary, 219
secondary, 219
Hyper-Tet. See tetanus immune human globulin
hyperthyroidism, 230
hypertonic solution(s), 137, 138
as cathartics, 167
hyperuricemia, 157
hypervitaminosis A, 133
hypervitaminosis D, 133
hypnotics, 43, 153
classification, 125
definition, 125
interaction
with narcotics, 97
with tranquilizers, 51
nursing implications, 129
hypochloremia, 157
hypodermic syringe, 32
hypoglycemia, 231, 242
hypokalemia, 157, 161, 163, 168
hypomagnesemia, 157
hyponatremia, 157
hyposecretion, 229
hypotensive(s), interaction with MAO inhibitors, 9
hypothyroidism, 230

hypotonic solution(s), 137, 138
hypoventilation, 171
hypoxemia, 171
hypoxia, 171
HypRho-D. See Rh$_O$ immune globulin

ibuprofen (Motrin, Rufen), 112, 114
idoxuridine (Herplex, Herplex Liquifilm, Stoxil), 72, 73, 266
Iletin, 231, 236
Ilosone. See erythromycin
Ilotycin. See erythromycin
Imferon, 195
imipramine (Tofranil), 52
adverse effects, 49
interactants, 9
interaction with MAO inhibitors, 9
nursing implications, 49
route and dosage range, 49
use, 49
immune serum globulin (Gamimune, Gamma Globulin, Sandoglobulin), 83, 84
for viral infections, 73
immunity, 83
immunosuppression, with antineoplastic drugs, 253
Imodium, 169
impotence, with antihypertensive therapy, 224
Inapsine, 100
Inderal. See propranolol
Inderide, 223
indigestion, 143
Indocin. See indomethacin
Indocin-SR. See indomethacin
indocyanine green (Cardio-Green), 279
indomethacin (Indocin, Indocin-SR), 109, 110
interaction
with coumarin anticoagulants, 9
with insulin, 9
infant formula(s), 274
infants. See children
infection(s)
fungal, 80
mixed, 68
skin, 80
superimposed, 69
infertility, 229–230

inflammatory joint disease(s), 117
influenza virus vaccine, 84
infusion pump(s), 139, 140
INH. See isoniazid
inhalations, 6
inhibition, definition, 10
injection(s), 8
deltoid, 35–36
dorsogluteal, 34
equipment, 31
intracutaneous, 8
intradermal, 7, 8
sites, 33
intramuscular, 7, 8, 35
sites, 34–36
syringes for, 31
intravenous, 7, 8
method, 31–32
mixed, 32–33
parenteral, 8
rectus femoris, 35
sites, 33–36
in children, 273
special considerations, 31–36
subcutaneous, 7, 8, 35
sites, 33
syringes for, 31
vastus lateralis, 35
ventrogluteal, 34–35
Z-track, 193–194
Innovar, 100
insulin, 231
dietary therapy with, 242
human (Humulin, Novalin), 231
injection sites, 242
interactants, 9
nursing implications, 242
preparations, 231
units, 242
insulin syringes, 31–32, 242
insulin zinc suspension (Lente), 231, 237
extended (Ultralente), 231, 237
Intal, 178, 180
intermittent positive-pressure breathing, 177
intestinal amebiasis, 75
intravenous therapy
complications, 140
drops per minute, formula for determination, 137
for fluid and electrolyte replacement, 137–140
macrodrip infusion, 137
microdrip infusion, 137
nursing implications, 139–140
piggyback infusion, 139

intravenous therapy (*continued*)
  volume-controlled
      administration, 139
intravenous tubing, 137, 138
intrinsic factor, 193
Intropin, 215
iodine, 136
  antithyroid effect, 230
  radioactive, 230, 240, 279
iodine 131, 245, 280
iodine compounds, as diagnostic
      agents, 279
iodochlorhydroxyquin +
      hydrocortisone
      (Vioform-Hydrocortisone), 80
Ionamin, 100
iopanoic acid (Telepaque), 280
ipecac syrup, 153, 154
Ircon, 195
iron, 136, 193
  administration, 193
  nursing implications, 193–194
iron dextran (Imferon), 195
irrigations, 6
irritants, 77
Ismelin. *See* guanethidine
IsoBid. *See* isosorbide
isoetharine (Bronkosol), 177, 179
isoniazid (INH), 62, 68
  interactants, 9
isophane insulin zinc suspension
      (NPH), 231, 236
isopropamide + prochlorperazine
      (Combid), 148
isopropyl alcohol, 87
  adverse effects, 88
  nursing implications, 88
  route and dosage range, 88
  use, 88
isoproterenol (Isuprel,
      Medihaler-Iso), 177, 179, 205
Isoptin. *See* verapamil
Isopto Carpine, 265
Isordil, 211, 212
isosorbide (IsoBid, Isordil,
      Sorbitrate), 211, 212
isotonic solution(s), 137, 138
  as cathartics, 167
isoxsuprine (Vasodilan), 213
Isuprel. *See* isoproterenol

kanamycin (Kantrex), 64–65, 163
  interaction with muscle

relaxants, 9
Kantrex. *See* kanamycin
kaolin, 146
kaolin-pectin (Kaopectate), 146,
      169
kaolin + pectin, 169
Kaon. *See* potassium
Kaopectate, 146, 169
Kay-Ciel. *See* potassium
Kayexalate. *See* sodium polystyrene
      sulfonate
Keflex, 61
Keflin, 60
Kefzol, 61
Kenalog. *See* triamcinolone;
      triamcinolone acetonide
keratitis, 266
keratolytics, 77
Ketalar, 99
ketamine (Ketalar), 99
ketoconazole (Nizoral), 70
kidney disease, 161
Klor-vess. *See* potassium
Klotrix. *See* potassium
K-Lyte. *See* potassium
K-Phos. *See* potassium
K-Tab. *See* potassium
Kwell. *See* lindane

labatolol (Normodyne, Trandate),
      221
lactation, drugs for suppressing,
      277
Lactinex, 170
lactobacillus (Lactinex), 170
lactulose (Chronulac), 166
Lanoxin, 204
Larodopa. *See* levodopa
Lasix, 160
laxative habit, 168
laxatives, definition, 165
Lente, 231, 237
Leukeran, 246
levarterenol, 204, 215–217
  as vasoconstrictor, 215
levodopa (Dopar, Larodopa), 121,
      123
levodopa + carbidopa (Sinemet),
      122, 123
levonorgestrel + ethinyl estradiol
      (Nordette, Triphasil), 232
Levophed. *See* norepinephrine
Levothroid, 235

levothyroxine (Levothroid,
      Synthroid), 235
Librax, 46
Libritabs. *See* chlordiazepoxide
Librium. *See* chlordiazepoxide
Lidex, 79
lidocaine (Xylocaine), 101
  as cardiac depressant, 205–208
Limbitrol, 49
Lincocin, 66
lincomycin (Lincocin), 66
lindane (Kwell, Scabene), 73, 75
Lioresal. *See* baclofen
liquid phenol, 77
Liquifilm Tears, 265
Liquifilm Wetting Solution, 265
Lithane. *See* lithium
lithium (Eskalith, Lithane,
      Lithobid), 44, 45
  interaction with diuretics, 51
Lithobid. *See* lithium
liver disease, 157, 161
loading dose, 55
Loestrin, 232
Lomotil. *See* diphenoxylate +
      atropine
lomustine (CCNU, CeeNU), 247
Loniten, 223
Lo/Ovral, 232
loperamide (Imodium), 169
Lopressor, 223
Lopurin. *See* allopurinol
lorazepam (Ativan), 44, 47
lotion(s), 6
Lotrimin, 70
low back problems, 117
Ludiomil. *See* maprotiline HCl
Lugol's solution, 230
Luminal. *See* phenobarbital
luteinizing hormone, 230

Maalox, 144
Maalox Plus, 144
Macrodantin, 57
mafenide acetate (Sulfamylon), 56
magaldrate (Riopan), 143, 144
magnesium, 136
magnesium chloride, as cathartic,
      167
magnesium citrate, 166
magnesium compounds, as
      antacids, 143
magnesium hydroxide mixture
      (Milk of magnesia), 144

malaria, 73
malt extract, 146
Mandelamine. *See* methenamine mandelate
Mandol, 61
mannitol (Osmitrol), 158, 265
Maolate, 117
maprotiline HCl (Ludiomil), 52
    adverse effects, 49–50
    nursing implications, 49–50
    route and dosage range, 49
    use, 49
Marcaine, 100
Marezine. *See* cyclizine
marijuana, for nausea and vomiting, 253
Matulane, 248
Maxzide, 160
measles, mumps, rubella virus (M-M-R-II), 84
measurement(s)
    conversion, 13, 38–39
    systems, 11–13
mebendazole (Vermox), 74
mechlorethamine (nitrogen mustard, Mustargen), 247
meclizine (Antivert, Bonine), 155, 267
meclofenamate (Meclomen), 112
Meclomen, 112
medication, preparation for administration, 29–30
medication errors, 31
Medihaler-Epi, 177, 178
Medihaler-Iso. *See* isoproterenol
Medrol. *See* methylprednisolone
medroxyprogesterone (Amen, Curretab, Depo-Provera, Provera), 239
Mefoxin, 61
melanocyte-stimulating hormone, 230
melphalan (Alkeran), 247
menadione (vitamin K₃), 135, 199
menotropins (Pergonal), 229–230, 233
meperidine (Demerol), 93, 96
    interaction with MAO inhibitors, 9
Mephyton. *See* phytonadione
meprobamate (Equanil, Miltown), 44, 47
meprobamate + aspirin (Equagesic), 95
mercurials, 161
Merthiolate, 79
Mestinon, 148

metal(s), interaction with tetracyclines, 10
Metamucil. *See* psyllium, psyllium seeds
Metaprel, 177, 179
metaproterenol (Alupent, Metaprel), 177, 179
metaraminol (Aramine), 215
    interaction with MAO inhibitors, 9
methadone (Dolophine), 93, 96
methamphetamine (Desoxyn), 107
methantheline bromide (Banthine), 150
methenamine hippurate (Hiprex), 57
methenamine mandelate (Mandelamine), 58, 67
Methergine, 276
methicillin (Staphcillin), 59
methimazole (Tapazole), 235
methocarbamol (Robaxin), 117, 119
methohexital (Brevital), 99
methotrexate (Folex, Mexate), 249
    interactants, 9
methylcellulose (Tearisol), 167, 264
methyldopa (Aldomet), 222, 224
    interactants, 9
    interaction with MAO inhibitors, 9
methyldopa + hydrochlorothiazide (Aldoril), 222
methylergonovine (Methergine), 276
methylphenidate (Ritalin, Ritalin-SR), 105, 106
    interaction with guanethidine, 9
methylprednisolone (Medrol, Solu-Medrol), 236
    in eye treatment, 266
methyltestosterone (Oreton Methyl), 240
methyltestosterone + estrogen (Estratest), for breast engorgement, 277
methysergide maleate (Sansert), 216, 217
Meticortelone. *See* prednisolone
Meticorten, 236
metolazone (Diulo, Zaroxolyn), 158–159, 222
metoprolol tartrate (Lopressor), 223
metric system, 11–12
metronidazole (Flagyl), 74
    interaction with alcohol, 9
Metubine Iodide. *See* dimethyltubocurarine

Mexate. *See* methotrexate
Mezlin, 59
mezlocillin (Mezlin), 59
miconazole (Monistat), 71
miconazole nitrate (Monistat 7, Monistat Derm), 71
Micro-K. *See* potassium
Micronase, 237
Micronefrin, 177
Micronor, 232
Midamor, 159
migraine, 217
milk, interaction with tetracyclines, 10
milk allergy, 274
milk of magnesia, 144
Miltown. *See* meprobamate
mineral oil, 168
    cathartic, 166
minerals, 135–136
    nursing implications, 136
minimal brain dysfunction, 105
Minipress, 219, 223
Minocin, 64
minocycline (Minocin), 64
minoxidil (Loniten), 223
miotics, 263
mite infestations, 73–75
Mitomycin (Mitomycin–C, Mutamycin), 251
Mitomycin-C, 251
mixed numbers, 16–17
    adding and subtracting with, 18–19
    multiplication of, with fractions, 19
M-M-R-II. *See* measles, mumps, rubella virus
Modicon, 232
Moduretic, 159
molybdenum, 136
Monistat, 71
Monistat 7, 71
Monistat Derm, 71
monoamine oxidase inhibitors, 48, 51
    adverse effects, 51
    interactants, 9
    interaction with sulfonylureas, 10
Monocid, 61
morphine, 91, 92, 96
    antitussive effect, 186
    interaction with MAO inhibitors, 9
    synthetic derivatives, 92–94, 96
motion sickness, 153–156, 187, 267, 268

Motrin. *See* ibuprofen
movement, 117
moxalactam (Moxam), 62
Moxam, 62
mucolytics, 183
Mucomyst, 184
multiple sclerosis, 117
multivitamin(s), 135
   for children, 274
Murine Ear Drops, 267
muscle(s)
   contraction, 117
   flaccid, 117
   spasms, 117
   sprains, 117
   strains, 117
   tone, 117
muscle relaxant(s). *See also* skeletal
      muscle relaxants
   interaction
      with MAO inhibitors, 9
      with narcotics, 97
   nondepolarizing
      interactants, 9
      interaction with quinidine, 10
mustard gas, 245
Mustargen, 247
Mutamycin-C, 251
Myambutol, 62
Mycelex, 70
Mycelex-G, 70
Mycifradin. *See* neomycin
Mycolog, 66
Mycostatin. *See* nystatin
Mydriacyl, 265
mydriatics, 263
Mylanta, 144
Myleran, 246
Mylicon, 146
myocardial infarction, 197, 201
Myochrysine. *See* gold sodium
      thiomalate
myometrium, 275
myoneural junction, 117
Mysoline. *See* primidone

nadolol (Corgard), 211, 213
nafcillin (Unipen), 59
nalbuphine (Nubain), 93, 97
Naldecon, 217
Nalfon, 111
nalidixic acid (NegGram), 58, 67

naloxone (Narcan), 94
Naprosyn. *See* naproxen
naproxen (Anaprox, Naprosyn),
      112, 114
Narcan, 94
narcolepsy, 105
narcotic antagonist(s), 94, 97
   nursing implications, 97
narcotics, 43. *See also* analgesics,
      narcotic
   interactants, 97
   interaction
      with alcohol, 9
      with tranquilizers, 51
Nardil, 48
Natacyn, 264
natamycin (Natacyn), 264
National Formulary, 3–4, 11
nausea, 153, 156
   with chemotherapy, 253
Nebcin, 65
nebulization, 177, 180
necrosis, 140
needle(s), types of, 31
NegGram. *See* nalidixic acid
Nembutal, 126
Neobiotic. *See* neomycin
Neoloid, 166
neomycin (Mycifradin, Neobiotic),
      65
   interaction with muscle
      relaxants, 9
neoplasm(s), 245
Neosar, 247
Neosporin, 66
neostigmine (Prostigmin), 120, 148,
      150
Neo-Synephrine, 187
nephrotoxicity, 68
nerve block, 87
Nesacaine, 100
netilmicin (Netromycin), 65
Netromycin, 65
neuromuscular blocking agent(s),
      122
   antidotes, 120
neurosis, drug therapy, 44
niacin (nicotinic acid), 133, 134
nicotine, 217
nicotinic acid. *See* niacin
nifedipine (Procardia), 211, 213
Nilstat. *See* nystatin
nitrates, 211
nitrites, 211
Nitro-Bid. *See* nitroglycerin
Nitrodisc. *See* nitroglycerin

Nitro-Dur. *See* nitroglycerin
nitrofurantoin (Furadantin), 57
nitrofurantoin macrocrystals
      (Macrodantin), 57
nitrogen mustard, 247
nitroglycerin (Nitro-Bid, Nitrodisc,
      Nitro-Dur, Nitrol, Nitrostat,
      TNG, Transderm-Nitro,
      Tridil), 214
   interaction with alcohol, 9
   patches, 215
   sublingual, 211
Nitrol. *See* nitroglycerin
Nitropaste, 214–215
Nitrostat. *See* nitroglycerin
Nizoral, 70
Noctec. *See* chloral hydrate
nocturia, 162
nomogram(s), 272–273
non-barbiturate sedatives and
      hypnotics, 125
   dependence, 128
   interaction with alcohol,
      128
nonsalicylate analgesics, 97–98
Nordette, 232
norepinephrine (Levophed), 204,
      205, 230
   as vasoconstrictor, 215
norethindrone (Norlutate,
      Norlutin), 232, 239
norethynodrel + mestranol
      (Enovid), 232
Norgesic, 95
norgestrel, 232
norgestrel + ethinyl estradiol
      (Lo/Ovral, Ovral), 232
Norinyl, 232
Norinyl 2mg, 232
Norlestrin, 232
Norlutate. *See* norethindrone
Norlutin. *See* norethindrone
normal flora, 69
Normodyne, 221
Norpace. *See* disopyramide
Norpace CR. *See* disopyramide
Norpramin. *See* desipramine
Nor-Q.D., 232
nortriptyline, 52
Novalin, 231
Novocain, 101
NPH, 231, 236
Nubain. *See* nalbuphine
Nupercainal, 100
nystatin (Mycostatin, Nilstat), 69,
      71

nystatin + neomycin sulfate + gramicidin + triamcinolone (Mycolog), 66

obesity, 105
obstetrics, definition, 275
ointment(s), 6
  eye, 266
    allergic reactions to, 267
oliguria, 98, 157
olive oil, 168
Omnipen, 59
Oncovin, 251
onset of action, 5
Ophthaine, 265
opiate(s), 91
  in obstetrics, 277
opiate dependence, 97
opium, 91
  as antidiarrheal, 169
  products, 96
oral contraceptives, 231–232, 243
  interactants, 243
oral hypoglycemics, 231, 237
Oretic, 158
Oreton Methyl, 240
Orimune Trivalent, 84
Orinase. See tolbutamide
Ornade, 188
orphenadrine (Disipal), 123
  interaction with chlorpromazine, 9
Ortho-Novum, 232
Ortho-Novum 2mg, 232
orthostatic hypotension, 123, 224
Osmitrol, 158, 265
Osmoglyn, 265
otic medications. See ear medications
otitis externa, 267
otitis media, 267
ototoxicity, 68, 162, 163
ovaries, 231–232
Ovcon, 232
overhydration, 136, 162
Ovral, 232
Ovrette, 232
ovulation, drugs that stimulate, 232
Ovulen, 232
oxacillin (Bactocill, Prostaphlin), 59
oxazepam (Serax), 44, 47
oxtriphylline (Choledyl), 179
oxybutinin (Ditropan), 149

oxycodone + acetaminophen (Percocet, Tylox), 94
oxycodone + aspirin (Percodan), 93
oxygen, 171-172
  administration, 171
  hyperbaric, 171
  nursing implications, 171–172
oxymetazoline (Afrin), 187, 216
oxytetracycline (Terramycin), 63
oxytocics, 275–277
  definition, 275
  nursing implications, 277
oxytocin (Pitocin, Syntocinon), 230, 275, 276
  synthetic, 275

pain, 91
pancreas, 231
Pancrease, 145–146
pancreatic enzyme deficiency, 274
pancuronium (Pavulon), 119, 122
para-aminosalicylic acid. See aminosalicylic acid
paradoxical hypertensive crisis, 51–52
paradoxical states, 51
Parafon Forte, 95
Paral. See paraldehyde
paraldehyde (Paral), 128, 129
Parasal. See aminosalicylic acid
parasympathetic nervous system, 203
parasympatholytic drug(s), 150
parasympathomimetic drug(s), 147
parathormone, 230
parathyroid glands, 230
paregoric (Camphorated opium tincture), 169
parkinsonism, 44
Parkinson's disease, 122–123
Parlodel. See bromocriptine mesylate
Parnate, 51, 52
paroxysmal atrial tachycardia, 203
PAS. See aminosalicylic acid
Pathocil, 59
pathogen(s), identification, 55
Pavulon, 119, 122
PBZ, 189
PBZ-SR, 189
pectin, 170
pediatrics, 271
  drugs used in, 273–274
Pediazole, 64

pediculicides, 75
pediculosis, 73–75
Peditrol, 139
penicillamine (Cuprimine, Depen Titratabs), 282
penicillin G benzathine (Bicillin Long-Acting), 60
penicillin G potassium (Pentids), 58
penicillin G procaine (Crysticillin, Duracillin, Wycillin), 60
penicillins, 55, 58–60, 67
  adverse effects, 67
penicillin V potassium (Pen-Vee-K, V-Cillin-K, Veetids), 60
pentaerythritol (Peritrate), 214
pentazocine (Talwin), 94, 96
pentazocine + naloxone (Talwin NX), 94
Pentids, 58
pentobarbital (Nembutal), 126
Pentothal, 99
Pen-Vee-K, 60
Pepto-Bismol, 143, 153
percents, 24–25
  finding, 24
  multiplying by, 25
Percocet, 94
Percodan, 93
PerDiem, 167
Pergonal, 229–230, 233
Periactin, 188
Peri–Colace, 167
peripheral vascular disease, 211, 214
Peritrate, 214
pernicious anemia, 193
Persantine, 197, 211, 212
Pertofrane. See desipramine
petechiae, 241
pH, 136
pharmacology, definition, 3
pharmacopeias, 3
phenacetin, 97
  adverse effects, 97
  hypersensitivity reactions, 97–98
Phenaphen. See acetaminophen
phenazopyridine (Pyridium), 95
phenelzine sulfate (Nardil), 48, 51–52
Phenergan. See promethazine
phenobarbital (Luminal), 126
  anticonvulsant effect, 257
  interaction
    with coumarin anticoagulants, 9
    with phenylbutazone, 9

phenobarbital + hyoscyamine + atropine + scopolamine (Donnatal), 149
phenolphthalein, 165
phenolsulfonthalein (Pheno-Red), 279
Pheno-Red, 279
phenothiazines, 43–44, 45–46
    adverse effects, 44
phentermine (Fastin, Ionamin), 106
phentolamine (Regitine), 219
phenylbutazone (Butazolidin), 109, 110, 114
    interactants, 9
    interaction
        with coumarin anticoagulants, 9
        with phenytoin, 10
phenylketonuria, 274
phenylpropanolamine + phenylephrine + phenyltoloxamine citrate + chlorpheniramine maleate (Naldecon), 217
phenyramidol, interaction with phenytoin, 10
phenytoin (Dilantin), 208, 259
    adverse effects, 260–261
    anticonvulsant effect, 257
    interactants, 9, 10
Phospholine, 264
phosphorus, 136
phosphorus 32, 245
photophobia, 266
photosensitivity, with anti-infectives, 69
Physician's Desk Reference, 4
phytonadione (vitamin K$_1$, AquaMEPHYTON, Mephyton), 135, 199, 274
piggyback infusion set-up, 139
pill(s), 6
    preparation for administration, 30
pilocarpine (Isopto Carpine), 265
piperacillin (Pipracil), 60
piperazine salts (Antepar), 74
Pipracil, 60
piroxicam (Feldene), 112–113
Pitocin. See oxytocin
Pitressin. See vasopressin
Pitressin Tannate in Oil. See vasopressin
pituitary gland, 229–230
    anterior lobe, 229
    posterior lobe, 229, 230
placebo, definition, 5n

placebo effect, 5
Placidyl, 127
Plaquenil, 114
plasma expanders, 191
Platinol, 246–247
pneumococcal vaccine (Pneumovax, Pnu-Immune), 85
Pneumovax, 85
Pnu-Immune, 85
poisoning, 157
poliomyelitis, 117
poliovirus vaccine (Orimune Trivalent, Sabin), 84
Polycillin, 59
Polymox, 59
polymyxin B (Aerosporin), 66
    interaction with muscle relaxants, 9
polymyxin B + bacitracin + neomycin (Neosporin), 66
polyvinyl alcohol (Liquifilm Tears, Liquifilm Wetting Solution), 265
Poly-Vi-Sol, 274
Pontocaine. See tetracaine
potassium (K-Lyte, K-Phos, K-Tab, Kaon, Kay-Ciel, Klor-vess, Klotrix, Micro-K, Slow-K), 136, 137, 241
    deficiency, 163
    supplementation, 162
potassium iodide solution (SSKI), 183, 185, 230
potentiation, definition, 10
Povan, 74
prazepam (Centrax), 44, 48
prazosin (Minipress), 219, 223
preanesthetic agents, 98, 100
    nursing implications, 101
Precef, 61
prednisolone (Delta-Cortef, Meticortelone, Sterane), 236
    in eye treatment, 266
prednisone (Deltasone, Meticorten), 236
pregnancy, 157
    edema of, 161
Pregnyl, 232, 234
Premarin, 238
premedication, 98
pressors, 215
    interaction with MAO inhibitors, 9
primaquine, 74
Primatene Mist, 177
primidone (Mysoline), 260
    interaction with coumarin anticoagulants, 9

Pro-Banthine. See propantheline bromide
probenecid (Benemid), 113, 114
    interactants, 10
    interaction with sulfonylureas, 10
procainamide (Pronestyl), 206, 208
procaine (Novocain), 101
procarbazine (Matulane), 248
Procardia, 211, 213
prochlorperazine (Compazine), 43, 153
Profasi HP. See human chorionic gonadotropin
progesterone, 231
    adverse effects, 239
    nursing implications, 239
    route and dosage range, 239
    use, 239
progestin(s), 239
    for breast engorgement, 277
    in oral contraceptives, 231–232
prolactin, 230
Prolixin. See fluphenazine HCl
Proloid, 235
Proloprim, 58
promethazine (Phenergan), 155, 156
    interaction with phenylbutazone, 9
prompt insulin zinc suspension (Semilente), 231, 236
Pronestyl, 206, 208
propantheline bromide (Pro-Banthine), 149, 150
proparacaine (Ophthaine), in eye treatment, 265
proportion, 26
    extremes, 26
    means, 26
propoxyphene HCl (Darvon), 94, 96
propoxyphene HCl + aspirin + caffeine (Darvon compound), 94
propoxyphene napsylate + acetaminophen (Darvocet-N), 94
propranolol (Inderal), 123, 207, 208
    for cardiac pain, 211
propranolol HCl + hydrochlorothiazide (Inderide), 223
propylthiouracil, 235
prostaglandin(s)
    nursing implications, 277
    in obstetrics, 275
prostaglandin inhibitors, in obstetrics, 277

Prostaphlin, 59
Prostigmin. *See* neostigmine
Prostin F$_2$ Alpha, 276
protamine sulfate, 199
protamine zinc insulin suspension
    (PZI), 231, 237
protectives, 80
Proventil. *See* albuterol
Provera, 239
pseudoephedrine (Sudafed), 187
    as vasoconstrictor, 217
psychic energizers, 51
psychosis, drug therapy for, 43–44
psychostimulants, 51
psychotropic drug(s), 43–53
    antihypertensive effect, 219
    classification, 43
    definition, 43
    nursing implications, 44–51
psyllium (Metamucil), 166
psyllium seed, 167
psyllium + senna (PerDiem), 167
pulmonary thrombosis, 197
Pure Food and Drug Act, 3
purgatives, definition, 165
Pyopen, 59
pyrantel pamoate (Antiminth), 74
Pyribenzamine, 189
Pyridium, 95
pyridostigmine (Mestinon), 148, 150
pyridoxine (vitamin B$_6$), 135
pyrimethamine (Daraprim), 74
pyrvinium pamoate (Povan), 74
PZI, 231, 237

Questran. *See* cholestyramine
Quibron, 180
Quinaglute, 207
quinidine, 208
    interactants, 10
quinidine gluconate (Duraquin,
    Quinaglute), 207
quinidine sulfate (Quinoral), 207
Quinoral, 207

radiation therapy, 245
    adverse effects, 253
radioactive isotope(s), 245, 279, 280
radiopaque materials, 279
radium 226, 245
ranitidine (Zantac), 145

ratio, 25
    changing to decimal or percent,
        25
    changing to fraction, 25
Rauwolfia alkaloids, 219, 224
rebound hypertension, 224
rebound insomnia, 129
Regitine, 219
Rela. *See* carisoprodol
renal insufficiency, 201
reserpine (Serpasil), 223
    adverse effects, 46
    interactants, 10
    interaction with MAO inhibitors,
        9
    nursing implications, 46
    route and dosage range, 46
    use, 46
reserpine + hydralazine +
    hydrochlorothiazide
    (Ser-Ap-Es), 223
resorcinol, 77
respiration, definition, 171
respiratory stimulants. *See*
    stimulant(s), respiratory
Restoril, 128
rheumatic heart disease, 197
rheumatism, 109–114
Rh$_O$ immune globulin
    (Gamulin-Rh, HypRho-D,
    RhoGam), 83, 84
RhoGam. *See* Rh$_O$ immune globulin
riboflavin (vitamin B$_2$), 134
Rifadin, 63
rifampin (Rifadin, Rimactane), 63
Rimactane, 63
Riopan. *See* magaldrate
Ritalin. *See* methylphenidate
Ritalin-SR. *See* methylphenidate
ritodrine (Yutopar), 276
Robaxin. *See* methocarbamol
Robitussin. *See* guaifenesin
roman numerals, 15
Romilar, 186
rubella virus vaccine, 84
Rubramin-PC. *See* cyanocobalamin
Rufen. *See* ibuprofen

Sabin, 84
salicylate(s), 97, 109, 114
    interaction
        with probenecid, 10
        with sulfonylureas, 10
salicylic acid, 77

dermatologic use, 78
salicylism, 98
salt restriction, 162
Sandoglobulin. *See* immune serum
    globulin
Sansert, 216, 217
saturated solution of potassium
    iodide (SSKI), 183, 185, 230
Scabene. *See* lindane
scabicides, 75
scabies, 73–75
scopolamine (Hyoscine), 149, 150
secobarbital (Seconal), 126
Seconal, 126
sedative(s), 43, 153
    as antidiarrheals, 169
    antihypertensive effect, 219
    classification, 125
    definition, 125
    interaction
        with narcotics, 97
        with tranquilizers, 51
    nursing implications, 129
    in obstetrics, 277
sedative-hypnotics, 98
Seffin, 60
seizure(s)
    absences, 261
    aura, 260
    classification, 257, 261
    clonic, 257
    generalized, 257
    grand mal, 257
    partial, 257
    petit mal, 257
    psychomotor, 261
    tonic, 257
    unilateral, 257
selenium, 136
Semilente, 231, 236
senna (Senokot), 165, 167
Senokot. *See* senna
Sensorcaine, 100
Septra, 56
Septra DS, 56
Ser-Ap-Es, 223
Serax. *See* oxazepam
Serophene. *See* clomiphene citrate
Serpasil. *See* reserpine
serum(s), antitoxic, 83
sex hormones. *See also specific
    hormone*
    antineoplastic effect, 245
    nursing implications, 242–243
side-effect(s), 8–10
Silain, 146
Silvadene, 56

silver nitrate, 77, 274
silver sulfadiazine (Silvadene), 56
simethicone (Mylicon, Silain), 146
Sinemet, 122
Sinequan, 49
skeletal muscle relaxants, 98,
    117–124
  centrally acting, 117–122
  nursing implications, 123
  peripherally acting, 122
skin disease(s), 77
skin irritation
  drugs that cause, 77
  drugs that prevent or lessen,
    77–81
sleep, 125
  disruptions, caused by
    sedative-hypnotics, 129
sleeping pills, 125
Slo-bid. *See* theophylline
Slow-K. *See* potassium
smelling salts, 173
smoking, 181, 186
sodium, 136
  in antacids, 145
sodium bicarbonate
  as electrolyte, 137
  with uricosuric drugs, 114
sodium biphosphate, as cathartic,
    167
sodium butabarbital (Butisol), 126
sodium phosphate, as cathartic, 167
sodium phosphate + sodium
    biphosphate (Fleet
    Phospho-Soda), 167
sodium polystyrene sulfonate
    (Kayexalate), 137, 140
sodium-restricted diets, 162
Solganal. *See* aurothioglucose
solid(s), 6
Solu-Cortef. *See* hydrocortisone
Solu-Medrol. *See*
    methylprednisolone
Solusets, 139
solution(s), 5-6. *See also* hypertonic
    solution(s); hypotonic
    solution(s); isotonic
    solution(s)
Soma. *See* carisoprodol
somatotropic hormone, 230
Sorbitate. *See* isosorbide
spectinomycin (Trobicin), 65
spirit(s), 6, 88
spironolactone (Aldactone), 159
spironolactone +
    hydrochlorothiazide
    (Aldactazide), 159

SSKI. *See* saturated solution of
    potassium iodide
Stadol. *See* butorphanol
Staphcillin, 59
status epilepticus, 257
Sterane. *See* prednisolone
steroids, 230*n*
Stevens-Johnson syndrome, 67, 260
stimulant(s)
  definition, 105
  nursing implications, 105–107
  respiratory, 105, 107, 173
stomatitis, with chemotherapy, 253
stool softeners, 167, 168
Stoxil. *See* idoxuridine
Strepase, 197
streptokinase (Strepase), 197
streptomycin, 68
  interaction with muscle
    relaxants, 9
streptomycin sulfate, 65
streptozocin (Zanosar), 248
strong iodine solution (Lugol's
    solution), 230
succinylcholine (Anectine), 119, 122
sucralfate (Carafate), 145
Sudafed, 187, 217
sulfa drug(s). *See* sulfonamides
sulfamethoxazole (Gantanol), 56
sulfamethoxazole + trimethoprim
    (Bactrim, Bactrim DS,
    Septra, Septra DS), 56
Sulfamylon, 56
sulfanilamide + aminacrine (AVC),
    57
sulfaphenazole, interaction with
    phenytoin, 10
sulfasalazine (Azulfidine), 57
sulfathiazole + sulfacetamide +
    sulfabenzamide (Sultrin), 57
sulfinpyrazone (Anturane), 113,
    114, 197
sulfisoxazole (Gantrisin), 56
sulfisoxazole + phenazopyridine
    (Azo Gantrisin), 56
sulfobromophthalein
    (Bromsulphalein), 279
sulfonamide(s), 55–57, 67
  allergic reactions to, 67
  fluid intake and output with, 69
  interactants, 10
  interaction
    with methotrexate, 9
    with sulfonylureas, 10
    with tolbutamide, 10
sulfones, 67
sulfonylureas

interactants, 10
interaction with alcohol, 9
sulindac (Clinoril), 113, 114
Sultrin, 57
Sumycin, 63
suppositories, 6
Surfak, 167
suspension(s), 6
Symmetrel. *See* amantadine HCl
sympathomimetic drug(s), 205
  interactants, 10
  interaction with MAO inhibitors,
    9
Synalar, 79
Synalgos-DC, 92
Synthroid, 235
Syntocinon. *See* oxytocin
syringe(s), 31
  mixing medications in, 32–33
  types, 31–32

tablet(s), 6
  enteric-coated, 6
  preparation for administration,
    30
Tagamet. *See* cimetidine
Talwin. *See* pentazocine
Talwin NX, 94
Tapazole, 235
tardive dyskinesia, 44, 50
tar substances, 77
Tearisol. *See* methylcellulose
Tedral, 180
Tegretol, 258
Teldrin, 188
Telepaque, 280
temazepam (Restoril), 128
Tenormin, 220
Tensilon, 120
Tenuate, 106
Tenuate Dospan, 106
Tepanil, 106
Tepanil Ten-Tab, 106
teratogenic effect(s), definition, 10
terbutaline (Brethaire, Brethine,
    Bricanyl), 177, 179
terpin hydrate, 185
Terramycin, 63
Tessalon, 185
Tes-tape, 242
testes, 232
testosterone, 232
testosterone cypionate
    (Depo-Testosterone), 240

testosterone enanthate + estradiol valerate (Deladumone), for breast engorgement, 277
testosterone + estradiol (Deladumone OB), 276
tetanus, 122
tetanus immune human globulin (TIG, Hu-Tet, Hyper-Tet), 84
tetracaine (Pontocaine), in eye treatment, 263–265
tetracycline(s), 63–64, 68
   interactants, 10
   and oral contraceptives, 243
tetracycline HCl (Achromycin, Sumycin), 63
tetrahydrozoline (Tryzine, Visine), 217
theobromine, 105
Theo-Dur. See theophylline
Theolair. See theophylline
theophylline (Elixophyllin, Slo-bid, Theo-Dur, Theolair), 105, 161, 177–180
theophylline + ephedrine + phenobarbital (Tedral), 180
theophylline + guaifenesin (Quibron), 180
thiamine (vitamin B$_1$), 133, 134
thiazide diuretic(s), 158–159, 161, 219
   interactants, 10
thiethylperazine (Torecan), 155
thimerosal (Merthiolate), 79
thiopental (Pentothal), 99
thioridazine, 44
   interaction with diphenhydramine, 9
thiotepa, 248
thiouracil drug(s), 230
Thorazine. See chlorpromazine
thrombocytopenia, 253, 260
thromboembolism, 243
thrombolytic drug(s), 197
thrombosis, 140
thrombus, definition, 197n
thyroglobulin (Proloid), 235
thyroid gland, 230
thyroid hormone, 234
thyroid-stimulating hormone, 230
thyrotoxicosis, 240
D-thyroxine, interaction with coumarin anticoagulants, 9
Ticar, 60
ticarcillin (Ticar), 60
TIG. See tetanus immune human globulin
Tigan, 155–156

timolol (Timoptic), 265
Timoptic, 265
Tinactin, 79
tincture(s), 6, 88
Titralac. See calcium carbonate
TNG. See nitroglycerin
tobramycin (Nebcin), 65
tocainide (Tonocard), 207
Tofranil. See imipramine
tolazamide (Tolinase), 237
tolbutamide (Orinase), 237
   interactants, 10
Tolectin, 113
Tolectin DS, 113
tolerance, definition, 8–10
Tolinase, 237
tolmetin (Tolectin, Tolectin DS), 113
tolnaftate (Aftate, Tinactin), 79
Tonocard, 207
topical application(s), 6
Topsyn, 79
Torecan, 155
total parenteral nutrition, definition, 136
toxin(s), 83
toxoid, 83
trade name, 4
Trandate, 221
tranquilizer(s)
   and antidepressants, 52
   convulsions with, 51
   idiosyncrasy, 51
   interactants, 51
   interaction with alcohol, 9, 51
   major, 43–44, 45–46
      adverse effects, 44-51
      definition, 43
      hypersensitivity reactions with, 50
      photosensitivity with, 50
   minor, 44, 46—48
      definition, 43
      dependence, 51
tranquilizers, 98
   antihypertensive effect, 219
Transderm-Nitro. See nitroglycerin
transmitter, nervous system, 147
Tranxene, 46
tranylcypromine (Parnate), 51–52
trazodone (Desyrel), 50
Tremin. See trihexyphenidyl
triamcinolone (Aristocort, Kenalog), 236
triamcinolone acetonide (Kenalog, Aristocort), 80
   in eye treatment, 266
triamterene (Dyrenium), 160

triamterene + hydrochlorothiazide (Dyazide, Maxzide), 160
Triavil, 49
triazolam (Halcion), 128
tricyclic antidepressant(s), 48–49, 52
   and oral contraceptives, 243
Tridil. See nitroglycerin
triethanolamine (Cerumenex), 267
trifluoperazine, 43
   interaction with chlorpromazine, 9
trifluridine (Viroptic), 265, 266
trihexyphenidyl (Artane, Tremin), 122, 123
trimethobenzamide (Tigan), 155–156
trimethoprim (Proloprim, Trimpex), 58
Trimox, 59
Trimpex, 58
Tri-Norinyl, 232
tripelennamine (Pyribenzamine, PBZ, PBZ-SR), 189
Triphasil, 232
triprolidine + pseudoephedrine (Actifed), 187, 189
Tri-Vi-Sol, 274
Trobicin, 65
tropicamide (Mydriacyl), 265
Tryzine, 217
tuberculin syringe, 31–32
tuberculosis, 67
Tums, 143
Tussionex, 186
Tuss-Ornade, 185
Tylenol. See acetaminophen
Tylox, 94
tyramine(s), 51–52, 217

Ultracef, 60
Ultralente, 231, 237
Unipen, 54
United States Pharmacopeia, 3–4
urea (Ureaphil), 265
Ureaphil, 265
Urecholine. See bethanechol chloride
uric acid, 109
uricosuric drug(s), 113
   definition, 109
   nursing implications, 114
urinary tract antiseptics, 55, 57–58, 67

urinary tract antiseptics (*continued*)
    fluid intake and output with, 69
urine, monitoring, in diuretic
    therapy, 162

vaccine(s), 83–85, 274
    nursing implications, 85
Valisone, 79
Valium. *See* diazepam
valproic acid (Depakene, Depakote),
    260
Vancocin. *See* vancomycin
vancomycin (Vancocin), 66
    interaction with alcohol, 9
vasoconstrictors, 215–218
    local, 217
    nursing implications, 217
    systemic, 215–217
Vasodilan, 213
vasodilators, 211–215, 219
    coronary, 211
    nursing implications, 211–215
    peripheral, 211
vasopressin (Pitressin, Pitressin
    Tannate in Oil), 230, 234, 240
vasopressors, 215
V-Cillin-K, 60
Veetids, 60
Velban, 251
Velosef, 62
venous thrombosis, 197
Ventolin. *See* albuterol
VePesid, 250
verapamil (Calan, Isoptin), 211, 214
Vermox, 74
vial(s), 6
    multiple-dose, 6
Vibramycin, 63
vidarabine (Vira-A), 73, 266

Vi-Daylin, 274
vinblastine (Velban), 251
vincristine (Oncovin), 251
Vioform-Hydrocortisone, 80
Viokase, 145–146
Vira-A. *See* vidarabine
virilism, 243
Viroptic, 265, 266
virus infections, 71
Visine, 217
✓Vistaril. *See* hydroxyzine pamoate
vitamin(s), 274
    allergic reactions to, 133
    deficiency, 133, 135
    definition, 133
    fat-soluble, 133, 201
    minimum daily requirement, 133
    nursing implications, 133–135
    and oral contraceptives, 243
    overdoses, 133
    recommended daily allowance,
        133
    therapeutic formulations, 135
    water-soluble, 133
vitamin A (Aquasol A), 133, 134
    dermatologic use, 78
vitamin B_1. *See* thiamine
vitamin B_2. *See* riboflavin
vitamin B_6. *See* pyridoxine
vitamin B_{12}. *See* cyanocobalamin
vitamin B complex, 133
vitamin C (ascorbic acid), 133, 135
vitamin D (calciferol), 133, 134
    dermatologic use, 78
vitamin E, 133
vitamin K, 69, 133
    for children, 274
    deficiency, 98
    preparations, 199
vitamin K_1. *See* phytonadione
vitamin K_3. *See* menadione
Volutrols, 139
vomiting

with chemotherapy, 253
household remedies, 153
induced, 153

warfarin (Coumadin), 198
wheal, 187
Wycillin, 60
Wymox, 59

Xanax. *See* alprazolam
xanthines, 105, 177–180, 211
Xylocaine. *See* lidocaine

Young's rule, 271
Yutopar, 276

Zanosar, 248
Zantac, 145
Zarontin, 259
Zaroxolyn, 158–159, 222
Zephiran, 78
Zinacef, 61
zinc, 136
zinc oxide, 78
Zovirax, 72
Zyloprim. *See* allopurinol